YOUNG CHILDREN AND TRAUMA

YOUNG CHILDREN AND TRAUMA

Intervention and Treatment

WITHDRAWN

Edited by

JOY D. OSOFSKY

Foreword by Kyle D. Pruett

THE GUILFORD PRESS
New York   London

© 2004 The Guilford Press
A Division of Guilford Publications, Inc.
72 Spring Street, New York, NY 10012
www.guilford.com

Printed in the United States of America

This book is printed on acid-free paper.

Last digit is print number: 9 8 7 6 5 4 3 2 1

Library of Congress Cataloging-in-Publication Data

Young children and trauma : intervention and treatment / edited by Joy D.
Osofsky.
      p. cm.
  Includes bibliographical references and index.
  ISBN 1-59385-041-7 (hardcover : alk. paper)
  1. Posttraumatic stress disorder in children—Treatment. 2. Psychic trauma
in children—Treatment. I. Osofsky, Joy D.
  RJ506.P55Y686 2004
  618.92′8521—dc22
                                                     2004005191

To my husband, Howard, and three children,
Hari, Justin, and Michael, through whom I have learned
how very important love, nurturance, trust,
and protection are for healthy development.

To my VIP staff made up of truly extraordinary
individuals who have worked with me for the past
10 years as part of the Violence Intervention Program
for Children and Families in New Orleans and continue
to help children who would otherwise
"fall between the cracks" of the mental health system.

ABOUT THE EDITOR

Joy D. Osofsky, PhD, is a psychologist and psychoanalyst and Professor of Pediatrics, Psychiatry, and Public Health at Louisiana State University Health Sciences Center in New Orleans. Dr. Osofsky is also President of Zero to Three/National Center for Infants, Toddlers, and Families, and Director of the Violence Intervention Program for Children and Families and the Harris Center for Infant Mental Health at Louisiana State University Health Sciences Center. She is editor of *Children in a Violent Society* and two editions of the *Handbook of Infant Development;* coeditor of the four-volume *WAIMH Handbook of Infant Mental Health,* which received the American Publishers Association award as the best social science reference book in 2000; and editor of the *Infant Mental Health Journal.* Her 1995 *American Psychologist* article, "The Effects of Violence Exposure in Young Children," was chosen by the American Psychological Association as one of the top articles published in the journal in the past 50 years. Currently, Dr. Osofsky serves on the Pew Commission for Children in Foster Care and the Research Committee of the International Psychoanalytical Association, and consults with the 11th Circuit Juvenile Court in Miami–Dade County, Florida. Dr. Osofsky has conducted research, intervention, and clinical work with infants, children, and families at high psychosocial risk, and has studied adolescent mothers as well as infants, children, and families exposed to community and domestic violence and maltreatment. In 1998, Dr. Osofsky was awarded the Badge of Honor by the New Orleans Police Foundation for her work with children and families exposed to violence. In 2002, she was awarded the Medal of Honor by the Mayor of New Orleans for her work with the police and the community and the Nicholas Hobbs Award by Division 37 of the American Psychological Association for contributions to public policy.

CONTRIBUTORS

Marilyn Augustyn, MD, Division of Developmental and Behavioral Pediatrics, Boston Medical Center, Boston, Massachusetts

Shana M. Bellow, PhD, Department of Psychiatry and Neurology, Tulane University Health Sciences Center, New Orleans, Louisiana

Neil W. Boris, MD, Department of Community Health Sciences, Tulane University Health Sciences Center, New Orleans, Louisiana

Michelle Bosquet, PhD, Department of Child and Adolescent Psychiatry, Boston Medical Center, Boston University School of Medicine, Boston, Massachusetts

Nancy Freeman, LCSW, Institute for Mental Hygiene, New Orleans, Louisiana

Theodore J. Gaensbauer, MD, Department of Psychiatry, University of Colorado Health Sciences Center, Denver, Colorado

Betsy McAlister Groves, LICSW, Child Witness to Violence Project, Division of Developmental and Behavioral Pediatrics, Boston Medical Center, Boston, Massachusetts

Jill Hayes Hammer, PhD, Department of Psychiatry, Louisiana State University Health Sciences Center, New Orleans, Louisiana

Robert J. Harmon, MD, Department of Psychiatry, University of Colorado Health Sciences Center, Denver, Colorado

Sherryl Scott Heller, PhD, Department of Psychiatry and Neurology, Tulane University Health Sciences Center, New Orleans, Louisiana

Sarah Hinshaw-Fuselier, MSW, LCSW, PhD, Department of Human Development and Family Science, University of Texas, Austin, Texas

Donna J. Hitchens, MSW, JD, San Francisco Superior Court, San Francisco, California

Chandra Ghosh Ippen, PhD, Early Trauma Treatment Network, University of California, San Francisco, San Francisco, California

Stacy A. Klapper, PsyD, Department of Psychiatry, University of Colorado Health Sciences Center, Denver, Colorado

Julie A. Larrieu, PhD, Department of Psychiatry and Neurology, Tulane University Health Sciences Center, New Orleans, Louisana

Cindy Lederman, JD, Juvenile Division, 11th Judicial Circuit, Miami–Dade County, Florida

Marva L. Lewis, PhD, School of Social Work, Tulane University, New Orleans, Louisiana

Alicia F. Lieberman, PhD, Child Trauma Research Project, Department of Psychiatry, University of California, San Francisco, San Francisco, California

Karlen Lyons-Ruth, PhD, Department of Psychiatry, Cambridge Hospital/Harvard Medical School, Boston, Massachusetts

Joy D. Osofsky, PhD, Departments of Pediatrics, Psychiatry, and Public Health, Louisiana State University Health Sciences Center, New Orleans, Louisiana

Victoria T. Parton, BA, Department of Psychology, University of Texas, Austin, Texas

Nancy S. Plummer, BA, Department of Psychiatry, University of Colorado Health Sciences Center, Denver, Colorado

Lara Robinson, MPH, Department of Applied and Developmental Psychology, University of New Orleans, New Orleans, Louisiana

J. Michael Rovaris, LCSW, Department of Psychiatry, Louisiana State University Health Sciences Center, New Orleans, Louisiana

Michelle R. Schuder, PhD, Department of Psychiatry, Massachusetts General Hospital/Harvard Medical School, Boston, Massachusetts

Anna T. Smyke, PhD, Department of Psychiatry and Neurology, Tulane University Health Sciences Center, New Orleans, Louisiana

Patricia Van Horn, PhD, JD, Child Trauma Research Project, Department of Psychiatry, University of California, San Francisco, San Francisco, California

Valerie Wajda-Johnston, PhD, Department of Psychiatry and Neurology, Tulane University Health Sciences Center, New Orleans, Louisiana

Charles H. Zeanah, Jr., MD, Department of Psychiatry and Neurology, Tulane University Health Sciences Center, New Orleans, Louisiana

FOREWORD

Every day, come what may, young children are drawn irresistibly to fathom the lives they lead. Their miraculous capacities to explore and understand render them unique as well as vulnerable. Their keen appetites for relationships, novelty, calm, excitement, and comfort draw them repeatedly to the edge of safety. Miscalculations, misunderstandings, and misattributions encountered at that edge enlighten young children as often as they bruise and wound. Ultimately, however, it is how children are loved and protected by the ones they hold most dear that makes their days, and often their lives, matter.

It is here, in the primacy of intimacy and trust, that trauma works its toxic and corrosive mischief. We have come to understand that the child's first self-image is mirrored in the eyes of his or her parents. If he is idealized, he will see himself rendered in vitality and beauty. If she is in danger, she will see fear and doubt. If he is resented, he will see bitterness. Frightening self-images may emerge that can take even the young child beyond the limits of trust and endurance, or the emotional reach of his or her loved ones. This is precisely what makes trauma a family affair—whether in perpetration or resolution. Those who ignore this maxim are generally less than helpful in the attempts they make to intervene on behalf of the traumatized child and family.

This highly relevant and useful volume assembles our best current understandings of the young child at the edge of safety and beyond. It welcomes us to embrace the complexity of the traumatic experience for the young child, from the biological and psychological context in which it occurs, all the way through to the ultimate processing of the experience into memory, recall, and beyond. We see in the contributors' and editor's prismatic insights the emergence of a kind of social neuroscience interwoven with clarifications from the unique and trustworthy lens of developmental psychopathology.

As we are just at the beginning of this odyssey, this particular gathering of guides is especially helpful because of the clarity of their vision, the breadth of their experience, and the rigor of their science—all tempered with the humility of their assumptions. It is my fervent hope, given their excellence, that they will be in this for the long haul. Understanding the changeling that is trauma is not for the impatient or "short memoried." And this is no easy commitment. As the therapists, evaluators, diagnosticians, jurists, and other interveners in the lives of traumatized children tell us throughout this volume, they must be especially well prepared and supported to enter what Donald Cohen (2001) called the "furnace of clinical engagement."

Young Children and Trauma is invaluable to those who seek sage guidance through the realm of affective chaos that so often defines trauma from the child's and his or her family's viewpoint. It will be a great comfort to those very families to know that such skill, devotion, and good science has been assembled in these pages to guide those who hope to help them and their children through these dark and roadless passages.

KYLE D. PRUETT, MD
Yale Child Study Center,
Yale University School of Medicine

REFERENCE

Cohen, D. J. (2001, February 27). *Into life: Autism, Tourette's syndrome and the community of clinical research*. Sterling Lecture, Yale University, New Haven, CT.

SCOPE OF THE PROBLEM

The effects of exposure to violence and traumatization in young children remain complex in that many different issues need to be addressed, such as how the children themselves may react, how their caregivers may be affected, and the subtle and not so subtle effects on the interveners and treaters, as young children are so vulnerable. The purpose of this volume is to provide information—in as "user friendly" a way as possible—about the current available knowledge on young children and trauma from a variety of perspectives. Parts I, II, and III each have a brief section introducing the main ideas to be discussed in the chapters: Part I includes theoretical discussions framing the area for the reader; Part II presents several different approaches to assessment, diagnosis, and treatment; and Part III considers innovative ways to reach young traumatized children by partnering with juvenile courts, law enforcement, and child welfare. Finally, Part IV includes two chapters, one with an overview of current research in this area and the other considering additional clinical perspectives.

In my introduction to Part I, "Background and Perspectives: Providing the Foundations for Understanding," I provide a brief overview of the effects of trauma on infants, young children, and their parents or caregivers, and outline the issues pertaining to assessment and treatment. Theoretical and background issues related to traumatized young children are presented in the three chapters in Part I. In Chapter 1, Marva L. Lewis and Chandra Ghosh Ippen frame our understanding of the very important cultural issues related to young children and trauma, as well as how trauma is conceptualized from different cultural perspectives. Theoretical and diagnostic perspectives are presented in Chapter 2 on attachment and disruption by Sarah Hinshaw-Fuselier, Sherryl Scott Heller, Victoria T. Parton, Lara Robinson, and Neil W. Boris. In Chapter 3, Michelle R. Schuder and Karlen Lyons-Ruth deal with issues of "hidden trauma" in infancy and how attachment and fearful arousal can lead to problems in physiological functioning related to extreme stress reactions.

In the past decade, there has been enormous growth in our understanding of assessment, diagnosis, and treatment of young traumatized children. In Part II, state-of-the-art strategies are presented that allow interveners and clinicians to gain an understanding of the impact of trauma on young children and their families in order to plan for and frame treatment approaches. In Chapter 4, Alicia F. Lieberman and Patricia Van Horn present their approach to assessment and treatment of young children exposed to domestic violence. In Chapter 5, Stacy A. Klapper, Nancy S. Plummer, and Robert J. Harmon discuss diagnostic and treatment issues focusing on the ways that children with different temperaments, personalities, and psychological resources react to trauma, especially severe abuse and neglect. In Chapter 6, Julie A. Larrieu and Shana M. Bellow focus on the problematic behaviors, perceptions, and relationship disruptions typically manifested by maltreating parents and their young children and present a comprehensive assessment procedure. In Chapter 7, Betsy McAlister Groves and Marilyn Augustyn present an approach to identification, assessment, and treatment in a pediatric setting, a very important but not yet widely accepted location in which trauma can be identified in young children much earlier than in mental health settings. Theodore J. Gaensbauer, through the use of a sensitive case presentation of a different type of trauma for children, presents in Chapter 8 his perspective on evaluation and treatment for a broad range of trauma in young children.

Part III deals with innovative work that has been going on with both traditional and nontraditional "first responders" in order to reach traumatized children earlier and to develop interventions in nontraditional settings. Chapters 9 and 10 present different approaches for working with young traumatized children in juvenile court, one in Miami dependency court by Joy D. Osofsky and Judge Cindy Lederman, the other in San Francisco by Patricia Van Horn and Judge Donna J. Hitchens. Chapter 11, by Anna T. Smyke, Valerie Wajda-Johnston, and Charles H. Zeanah, Jr., reviews important work with young traumatized children in the child welfare system, a place where so many of these children present. In Chapter 12, I and Jill Hayes Hammer, Nancy Freeman, and J. Michael Rovaris discuss our work with law enforcement in New Orleans and how to build a partnership between police and mental health professionals to intervene on behalf of young traumatized children.

In Part IV, "Directions for the Future," first Michelle Bosquet presents (in Chapter 13) a comprehensive overview of the existing and newly emerging research in the area of trauma and young children. Clearly, this is an area that is sorely in need of much more careful study of approaches, assessment, and treatments. In Chapter 14, I conclude with a consideration of additional clinical perspectives and issues not presented previously in the volume.

I am very appreciative of the enormous effort made by all of the contributors to this volume. I am even more grateful for their ongoing commitment to help young underserved traumatized children, who often have no voice and depend on these experts and other nontraditional responders and protectors like them. It is my hope that readers will find the book helpful as they reach out to traumatized children and families in different settings.

JOY D. OSOFSKY

ACKNOWLEDGMENTS

This book evolved from my experience working with young traumatized children and families exposed to community and domestic violence, abuse, and neglect, and those who grow up in dysfunctional families. Traumatized young children rarely have a voice in response to the trauma they suffer, and many suffer tremendously, often at the hands of those who are supposed to love, nurture, and protect them. In this book, my colleagues and I have written about the experiences of these children in the different settings where their experiences come to light—the child welfare system, juvenile courts, law enforcement, mental health clinics—in order to give them that crucial *voice*. Those of us who deal with treating trauma, particularly traumatized children, learn very quickly that we can do this work most effectively if we have support from colleagues and coworkers because the work can be so taxing. All of the contributors to this book believe strongly that it is important to inform others about the suffering of traumatized young children, and in their chapters, they demonstrate ways to better understand these children through research and evaluation and ways to help them through treatment. I am very grateful to all of the contributors and respect and appreciate their work, effort, and sensitivity.

There are a number of individuals who played key roles and provided inspiration for the work that has resulted in this book. First, without the confidence, trust, and support of Irving Harris, those of us at the Harris Center for Infant Mental Health at Louisiana State University Health Sciences Center would not be able to do the work that we do. Many of the contributors to this volume have also been touched by his wisdom and generosity. I thank colleagues at Zero to Three/National Center for Infants, Toddlers, and Families for believing that we can make a difference for traumatized infants and young children. My dedicated colleagues at the Violence Intervention Program for Children and Families and the Harris Center for Infant Mental Health have formed the teams that have provided me with the support and motivation we all need to do this difficult work. The Advisory Committee to the Department of Psychiatry at Louisiana State University Health Sciences Center has always believed in this work and provided support to my teams. And for the past 9 years, Chef Emeril Lagasse and his staff have sponsored a benefit dinner that has helped to raise the funds we need to support our work.

For the past decade, I have been inspired in my approaches to work with traumatized young children by collaborating with the New Orleans Police Department and several juvenile judges. Work with these groups of professionals is represented in chapters in this book.

I am very grateful for the availability and support of Kerry Wiltz, in the Department of Psychiatry at Louisiana State University Health Sciences Center, for her invaluable assistance in communicating with authors and publishers and helping with the organization of this volume. Without her help, I would not have been able to finish this book so efficiently.

Once again, I thank my family: My husband, Howard, has always been at my side as I have undertaken this very difficult work with traumatized children and families. He has been there to listen patiently about my concerns and worries and to provide support. I am also blessed with three wonderful and supportive children—Hari, Justin, and Michael—who have grown into young adults who share my passion for public service and helping others.

Finally, I thank Kathryn Moore, Senior Editor at The Guilford Press, who never wavered in her support for this project and was extremely helpful in conceptualizing the final product. I appreciate her flexibility in being open to the different types of material presented in this book.

CONTENTS

PART I

BACKGROUND AND PERSPECTIVES

*Providing the Foundations
for Understanding*

DIFFERENT WAYS OF UNDERSTANDING YOUNG CHILDREN AND TRAUMA

The Court's Babies
Battered from birth or
victims of the care-less touch,
Brain wires tangled
from all love deprived,
No tears, no joy.
Generations of hate passed on
  from stalled infant minds
  in prison cribs.

Black robes so thin
we often cannot shield;
And the soapbox promise
in red, white, and blue!
A promise kept,
Or merely grand words,
  like babies in court,
    vacant?
            —WILLIAM E. GLADSTONE,
        Senior Circuit Judge, Florida (June 21, 2003)

Judge Gladstone's poignant and sensitive thoughts expressed through his poem, "The Court's Babies," brings to mind many complex feelings that include sadness, anger, fear, uncertainty, and a sense that the onlookers, like the babies, are overcome by helplessness and hopelessness. It is an unfortunate reality that many infants and young children are neglected and abused by the adults in their lives who are supposed to love and nurture them. For these unfortunate youngsters, child protection services or even the juvenile court may become their last resort—one that comes into play when they do

3

not have sensitive, caring adults in their lives to help them grow and develop into physically and emotionally healthy children and adults.

For those of us who continually come in contact and work with traumatized young children and their families as mental health providers, judges, police officers, lawyers, child protection workers, doctors, nurses, and many others, we need more information to be able to respond more sensitively and effectively to these children's many needs. Children who have been traumatized frequently have no *voice*, and we must help provide words as well as actions to better their lives.

Generally, during their first few years of life, most healthy children learn to trust that parents and other caring adults in their environment will be available, reliable, consistent, and protective. For traumatized young children, however, these behaviors and attitudes that are so important for their physical, cognitive, social, and emotional development are lacking. Since early relationships form the basis for all later relationships, the negative experiences of abused and neglected young children often lead to difficulties in forming positive relationships later in their lives. Further, with these negative early experiences, a child's sense of self and, ultimately, self-esteem may be impacted negatively. If such children are treated poorly, they may come to expect that they will be continue to be treated badly. Such early experiences can result in the children acting out aggressively, which may provoke more negative behaviors in others, or (alternatively) such vulnerable children may become withdrawn and depressed. We need much more information about ways to understand the effects of such events on young children and about ways to support them when they have lost their "secure base" and trust in their environment, a trust that is crucial for healthy development.

It is also important to recognize that, frequently, when a young child is traumatized, the parent or caregiver is also traumatized. Parenting under "normal" circumstances is a complex process. The added stress associated with parenting traumatized young children as well as coping with violence as an everyday event affects both the parent's and the child's capacity to form healthy attachment relationships. Parents living in such circumstances may become depressed and unable to provide for their young children's needs. Further, parents who witness violence or are themselves victims of violence are likely to have difficulty being emotionally available, sensitive, and responsive to their children. Exposure to violence and traumatization may also interfere with normal developmental transitions for both the parents and the children. Community or domestic violence exposure may lead parents to be overly protective and unable to encourage normal autonomy, which is important for development. With exposure to violence, children can lose trust in the safety of the environment as well as the people surrounding them in the environment (Erikson, 1950). Thus, supports outside of the family may be very important for parents and children exposed to violence. All of these factors, although understandable, may influence young children to be less responsive to others and even to feel that they have done something "bad" to contribute to this state of affairs. Thus, often it is necessary for parents to cope with their own traumatization before they are able to deal effectively with their children's needs.

EFFECTS OF TRAUMA ON INFANTS AND TODDLERS

While children are affected by violence exposure at all ages, less is known about the consequences of such exposure at younger ages, especially as it relates to long-term effects. In fact, many people assume that very young children are not affected at all, erroneously believing that they are too young to know or remember what has happened. In the past decade, there has been increasing research and clinical work carried out on the effects of both chronic community violence and domestic violence exposure on younger children. Further, there is more awareness of the importance of prevention and early intervention to address these issues as early as possible in children's lives in order to help them cope with trauma and to prevent more serious problems.

An understanding of developmental issues is important in any response to trauma. First, reactions vary at different ages because children understand and internalize the experience depending on their cognitive and emotional capacities. Understanding and processing death varies across different ages. A 2- or 3-year-old toddler will not incorporate the same sense of finality as an 8- or 9-year-old latency-age child. Little children, especially toddlers, with their sense of omnipotence, may feel responsible as if they may have caused something bad to happen. This situation can come up often in cases of exposure to domestic violence. It is important to recognize that infants' and toddlers' reactions and behaviors resonate with those of their caregivers.

Even in the earliest phases of infant and toddler development, existing research as well as clinical reports indicate clear associations between exposure to violence and emotional and behavior problems. Infants and toddlers who witness either violence in their homes or a violent incident in their community show increased irritability, immature behavior, sleep disturbances, emotional distress and crying, fears of being alone, physical complaints, and loss of skills, such as regression in toileting and language (Drell, Siegel, & Gaensbauer, 1993; Osofsky & Fenichel, 1994; Zeanah & Scheeringa, 1996). In addition, temper tantrums and clinging, manifested in inability to separate from parents or familiar caregivers, are common responses. As will be elaborated in the chapters in this volume, these behaviors are assessed in infants and toddlers by interviewing the parent or caregiver and through direct observation of the young child with the caregiver. Exposure to trauma, especially violence that impacts directly on the family,

interferes with children's normal development of trust and later explor-
atory behaviors that lead to the development of autonomy (Osofsky &
Fenichel, 1994). When young children are severely traumatized, the symptoms noted are similar to posttraumatic stress disorder (PTSD) in adults,
including repeated reexperiencing of the traumatic event, avoidance, numbing of responsiveness, new fears, and increased arousal (Drell et al., 1993;
Osofsky, 1995; Osofsky, Cohen, & Drell, 1995). For example, these young
children often are afraid to be near the scene of the violent event they had
witnessed, are afraid to go to sleep, and may wake up with nightmares.
They show little or blunted emotions rather than the normal range from
happy to sad and show little enthusiasm and fun in play. They are most often very serious and even "spacey" or disorganized at times and smile very
little. Preschool children exposed to violence are less likely to explore and
play freely and are less motivated to master their environment (Osofsky,
1995). Several studies support a link between exposure to community and
domestic violence and aggression, anxiety, or depressive symptoms in
lower-socioeconomic-class children ranging in age from 6 to 15 years living
in violent urban neighborhoods (Gorman-Smith & Tolan, 1998; Cooley-
Quille, Turner, & Beidel, 1995; Schwab-Stone et al., 1995). Children exposed to family violence often show a greater frequency of externalizing
(aggressive) and internalizing (withdrawn, anxious) behavior problems in
comparison to children from nonviolent families. Overall functioning, attitudes, social competence, and current and later school performance are often affected negatively. Selma Fraiberg and associates' (Fraiberg, Adelson,
& Shapiro, 1975) groundbreaking work on "ghosts in the nursery" lends
insight in understanding both the immediate effects on young children and
their families and their subsequent reactions. For children exposed to trauma, retraumatization can play a very significant role in how individuals
and families may react. If they have experienced previous recent losses, or if
there is another dramatic event that impacts on them, such as a fire in their
school, their reactions may be much stronger than they might have been
previously due to retraumatization. Fraiberg et al. (1975) emphasized how
the unresolved issues of the parents can interfere and confound their ability
to provide loving, supportive relationships with their baby. In this case, the
unresolved traumatization easily leads to further traumatic reactions. Thus
when trauma affects young children or adults, they may be reminded about
earlier traumatic events, which may contribute to more severe reactions.
Children's reactions may vary with the level of exposure and be influenced
by relationships with people who are affected, which is why parents and
primary caregivers play such an important part in both the expected response and the recovery for young children.

In sum, the psychological outcomes of violence and trauma on children include threats to their sense of basic trust and secure attachment. Often their healthy curiosity is inhibited, as is their exploration of their envi-

ronment. When their sense of a secure base (Bowlby, 1988; Ainsworth, Blehar, Waters, & Wall, 1978) is shaken, they may experience adults as failing to protect them or even harmful. In some cases they will express their frustration and confusion in aggressive, acting-out behaviors, and in other cases they may turn inward and not expect to depend on others. Thus it is crucial that parents and other caregivers be able to listen to their children and hear their concerns. They also need to help them feel safe. If parents are traumatized, it is important for them to find support for themselves and to reach out to others for support for their children.

Several of the factors that made it so very difficult for young children in the aftermath of the September 11, 2001, trauma is that infants and toddlers depend on adults to protect them and keep them safe. Many adults were experiencing a need to be protected themselves and were fearful about whether or not they or their children would ever be safe again. Further, young children depend on adults to help them make sense of their world. In this case, adults, the media, and even many national leaders were having difficulty making sense of the world. So young children and their parents were left with a mutual loss of trust as well as many new fears, outcomes we frequently see in traumatized young children (see Coates, Rosenthal, & Schechter, 2003, for a fuller discussion).

INTERVENTIONS AND TREATMENT FOR YOUNG TRAUMATIZED CHILDREN

Reactions to trauma are difficult to predict. They may occur immediately after the event or days and even weeks later. They may remind young children (or adults) about earlier trauma experiences as well as losses, making the reactions more severe. Children's reactions to the traumatic event will be affected by those of their parents. Reactions can also vary depending on each child's level of exposure to the trauma and his or her relationship to the people who are affected.

One level of intervention is through the parents, extended family, and caregivers. Parents may become very distressed as they observe their young children's traumatic reactions. Thus, it is important for parents to deal with their own traumatization in order to help support their children. Parents can help their children by being available to them, not just physically but emotionally. They need to be able to both hear and "hold" their concerns and worries. Even if they are not sure that they can guarantee theirs or their children's safety, they need to be able to reassure them that they will do their very best to keep them safe and, with that, they need to describe concrete ways that they or others are ensuring their safety. Parents may want to minimize their young child's feelings for various reasons. They may be inclined to think that he or she is too young to experience such feelings, or they may not want to hear their child's expressions of great fear, which makes them feel even more insecure themselves. It is most important for parents in helping their children to follow their lead: if the youngsters want to talk, parents should be available to listen; if they want to be held, parents should pick them up. In order for parents to be able to support their children, they need to help them maintain or return to a regular schedule, allow them to show feelings including fear, and help them identify their feelings of fear, worry, and sadness. Parents may need to have help themselves in working through and better understanding their own traumatization in order to gain needed support.

When the traumatization goes beyond the support, love, and care that a parent can offer a child, professional intervention and treatment is important to help heal the child before the unaddressed traumatization can lead to even more serious problems. While some therapeutic approaches focus primarily on verbalization, with young children behavioral observations during play and during infant–parent interactions are the main means of understanding the young child's conflicts and internal world. For most dyads, even those that are extremely troubled, there are strong positive forces on each side of the relationship. The work of the psychotherapy is to uncover, discover, and support these strengths, recognize and work with the weaknesses, and build a stronger, more positive relationship. The psychotherapeutic work with infants, toddlers, and parents begins with an assessment that is based on interviews with the parents or caregivers and observations of the parent and child. The process of the assessment designed to understand the dynamics of the earliest relationship is in itself an intervention. Often work with the infant–parent dyad that includes learning more about the "ghosts" in the relationship and putting the internal world, understood through observations, into words is an important agent of change. A number of different strategies will be elaborated throughout this book.

ACKNOWLEDGMENT

The chapter-opening poem, "The Court's Babies," is reprinted by permission of Judge William E. Gladstone.

REFERENCES

Ainsworth, M. D. S., Blehar, M. C., Waters, E., & Wall, S. (1978). *Patterns of attachment: A psychological study of the strange situation.* Hillsdale, NJ: Erlbaum.

Bowlby, J. (1988). *A secure base.* New York: Basic Books.

Coates, S. W., Rosenthal, J. L., & Schechter, D. S. (2003). *September 11: Trauma and human bonds.* Hillsdale, NJ: Analytic Press.

Cooley-Quille, M. R., Turner, S. M., & Beidel, D. C. (1995). Emotional impact of children's exposure to community violence: A preliminary study. *Journal of the American Academy of Child and Adolescent Psychiatry, 34,* 1362–1368.

Drell, M. J., Siegel, C. H., & Gaensbauer, T. J. (1993). Post-traumatic stress disorders. In C. Zeanah (Ed.), *Handbook of infant mental health* (pp. 291–304). New York: Guilford Press.

Erikson, E. H. (1950). *Childhood and society.* New York: Norton.

Fraiberg, S., Adelson, E., & Shapiro, V. (1975). Ghosts in the nursery: A psychoanalytic approach to the problems of impaired mother–infant relationships. *Journal of the American Academy of Child Psychiatry, 14,* 378–421

Gorman-Smith, D., & Tolan, P. (1998). The role of exposure to community violence and developmental problems among inner city youth. *Development and Psychopathology, 10,* 99–114.

Osofsky, J. D. (1995). The effects of exposure to violence on young children. *American Psychologist, 50,* 782–788.

Osofsky, J. D. (Ed.). (1997). *Children in a violent society.* New York: Guilford Press.

Osofsky, J. D., Cohen, G, & Drell, M. (1995). The effects of trauma on young children: A case of two-year-old twins. *International Journal of Psychoanalysis, 76,* 595–607.

Osofsky, J. D., & Fenichel, E. (Eds). (1994). *Caring for infants and toddlers in violent environments: Hurt, healing, and hope.* Arlington, VA: Zero to Three/National Center for Clinical Infant Programs.

Schwab-Stone, M. E., Ayers, T. S., Kasprow, W., Voyce, C., Barone, C., Shriver, T., & Weissberg, R. P. (1995). No safe haven: A study of violence exposure in a urban community. *Journal of the American Academy of Child and Adolescent Psychiatry, 34,* 1343–1352.

Zeanah, C. Z., & Scheeringa, M. (1996). Evaluation of posttraumatic symptomatology in infants and young children exposed to violence. In J. D. Osofsky & E. Fenichel (Eds.), *Islands of safety: Assessing and treating young victims of violence* (pp. 9–14). Washington, DC: Zero to Three.

CHAPTER 1

RAINBOWS OF TEARS, SOULS FULL OF HOPE

Cultural Issues Related to Young Children and Trauma

MARVA L. LEWIS
CHANDRA GHOSH IPPEN

> The soul would have no rainbow if the eyes had no tears.
> —MINQUASS PROVERB

Like war, violence, and plagues, trauma to children is universal. So what we know about the cultural issues related to young children and trauma begins with what we know about young children. Young children grow up embedded in the physical and social niches of caregiving environments (Lewis, 2000b; Super & Harkness, 1997). They grow and develop physically, cognitively, and emotionally within a network of human relationships. These human relationships are circumscribed by what we call culture.

Culture, the human-made part of the environment, imbues the everyday experiences of its members with meaning and purpose (Bracken, 2002). Thus, when children experience trauma, like every person within their cultural group, culture provides meaning to their lived experience of trauma. Whether the trauma occurs within the confines of the family home in the form of incest by a biological parent or outside of the home in the form of sexual abuse by a trusted priest, such an abused child is generally socialized to emotionally and cognitively respond to the event as trauma according to the guidelines of his or her culture. Each culture has specific social and religious rituals for its members' experience of loss, tragedy, and disaster. These beliefs and rituals are an integral part of the healing (Woodcock, 1995).

Historically and currently many forms of interpersonal violence, natural disasters, and human-made disasters have been part of the lives of young children. Just as child maltreatment is determined by cultural, social and community standards (Korbin, 1977), what constitutes trauma to children is also a culturally defined phenomenon.

The classic tale that includes images of young Oliver Twist being beaten with a cane by his high-status employer in Charles Dickinson's 19th-century England is a treasured part of Western culture. In contrast, the images of young adolescent girls being prepared for ceremonial female circumcision in a country in Central Africa are less familiar in the West but have been depicted in news reports and have been the issue of recent international debates. Yet another familiar scene depicted in movies and part of family albums in both European and American Jewish homes is that of a young male infant being held aloft before the circumcision ceremony. A *mohel* (ritual circumciser) performs the ceremony with beaming parents, grandparents, and friends as proud witnesses of what is viewed in Western cultures as a trivial and benign procedure (Goldman, 1997).

Across cultures and around the world there are cultural practices that inflict pain and could easily fit into a modern definition of trauma. Yet, the children subjected to these everyday cultural practices—the circumcised male child, the caned child, and the circumcised adolescent female—do not necessarily experience the events as trauma. To Western knowledge the physical pain is transitory. From a Western perspective, their responses to the event do not become part of a psychic structure that fits the criteria for posttraumatic stress disorder (PTSD).

The more severe forms of intentional trauma to which children are exposed, such as war, child abuse, physical assault, severe neglect and abandonment, domestic violence, and community violence, are typically the focus of both theory and interventions. Within the past decade there has been increasing recognition of the vulnerability of children who simply witness or have knowledge of acts of interpersonal violence to develop PTSD symptoms (Garbarino, Dubrow, Kostelny, & Pardo, 1992; Lewis, Osofsky, & Moore, 1997). Research has found that young, inner-city, ethnic minority children are exposed to high rates of trauma, including witnessing a homicide or serious assault involving a weapon and being the direct victim of violence (Bell & Jenkins, 1993; Groves, Zuckerman, Marans, & Cohen, 1993; Osofsky, 1995).

There are increasing numbers of studies documenting the psychological effects of single-incident and chronic forms of trauma on infants and young children leading to reactive attachment disorders (Kaufman & Henrich, 2000) and PTSD (Scheeringa & Gaensbauer, 2000). More recently the distinct needs and experiences of children living in war zones and experiencing the trauma of refugee status have come to the attention of developmental practitioners (Baker & Shalhoub-Kevorkian, 1999; De Levita, 2000; Malakoff, 1994; Parson, 2002; Zea, Diehl, & Porterfield, 1997).

Given this reality, clinicians and researchers working with certain cultural and socioeconomic groups are likely to encounter children with high rates of trauma exposure and, therefore, must be prepared to assess for trauma and its sequela.

THE CONCEPTUAL DISTINCTION OF CULTURE, RACE, AND ETHNICITY

To best understand the cultural dimensions of trauma, it is important to differentiate the term "culture" from the terms with which it is commonly confused—"race" and "ethnicity." Though there are overlapping areas in the meanings of these terms, they are often used interchangeably by researchers and clinicians. This practice has led to conceptual as well as methodological confusion in research on young children and their families (Lewis, 2000a).

Culture refers to the traditions, values, customs of child-care and socialization practices and includes rituals and artifacts that symbolize the group's belief systems. Culture provides the psychic structure for relationships among members of a social group while simultaneously helping them to make meaning of the physical world. Individuals are socialized into a culture that is learned and transmitted primarily through language and everyday interactions.

Ethnicity is defined as the subjective social identity of an individual within a larger group (Lewis, 2000b). Race, a term distinct to the United States' and South Africa's sociopolitical histories, refers to what began as an anthropological category used to classify groups of people based on phenotypic features, primarily skin color. Typically, individuals identify their country of origin and their ethnicity. Their culture may be yet a different source. Thus, a child growing up in the United States and whose phenotypic features (skin color) are dark (black) may be externally categorized by the United States census as a "black American." Yet, this child's ethnicity may be Jamaican American and, as part of a fourth-generation immigrant family, his or her cultural heritage is "American."

Sadly, as we write this chapter the United States is at war in Iraq, a country where ethnicity as well as religious sectariansim have contributed to centuries-old conflicts. Arabs (who may be either Shi'ite or Sunni Muslims) and Kurds (who are Sunni) represent distinct ethnic groups within that country. Though they share some cultural values, there are distinct sociopolitical differences, and various historical traumas have solidified their ethnic identities and continued the conflict (Weinhold & Weinhold, 2000). The Kurds (some 15–20%) are concentrated in the northern highlands, and the Arabs predominate in the southern and central regions. About 95% of Iraqis are Muslims, of which 60–65% are Shi'ite, the rest Sunni.

It is the emotional intensity of ethnicity that we discuss later which we argue provides the psychological foundation for intergenerational legacies of risk factors for further trauma in young children's lives. Simultaneously, we argue that ethnic identity may be a source of psychological protection for young children faced with overwhelming trauma.

In this chapter, we focus on culture as a source of protection as well as a risk factor in the lives of young children traumatized by various types of natural and human-made events. We argue there are sources of protection within culturally derived systems, customs, and everyday practices that give meaning to the myriad of traumatic events occurring in the lives of children (Bagilishya, 2000; Rechtman, 2000; Salzman, 2001; Tully, 1999; Wessells, 1999). These sources include temporal, cognitive, and cultural patterned behaviors that serve as antidotes to what would otherwise be overwhelming experiences of traumatic events for children (Bracken, 2002; Peddle, Monteiro, Guluma, & Macaulay, & Thomas, 1999; Tully, 1999).

The concept of trauma as a cultural construct is examined first. A model is presented that describes the relationships among the various complex factors distinct to young children and their cultural groups. We use a theoretical framework of caregiver–child attachment to highlight the importance of these cultural factors. A second conceptual framework is presented to elucidate the emotional intensity and intergenerational legacies of child socialization in a variety of cultural groups, a discussion that includes the concepts of ethnic identity, historical trauma, and collective trauma response (Brave Heart, 2000). We examine how these legacies may raise socioeconomic issues in children that are related to continuing ethnic conflicts and stigmatization.

The following section addresses issues related to assessment of culture and trauma to the child, the caregiver, and the quality of their relationship. We then consider what we know about treatment of trauma in young children with an emphasis on cultural aspects of the treatment process. Finally, we discuss what we need to know and directions for research and practice.

THE CULTURAL CONSTRUCTION OF TRAUMA

The cultural context phenomenologically shapes the lived experience of both children's development and their experience of trauma. The meaning of trauma is often culture specific. Each culture has its own social and religious rituals for the experience of loss and disaster (Munet-Vilaró, 1998). These beliefs and rituals are an integral part of the social system of everyday lives. These beliefs and rituals are often predicated on the religious beliefs of the group.

Perceptions of trauma vary across members of the developmental niche: society, caregivers, parents, and children. It is the continuity and discontinuity of these perceptions of the trauma that help us to understand the risk to young children.

Cultural norms and practices provide the moral foundation for the formation of laws, policies, and practices within a society and for their institutions. Societal definitions of trauma include the legal definitions, and policies to define what is a stress, trauma, disaster, or tragedy (Zakour, 2000). These laws and policies are then translated by the variety of helping and support agencies that work directly with victims of trauma.

Cultural Determinants of Young Children's Experience of Trauma

There are common cultural threads that occur across all type of traumas experienced by young children. These common threads are based on the child's socialization into the cultural group. They include the developmental status of the child at the time of the event, individual PTSD responses, customs, and traditions available or directed at the event (grief, mourning, rituals).

There are many levels of cultural determinants of young children's experience of trauma. We present a graphic representation of these determinants in Figure 1.1. These determinants stem from the dominant or host culture's provision of social supports, laws, and policies in response to trauma as well as the definition of trauma provided by the culture of origin of the child's family.

At the societal level, protective factors for the child stem from formal recognition and cultural supports that affirm the individual experience of the traumatic event. "Was it real?" or "Did this event really occur?" are typical questions an individual may ask in the disorientation and chaos that follow a traumatic event. When there is societal acceptance and validation of the traumatic event, there are holidays, remembrances, rituals tied to the event, and even economic compensation provided by the government to the victims of the event. In the United States an example of this type of formal societal recognition of a traumatic event is that of the forced internment of all Japanese Americans in the aftermath of the bombing of Pearl Harbor on December 7, 1941. Entire families of American citizens of Japanese ancestry were removed from their homes on the west coast and placed into "detention camps" further inland. The families who experienced this traumatic event expressed feelings of rage, anger, powerlessness, fear, and shame. In

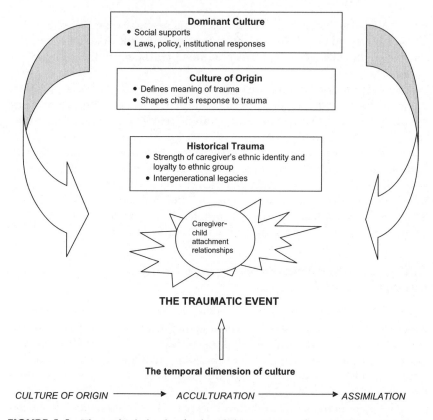

FIGURE 1.1. The multiple levels of cultural determinants of young children's experience of trauma.

recent years, the U.S. government has formally apologized to the interned families and their descendants as well as provided monetary compensation to them. Thus, the traumatic event has been validated as "real" for all who experienced it as well as for the later generations who had only heard about it.

The historical trauma experienced by the cultural group over generations and the strength of identification and loyalty to the group are also important emotional determinants.

At the center of the traumatic event are the child and the quality of his or her attachment relationship with the caregiver. The fundamental premise of John Bowlby's (1969, 1988) ethological definition of attachment is the availability of a responsive caregiver when the attachment system is activated. Trauma may activate or serve to mute the attachment-related behaviors of both the child and the caregiver.

Further, the context that provides the fabric of the experience of trauma of young children includes culturally determined characteristics of the caregivers. These characteristics include the subjective ethnic and racial identity of the caregiver, the caregiver's sense of empowerment, and cultural guidelines for the degree to which he or she may advocate for services for the child. Emotionally, the degree to which the individual caregiver has achieved resolution related to the traumatic event will impact the child's experience (Lewis, 1996). Especially relevant to our discussion is the caregiver's emotional history of loss including experiences of culture shock, oppression, discrimination, or torture as a member of an ethnic minority group. Consequently, these internal working models of ethnic minority–majority group relationships and residual complicated intense emotions may complicate the natural mourning process of culture loss (Rousseau, Mekki-Berrada, & Moreau, 2001). Culture shock refers to the wide range of experiences of loss and disorientation upon entering a new culture (Levy-Warren, 1987). We would argue that the social supports available for working through this shock, coupled with the timing with which those supports are offered, may have important implications for the idealization and strength of identification with the home culture. Bracken (2002) argues that posttraumatic anxiety is a problem with strong social and cultural dimensions and not simply an issue of individual psychopathology. We elaborate on this issue later in this chapter in the section on cultural issues and assessment.

The temporal aspects of culture include the concepts of acculturation and assimilation. These temporal aspects provide the conceptual foundation for understanding the experience of a traumatic event at the family level. We present these processes as two points on a continuum involving the culture of origin of the child's family and the acculturation process that occurs over time when the family moves to a new culture. We later return to these concepts in the section on cultural issues and assessment.

Culture as a Mediator of Trauma to Young Children

As noted earlier, culture provides meaning to the everyday experiences of children and their caregivers. Culturally patterned behaviors include rituals and traditions related to death, loss, and socialization practices (Woodcock, 1995).

In a comprehensive review of studies of children around the world "in particularly difficult circumstances," as defined by the United Nations, Aptekar and Stöcklin (1997) argue that though there may be multiple contributing factors, the cultural context serves as a potent mediator of traumas to young children. They state:

> But the cultural context may shape responses to extreme stress. The children's victimization cannot be measured in absolute terms. It is more than the degree to which they have been abused, neglected, or tortured. The sig-

nificance the child attaches to the trauma, which in large part is mediated by cultural factors, also determines how the child responds. Children's resilience and vulnerability cannot be explained merely by individual differences in temperament. . . . [T]his is largely because culture influences children's responses to trauma. (p. 379)

They propose three ways that culture interacts with children's reactions to extreme stress:

1. Culture mediates the possible range of child responses from PTSD to a relatively benign reaction, and finally to improved mental health.
2. Specific groups of children (e.g., street children) use culture as a means to cope. They actively use their knowledge of the socio-cultural environment as a means to transform their circumstances into opportunities.
3. Cultural stigmatization of groups of children occurs in particularly difficult circumstances.

Based on their review of cross-cultural studies of children diagnosed with PTSD symptoms, Aptekar and Stöcklin (1997) note that it is not the exposure to a single traumatic event but rather the multiple stresses that necessarily produces PTSD symptoms. They also argue that the formulation of a single event as the necessary diagnostic criteria for classification as a mental disorder by the American Psychiatric Association reflects a cultural bias. They propose that there is little information to distinguish different psychological reactions to single and multiple traumas. Multiple traumatic events are "considerably more likely to occur in the developing world, where war and disaster are common" (p. 384). They also note that from World War II to 1989 more than 21 million people, many of whom were children, were killed in wars in developing countries.

Similarly, with the high rates of urban community violence as well as violence related to war and genocide and its impact on children, the generational impact on caregivers locked in a cycle of chronic violence is an important focus (Bagilishya, 2000). Later in this chapter, we elaborate on these issues and assessment of children and their caregivers.

Next we discuss the manner through which culture may serve as a source of protection to children exposed to trauma as well as how culture and ethnicity may serve as risk factors for trauma for children.

Distinctive Forms of Trauma to Young Children and Their Cultural Groups

Table 1.1 summarizes the distinctive ways the developmental status of young children and the cultural context shape their experience of trauma.

TABLE 1.1. Distinct Forms of Trauma Experienced by Young Children and Their Cultural Groups

Trauma experienced uniquely by children		Trauma experienced or perpetuated uniquely by cultural groups	
Traumas based on developmental status	Trauma experienced as part of a cohort	Historical trauma of a minority group based on culture, race, or ethnicity	Intergenerational legacies of conflicts between dominant and minority groups
• Child maltreatment physical abuse sexual abuse abandonment emotional abuse severe neglect • Witness to domestic violence • Ritual abuse • Victim, witness, or knowledge of community violence • Victim of interpersonal peer violence (including bullying) • Victim of sibling violence	• The bombing of Hiroshima and World War II • The Atlanta child murders • Children in the Branch Davidian Compound in Waco, Texas • The forced separation and placement in boarding school of Native American children • Hurricane Betsy • Earthquakes • The Oklahoma City bombing • The attack on the World Trade Center, September 11, 2001	• The genocide, dislocation, and resettlement of Native Americans over the past 400 years in North America • Africans enslaved by Europeans in the North Atlantic slave trade over a period of 300 years • The era of Jim Crow segregation in the United States and apartheid in South Africa that enforced racial segregation of blacks and whites • The centuries-old caste system of India and legally sanctioned social discrimination • The Holocaust: the planned genocide of European Jews • Violence to females in patriarchal, misogynist eras (e.g., the Victorian era, or practices of the Taliban in Afghanistan)	• Arab–Israeli wars • Prolonged Northern Ireland conflict between Protestants and Catholics • U.S. institutionalized racism, white supremacy • Kurdish and Iranian families in political exile • Genocide of 2 million Cambodians in the "killing fields"

Note. Anthony Pereira, Professor of Political Science and Latin American studies, Tulane University, provided helpful comments on this table.

There are also individual and interpersonal factors associated with the child's experience of trauma related to his or her proximity to the event. By virtue of their developmental status, young children are at increased risk for exposure to specific types of traumas, such as parental abuse and witnessing interfamilial violence. They are also dependent upon their caregivers as sources of safety and protection.

Children may also experience trauma as part of a group or generation who form a cohort that experiences a single or short-term event. For example, on September 11, 2001, a cohort of children were traumatized by the terrorist attack on the New York World Trade Center. There has been much research on the cohort effect over generations, including distinct cohorts of adults who experienced the stock market crash of 1929, the Great Depression of the 1930s, or the assassination of President John F. Kennedy on November 22, 1963. But little work exists on the cohort effects of children experiencing trauma. The early work of Robert Coles (1967), who studied the traumatic impact of racial desegregation on African American children in cities in the southern United States, and the work of Bruce D. Perry (1994), who studied the long-term effects on those children who survived the tragic events in the Branch Davidian Compound in Waco, Texas, are examples of this type of research.

These various forms of trauma have common, as well as idiosyncratic or distinctive features that have differential implications for the young child's development and relationship with his or her caregiver.

Trauma experienced by someone as an individual versus as a member of a group will have a different impact and may result in different emotional responses (Peddle et al., 1999; Rechtman, 2000; Velez-Ibanez & Parra, 1999; Tully, 1999). Trauma to a group experienced over generations has a different set of implications for the caregiver–child relationship and developmental experience (Baker & Shalhoub-Kevorkian, 1999).

Children's Developmental Status and Trauma

There are distinct forms of trauma experienced by an individual child as a function of his or her dependent status. Traumas based on developmental status include physical and sexual abuse, neglect, and witnessing interfamilial violence. These traumas may involve a single incident or repeated, chronic occurrences, but generally occur in the context of close, interfamilial relationships. Thus, a parent abuses a child, a cult ritually abuses their child victims, and a sibling targets a smaller child in the family for aggressive behavior. These interpersonal traumas directed at a single child or family of children directly negatively impact the formation of caregiver–child attachment relationships (Kaufman & Henrich, 2000; Osofsky, 1995).

The emotions in children associated with these types of individual or interpersonal traumas include intense fear, vigilance, stigma, shame, guilt, and helplessness (Deater-Deckard, Dodge, Bates, & Pettit, 1996; Lewis et al., 1997; Lewis, 2000a). The emotions are distinct in that they are all social and relational. We believe these trauma-based emotions become the precursors and residual fuel for the intergenerational ethnic and cultural conflicts we discuss later.

The *cohort traumas* experienced by children typically involve a single event, either an intentionally caused incident or a natural disaster that affects selected groups of children and their caregivers. Such events usually occur in a single instance or over a discreet or short period of time. The larger society responds with supports and widespread validation for victims of these traumas. There is an outpouring of public sympathy and resources ranging from crisis counseling to monetary reparations to the families.

The third and fourth type of cultural traumas presented in Table 1.1 that children are vulnerable to are based on the dominant or minority status of their group and on the legacies of intergenerational ethnic conflicts. The two columns on the right side of Table 1.1 summarize the distinct forms of trauma experienced or perpetuated by cultural groups. The traumas associated with the minority status of the ethnic group include a widespread, socially structured array of physical and psychological traumas. Genocide and forced relocation of Native Americans and Cambodians (Bit, 1991), the enslavement of African people, and the genocide of Jewish people in the Holocaust are examples of prolonged traumas experienced by groups of people based in part on their minority status. Traumatic acts such as genocide, rape, racism, and discrimination are typically supported by laws and policies and tied to the political and economic power of the dominant group. Birth into the minority group presents automatic subjection to trauma. Membership in the minority group is not by choice but tied to arbitrary criteria determined by the dominant group. Thus, language, phenotypic features such as skin color or eye shape, or religious heritage may serve as the irrational catalyst for racial or ethnic hatred and the infliction of trauma.

Within their families and neighborhoods children are socialized across generations into beliefs, values, and emotions associated with their ethnic, religious, or minority group status. They may also be socialized through institutes (school, literature, art) that they have a specific enemy, given guidelines for acceptable behavior, and taught specific emotional display rules.

We argue that emotions associated with the cultural group's unique trauma history set the psychological stage for intergenerational legacies of trauma and the historical trauma response (Brave Heart, 2000).

Intergenerational Legacies of Trauma: Historical Trauma Response

The diathesis stress model proposes that individuals may be predisposed (have organic vulnerability) to stress (Shalev, 1996); cultural groups may have similar vulnerabilities. The concepts of historical trauma and collective trauma response provide a conceptual framework to understand intergenerational legacies of trauma. In her work with Native Americans, Brave Heart (2000) identifies historical trauma responses (HTR) as an organizing conceptual framework. The manifestations of HTR in caregiver–child relationships may be in relation to socialization practices that highlight cultural histories, stories and myths related to the minority group status. More likely there may be silence and omission of sections of history related to painful memories and traumatic events of the group.

Brave Heart (2000) describes that one of the mental health outcomes of HTR is historical unresolved grief. Thus, complicated bereavement may be passed down through generations of children carrying on the legacy of pain.

Ethnicity as a Source of Protection and Vulnerability

Ethnic identity is the subjective part of culture. How an individual acts upon her identification with her ethnic group and these behavioral manifestations is the outward evidence of these intrapsychic processes (Phinney, 1996). Individuals are born into a specific ethnic group that has a range of historical cultural practices. These everyday cultural practices have presented guidelines for everyday living, and the child is socialized into the group. A normative part of developing and consolidating an identity as an adult includes the degree to which the adolescent embraces the identity of the group into which he or she was born and socialized (Phinney, 1996). This developmental choice is of particular importance for understanding the continuity and transmission of intergenerational legacies that fuel ethnic conflicts, hatred, and even wars.

The sense of identity begins with the first mental images of the body and develops progressively into more differentiated, symbolic, and continuous mental representations of the self and of animate and inanimate objects (Levy-Warren, 1987). The abstractions of "country," "nationality," and "home" are filled with images of people, things, sights, smells, and sounds, as well as values.

Ethnic identity includes cognitive, affective, and behavioral factors. Cognitive factors in adult caregivers include beliefs about children and their parenting role. Knowledge and attitudes about the normative practices related to child care according to the standards of the ethnic group are included in these factors. Thus, opinions as to whether a crying child should be held and comforted and how long the child should be held are determined, in part, by the degree to which the individual identifies with her ethnic group.

Ethnic identity includes strong affect and is associated with a variety of emotions. Pride, feelings of belonging, safety, security, homesickness, pleasure, excitement, dread, mourning, and sadness are only a partial list of the myriad emotions that are associated with strong ethnic identification. The feelings of ethnic or racial pride or shame and internalized negative stereotypes about the in-group and out-group are critical factors that may lead to interethnic conflict (Ryan & Bogart, 1997). An underexplored area of ethnic identity is how feelings of ethnic or racial shame may be associated with intraethnic as well as intrafamilial conflicts and stigmatization (Lewis, 2000a).

The next area of culture and ethnicity that helps us understand the impact of trauma on children and their families is the temporal dimension of acculturation and assimilation.

Acculturation and Assimilation as Mediating Cultural Processes

The processes of acculturation and assimilation are of particular relevance to understanding the role of culture as a mediator of children's trauma. These processes incorporate the concept of culture loss to the individual members. Many countries are typically composed of a variety of ethnic groups that have varying historical relationships. In this current technologically driven era of decreasing formal boundaries through Internet connections and global travel there is also increased movement by groups of individuals and families from various ethnic groups.

When families with young children move because of a desire for improved economic resources or are forced to relocate for political asylum due to war or famine, they typically enter the host country in a minority group status. Fundamental processes associated with their immigration are acculturation and assimilation. Both are processes of accommodation to the host (or dominant) culture and individuals vary in their degrees of cultural shock and loss of the culture of origin.

Acculturation. An important psychological process that impacts the caregivers of young children who have relocated includes the experience of loss. The loss of friends, family, work, home, neighborhood, and all that is physically familiar including even the weather and landscape, is the source of grief to newly immigrated caregivers. The decreased opportunity for language partners outside of the home is a constant reminder of the social isolation that is part of the process of acculturating to a new country. Levy-Warren (1987) argues that much of the successful adaptation of individuals to separation from their homeland and country depends on the individual's ability to engage in a healthy mourning process. As culture provides meaning to everyday experiences within the home country and the formation of individual and family identity, it also provides the means to experience the loss of that culture in the new country.

Assimilation. The most complex aspect of the process of acculturation is the process of assimilation. These two ends of a continuum involve a physical and an internal experience of loss as well as internal and external processes of separation. Assimilation is fundamentally a process of culture loss. The ethnic identification, beliefs, and practices from the culture of origin may be eroded in some instances through passive inattention or, in other instances, simply overpowered by the dominant culture. In some dominant societies and cultures, members of the minority group may be forcibly stripped of any outward signs of their culture. They may be forbidden on pain of death to speak their language, wear their traditional clothes, or practice their religious customs. Further, the loss of language may be based on the practical need to be able to function in the economic and educational institutions of the host country. Without a conscious commitment to retaining the language of origin, disuse of the home language may represent an unconscious "loss."

There is a further need to distinguish between culture loss and culture shock (Levy-Warren, 1987). Some of the external cultural factors affecting the separation reaction include age at relocation, presence of animate and inanimate objects from the lost culture, circumstances surrounding the relocation (especially the degree of choice and preparation for the move), and differences between the culture of origin and the new culture. There is a natural mourning process of culture loss and more pathological melancholic expressions of culture shock. In Figure 1.1 we note that the degree of societal supports available that reflect the culture of the minority group will be of clinical significance.

For young children under the age of 5 years, the move from one country to another is simply a physical or geographic move: "Culture at this time is almost entirely associated with the primary caretakers, so that the 'culture' for the child moves with the family" (Levy-Warren, 1987, p. 306).

These developmental and cultural contextual factors we have just presented provide the conceptual framework for the next section on cultural issues related to assessment and treatment of traumatized young children and their caregivers.

CULTURAL ISSUES AND ASSESSMENT

The young child's cultural background constitutes a key factor that we need to assess because psychological symptoms, resulting from trauma exposure, may be expressed differently in different cultures (Yamamoto, Silva, Ferrari, & Nukariya, 1997). As DeVries (1996) eloquently states, "culture plays a key role in how individuals cope with potentially traumatizing experiences by providing the context in which social support and other positive and uplifting events can be experienced" (p. 400). Cultures help the individual to regulate emotions, order behavior, and obtain support through rituals and customs that create meaning for traumatic events, norms, rules, and values that link the individual to the larger community, and a shared vision of the future (DeVries, 1996).

Alicia F. Lieberman and Patricia Van Horn (Chapter 4, this volume) clearly delineate key domains to assess when we are working with young children exposed to trauma. In this section, we focus on how the young child's cultural and socioeconomic context affects the assessment of these domains, and we provide guidelines for assessing these areas in a culturally competent manner. Still, it is with the caveat that membership in a cultural group does not define the individual or the individual's experience. For example, while it is important to know that adult immigrants from Nicaragua may have been affected by the war between the Contras and the Sandinistas, it is important not to presume that all Nicaraguans have witnessed war atrocities. Information regarding the experience of a cultural group provides the assessor with a line of inquiry, which, while important to examine, must be explored openly and flexibly.

Objective and Subjective Features of the Trauma, Secondary Adversities, and Other Stressors

Pynoos and colleagues (Pynoos, Steinberg, & Goenjian, 1996; Pynoos, Steinberg, & Piacentini, 1999) stress that when we are working with traumatized children, it is essential to gather information regarding each child's objective and subjective experience of the event, the type and frequency of traumatic reminders, current and future stresses, and secondary adversities. The clinician or researcher assessing these areas with culturally diverse children should be aware of the following considerations.

First, certain cultural groups are more likely to have a history of exposure to multiple traumas, compounded by multiple secondary adversities and life stressors. Immigrant children, particularly refugees, may experience multiple traumas (Johnson-Powell, 1997). Refugee camps, instead of serving as safe havens, may present additional dangers as they are generally located near the violent regions from which the refugees fled (Miller, 1996). Thus, refugee children may be exposed not only to war trauma but also to violence in the camps. When they leave their country, they may also face the loss of family members who are not able to emigrate, loss of their culture, and community violence if they are relocated to American inner-city areas. In lower-income ethnic minority children, particularly those residing in America's inner cities, multiple secondary adversities and life stressors may compound the effects of trauma exposure. Common secondary adversities include—but are not limited to—single-parent family status, discrimination, overcrowding, poor housing, dangerous and impoverished neighborhoods, illegal immigrant status, and poverty.

Indirect exposure to trauma through caregivers' recounting of graphic details represents an additional way that children may experience trauma. Young children may form mental images of traumas described by family members in their presence and may develop fears and other symptoms to accompany these mental images. Miller (1996) found that Guatemalan children in refugee camps, who had not been directly exposed to the war, told stories of Guatemalan soldiers who might kill them, spoke of tortures, massacres, and war, and drew pictures that incorporated images of senseless military violence.

Finally, as detailed earlier in this chapter, when a cultural group has been affected by significant traumas, the trauma may be transmitted intergenerationally (Baker & Shalhoub-Kevorkian, 1999; Brave Heart, 2000;

Danieli, 1985). Cultural values may affect whether this process of secondary traumatization occurs. Baker & Shalhoub-Kevorkian (1999), for example, suggest that Palestinian culture and mores valuing collectivism lead individual traumas to be experienced by society, in particular by neighbors, friends, and acquaintances. Young children reared in the shadow of a historical collective trauma may experience altered views regarding the safety of the world and interpersonal relationships, which may in turn impact their development (Lewis et al., 1997).

We suggest, then, that it is important to thoroughly assess the child, family, and cultural group's history of exposure to potentially traumatic events, keeping in mind that the family may have experienced multiple events and that they may be accompanied by life stressors and/or secondary adversities that pose just as significant a risk to the child's development. The assessor's knowledge of events that the family's cultural group may have undergone and his or her ability to directly inquire about the family's experience of these events will greatly enhance the quality and validity of the assessment. In our own work, we have found that without our directly inquiring about specific events, parents and children often fail to report them. This is particularly the case with young children, as parents may acknowledge that an event happened when directly asked but may fail to bring it up because they feel sure that the child does not remember it and/or was not affected by it, or because it was so common an occurrence that they may not view it as a potentially traumatic event.

However, it is not only the objective fact of whether an event has occurred to a child, family, or cultural group that affects the child's development but also the culture's and individual's perception of the event that determines its ultimate impact on the child's functioning and developmental trajectory. Cultural values and mores help us to define what is traumatic. For mental health professionals, the fourth edition of the *Diagnostic and Statistical Manual of Mental Disorders* (DSM-IV; American Psychiatric Association, 1994) serves as one cultural guide that helps define traumatic events. They are those that meet the criteria for a Criterion A stressor by involving (1) the actual or threatened death or serious injury, or threat to physical integrity of self or others, and (2) a response including intense fear, helplessness, horror, or disorganized or agitated behavior. But what is the impact of the event on people from cultures where such an event may be considered common? For example, in cultures where domestic violence is common, how does the cultural lens that tells us "this is what happens" affect the individual's perception of and reaction to the event? When the event occurs as part of a ritual, as in the case of genital mutilation, does that alter its meaning? These are questions we cannot answer—and, even if we could, the individual's perception of the event may differ from that of the larger cultural group. As part of the assessment process, it is important to focus on whether the cultural group views a given event as traumatic and whether, and to what degree, the individual shares the group's perception of the event.

Child Functioning

When we assess young children, we must remember that judgments regarding their functioning are influenced by their actual behavior and by the way the adults view the behavior and that both of these are affected by cultural factors (Weisz, 1989). In a series of studies, Weisz and colleagues (Weisz, 1989; Weisz et al., 1988; Weisz, Sigman, Weiss, & Mosk, 1993) showed that culturally mediated beliefs and associated childrearing and socialization practices shape the type of behavior children display when distressed and the kind of problems caregivers identify as distressing. They found different patterns of behaviors in American, Thai, and African children, related to the cultural values of these countries. Thai children were more likely to be referred to treatment for problems of overcontrolled behavior, whereas American children were more likely to be referred for problems of undercontrolled behavior. Thai adults also expressed less concern than Americans regarding the seriousness of both types of behavior. In community samples, African youth were rated significantly higher on overcontrolled behaviors than either Thai or American children, but the high scores were due to endorsement of somatic items. Weisz and colleagues discussed how cultural values, including the emphasis on politeness and obedience in Kenyan culture and Thai Buddhist principles, are related both to children's behavior and to the way their caregivers view their behavior.

Cultures also vary significantly in terms of the developmental tasks children are expected to accomplish by a certain age, the way childhood and infancy are viewed, what is considered appropriate child behavior at different ages, and traits or values parents want their children to develop (Okagaki & Sternberg, 1993). Cultural variability in these areas will affect the assessment of children's functioning. Variability will also influence the caregiving environment and the caregiver's view of the child's behavior (Garcia Coll, 1990). When we work with children from diverse cultural backgrounds, we may find that the school culture and family culture have different values. For example, a Native American family may value interdependence while the school values having children act autonomously. These differences can lead to conflicts as the child learns to navigate between the two worlds. Therefore, it is important to assess the cultural values of the different settings within which children must function and adjust.

Language represents a key aspect of child functioning that is shaped by the child's cultural experiences and which in turn shapes the child's view of the world and of herself. As young children from different language backgrounds enter day care or preschool, they often spend more time speaking English than they do their native language. This can lead to problems in communication between parents and children. We have worked with Latino children in the process of learning English and have found many cases where a child does not understand certain words in Spanish because she learned them only in English. Her caregivers, not knowing this, feel she is misbehaving by seemingly ignoring their directives when really it is more probable that she does not understand them. A good assessment of the child's linguistic abilities is important when working with children whose primary language is not English. Different languages may also play different roles for children. For example, English may become the language of academics and school while the child's native language may serve as the language of feelings (Canino & Spurlock, 2000). This becomes important when children are seen in treatment after experiencing a trauma. Although the child may appear to speak sufficient English to work with an English-speaking therapist, the child's memories and feelings related to the event may be encoded and better processed in her native language.

Caregiver Functioning

When working with diverse cultural groups, we must broaden our definition of caregiver beyond the mother and father. Research suggests that extended kin play a significant role in the parenting of ethnic minority children and that ethnic minority infants may be exposed to multiple caregivers and may experience caregiving environments other than those provided by two-parent families (Garcia Coll, 1990; Tolson & Wilson, 1990). Therefore, when we conduct the assessment we may need to involve other potential caregivers including grandparents, older siblings, godparents, and even fictive kin such as compadres and "play family," both as reporters and as potential participants in treatment.

Across different cultural groups, young children's functioning following a trauma appears to be strongly tied to the presence and functioning of their primary caregivers (Laor, Wolmer, & Cohen, 2001; Miller, 1996) and to their caregivers' reaction to and ability to make sense of the event (Pynoos, 1994). Chemtob and Taylor (2002) highlight the importance of caregiver functioning in helping children reestablish regulatory operations and a sense of safety. They state that caregivers' symptoms and emotional reactivity may reduce their psychological availability and empathy for the child, making them less effective at helping the child to modulate his or her reactions. We have found that children exposed to traumas often have caregivers who have been exposed to traumas. Inquiring about the caregiver's trauma history, current symptomatology, and reactions to traumas may provide critical information about factors that may be related to the child's functioning.

In our work with caregivers of children exposed to chronic violence, we found that part of the assessment process required that a medical examination of the primary caregiver be completed. Somatic complaints, sleep disturbances, and eating disorders were common among caregivers immersed in chronic trauma (Lewis, 1996). Waitzkin and Magana (1997) formulated a theory based on their clinical work with immigrants and refugees from Central America. They postulated that culture might serve as a mediator for severe stress and produce symptoms in the somatizing patient that cannot be explained by the presence of physical illness.

In addition, when working with ethnic minority groups, it may be important to identify how historical traumas that have affected the cultural group impact the caregiver.

The Child–Caregiver Relationship

Infant development and emotional functioning occurs in the context of relationships (Lieberman, Van Horn, Grandison, & Pekarsky, 1997). Therefore, it is essential to assess the quality of the child's relationships with significant caregivers. Assessment of this area is crucial in families where the child has experienced trauma, because trauma can disrupt relationships and because these relationships may mediate the effect of trauma exposure.

The caregiver–child relationship is shaped by the larger sociocultural context. Caregivers socialize the child to survive in society (Bronfenbrenner, 1979). They develop socialization goals based on the society's cultural values, their degree of acculturation, and their level of stress. Harrison, Wilson, Pine, Chan, and Buriel (1990) point out that the family ecology of ethnic minority children varies significantly from that of majority children. For example, ethnic minorities are more likely to encounter racism and discrimination. Thus, ethnic minorities develop different socialization goals that are more adaptive given their ecology. These goals influence their affective and social interactions, which in turn may lead children to develop different ways of exploring the environment, communicating, and thinking about the world and relationships (Garcia Coll, 1990; Harrison et al., 1990).

Across different cultures caregivers vary in the way they respond to infant's cries, the amount and type of stimulation they provide young children, their responsiveness, and their discipline strategies, and these differences are related to culturally based socialization goals (Garcia Coll, 1990). The same behavior may hold different consequences for child development depending on the cultural context in which it occurs. For example, in a study examining the relationship between physical discipline and aggressive child behavior, Deater-Deckard et al. (1996) found that parents' use of physical discipline in the nonabusive range was related to behavior problems at school for Caucasian but not African American children. They raised the issue of whether the meaning of physical discipline is the same in different ethnic groups and suggested that parenting behaviors may hold different meanings for children across the different cultures.

Key dimensions along which cultures vary include autonomy and relatedness (Harwood, 1992; Harrison et al., 1990). Okagaki and Sternberg (1993) found that while Anglo-American parents favored autonomy, immigrant parents from Cambodia, Mexico, the Philippines, and Vietnam valued conforming to external standards over autonomous behaviors. Harwood (2002) suggested that although these dimensions appear to capture some aspect of infant attachment behavior across cultural groups, other dimensions such as respectfulness might be equally important in other cultures. When we work with caregivers and young children of diverse cultural groups, we need to identify the socialization goals of both the culture and the caregiver so we can create ecologically valid interventions that are consistent with these goals. We can do this by openly inquiring about appropriate child behavior given the child's developmental level, the meaning and desired outcome behind a given caregiving behavior, and desirable and undesirable child behaviors.

The Sociocultural Context

In previous subsections we detailed ways in which the sociocultural context is related to the child's and family's experience of trauma and secondary adversities, child and caregiver functioning, and the child–caregiver relationship. We will now delineate specific areas of the sociocultural context that are important to assess. We organize these areas by asking questions in the following areas:

1. Where did the family come from?
2. How did they get here?
3. What is their environment like now?
4. How does their culture view and cope with the potentially traumatic event they have experienced?

1. *Where did the family come from?* At a basic level we must gather information regarding the family's country or countries of origin; however, this still offers a very limited view of the family's cultural background. Greater but still incomplete knowledge can be gained by inquiring about the specific region the family is from, whether they are from an urban setting versus a rural setting, and whether they are from a particular cultural group within that setting. Imagine, for example, the increasing depth of knowledge an assessor from another country might gain as she progresses from knowing that a person is from America, to knowing he grew up in a small rural town in Minnesota, to blending this information with the knowledge that he is African American.

2. *How did they get here?* The way a family came to be in the country or region where they are living also has significant consequences for child and family functioning. The journey itself may have been traumatic. Many Mexican immigrants, for example, die while attempting to cross the border, and others face abuse at the hands of "Coyotes," men they pay to smuggle them across the border. Some families are not able to migrate together. Parents may leave their young children in the care of a relative while they make the dangerous trip to the new country where they hope to obtain work and the ability to later send for their children. Children may be sent to the new country to live with relatives because it is "safer," but the parents are unable to join them immediately for either financial or legal reasons. Families may be separated during a war or in refugee camps and may have difficulty locating other family members. For young children, separation from primary caregivers constitutes a trauma because of the importance of the caregiver–child relationship.

Once in the new country, the family's legal status continues to affect their safety and their ability to access important resources. Illegal immigrants face a range of secondary adversities including constant worrying that they may be deported, employers who take advantage of them, and an inability to or fear of accessing needed resources.

The reasons for coming to the new country also impact the family in significant ways. Those who came voluntarily may view their migration as a chance to help themselves and their children move ahead or, as many Latinos express it, *seguir adelante.* In contrast, those whose migration was involuntary, as in the case of African Americans whose ancestors were brought across the Atlantic as slaves and Native Americans whose ancestors were forcefully resettled into reservations, are unlikely to view America as the "land of opportunity," especially after enduring years of racism and negative encounters with the white majority system (Tharp, 1991). This experience may also affect the way they view therapy, especially when it is mandated by a seemingly oppressive majority system.

3. *What is their environment like now?* The family's current environment serves as a new cultural context, which may influence the caregivers' socialization goals, child and caregiver functioning, and the caregiver–child relationship. As assessors we need to understand the degree to which this context is both similar to and different from the context they came from. Many immigrants face significant changes in social status. In their countries they may have been professionals living in their own home in a middle-class neighborhood, whereas in the United States they are only able to obtain work in the service sector and they rent an apartment with other families in a lower-income neighborhood. The values and customs of the new culture may differ significantly from that of their culture. When a family's culture is disrupted or lost because of immigration or war, this may be viewed as a significant stressor that negatively affects the family's ability to cope with

traumatic events (DeVries, 1996). While these are all possibilities, they must be assessed and not assumed. Many immigrants move to locations where they are able to live among people of their same cultural group and, in many ways, re-create the cultural environment they once had.

The new environment offers both risk and protective factors, which are helpful to identify. Risk factors will increase the family's overall level of stress and impinge on their ability to deal with the effects of the trauma, whereas protective factors may serve to support and buffer the child and family. Protective factors may include the opportunity to interact with others from their cultural group, religious organizations, neighborhood resources, and good day care and schools. Risk factors may include lack of access to health care, racism and discrimination, and neighborhood violence. Environments with high rates of community violence not only increase the likelihood that witnessing violence will retraumatize the child but also interfere with the child's ability to safely explore the world.

4. *How does their culture view and cope with the potentially traumatic event they have experienced?* A key component of a cultural formulation involves understanding the cultural explanation of an individual's illness (Lu, Lim, & Mezzich, 1995). With children exposed to trauma, we need to understand how their culture views the potentially traumatic event, what the cultural explanation for their symptoms might be, and whether there are any typical ways that the culture helps the child and family cope with the experience. With very young children a key component of this understanding includes assessing whether they are expected to be affected by experiencing potentially traumatic events. Assessing this allows the clinician to gain a better understanding of the family's motivation for participating in treatment and, when appropriate, enables the clinician to both respect this position and provide carefully timed developmental guidance regarding how the child has been affected by the event.

In some groups, particularly those who have experienced collective traumas such as war and natural disasters, individual members share a trauma history with their cultural group. Under these circumstances, the culture may offer specific rituals, customs, and legends that offer meaning, social support, and an ordered way to express and regulate emotions. DeVries (1996) discusses how the Digo, living on the East African (Kenyan and Tanzanian) coast, experienced tremendous stress following raids by the Masai. This stress was expressed through "trance dances," during which individuals could express their anxiety and fear by behaving like the aggressive Masai. Traditional healers gave these dances a label and incorporated them within traditional healing rituals where the dances were formalized and used to alleviate stress. This example illustrates one way that culture can provide a context for understanding the experience of trauma. However, we must remember that while a group may share the same trauma, loss, and migration history, the experience of each individual is unique.

As we work with culturally diverse families we must determine whether the culture offers any ways to help young children cope with traumatic events. When a child's parent dies, what is the cultural explanation of death? Are there specific explanations for why natural disasters occur? How do family members act after a young child has been harmed by another family member? These are some of the questions for which we might seek answers. We might also wonder whether in their culture it is appropriate to seek help from someone outside of the family and how they understand the process of therapy.

CULTURAL ISSUES AND TREATMENT

We know little about the effectiveness of treatment with ethnic minority children because most treatment outcome research involves predominantly Caucasian participants and very few studies have examined ethnicity as a moderator of treatment effectiveness (Weisz, 1989). Traditionally, poor ethnic minorities have been less likely to use mental health services (McMiller & Weisz, 1996; Sue, Fujino, Hu, Takeuchi, & Zane, 1991) and more likely to drop out of treatment (Kazdin & Weisz, 2003). Participation in treatment has been hindered by both practical barriers (e.g., lack of insurance, child care, and transportation) and culture-related barriers (e.g., lack of minority practitioners, culturally appropriate services, and knowledge among majority practitioners about cross-cultural issues; Miranda, Azocar, Organista, Muñoz, & Lieberman, 1996; Pumariega, 2001).

If we are to serve and retain ethnic minorities in treatment, we must begin by integrating case management approaches that help families overcome practical barriers. Offering concrete assistance, such as bus tokens and on-site childcare will greatly enhance the likelihood that poor ethnic minorities are able to participate in treatment. However, the level of case management needed to truly help these families may extend beyond these preliminary interventions. When we truly understand the family's ecological context, we often discover significant real-life problems. Many families do not have adequate housing or sufficient food. They may live in neighborhoods or in families where physical safety has not been established. Families may need information to navigate mainstream culture, including learning how to sign up for good schools, how to obtain a restraining order, and how to find an immigration lawyer. Any culturally valid treatment must address these realities. Although at times we may not feel that this is part of a "psychological treatment," it is central to the well-being of the child and family, and thus is a cornerstone of treatment.

Also central to any treatment is the ability to develop rapport with both the child and his or her caregivers. Young children are brought to treatment by their caregivers, and their caregivers may be less likely to attend when they feel that their perspective, values, or socialization goals are not understood. Adopting cultural customs and showing awareness of cultural values can facilitate the development of rapport. For instance, when we are working with Latino families, it can be useful to be warm and respectful and to address caregivers using formal language, as doing so is consistent with the traditional Latino values of *simpatía*, *respeto*, and *personalísmo* (Miranda et al., 1996). In many cultures, it is advantageous to involve the head of the family, perhaps the father or grandmother, in early sessions, as his or her approval and involvement in therapy not only makes it more likely that the family will participate but also creates a more ecologically valid context in which therapy can unfold.

Treatment components and modalities must be examined to determine whether they are consistent with the family's ecological context, culture, and socialization goals (Zayas & Solari, 1994). For instance, while affect regulation may be a major target of most trauma treatments (Lieberman & Van Horn, Chapter 4, this volume), affect regulation strategies (e.g., humor, sublimation of anxiety into productivity, symbolic representation) may vary from culture to culture (Pumariega, 2001). Culturally valid treatments are sensitive to cultural customs, rituals, and childrearing practices, and incorporate them whenever possible. When treatment goals or modalities run contrary to cultural expectations, the therapist must balance the goals of the therapy with respect for the family's culture by perhaps altering the treatment or by providing carefully timed developmental guidance that provides a culturally meaningful context for the intervention. This might be the case when a therapist would like the parent to play with the child in order to facilitate the co-construction of a trauma narrative in a specific cultural group where parents typically do not play with their children. Treatments conducted in the child's ecological setting (e.g., the home or school) may be more effective for ethnic minority children as treatment unfolds and interventions are developed within the cultural context (Tharp, 1991). Finally, as discussed before, low-income ethnic minorities are more likely to have experienced multiple traumas, secondary adversities, and intergenerational traumas. Treatments for diverse cultural groups must be sensitive to issues of multiple traumatization, as such a history is likely to have consequences for the child's sense of safety, beliefs about the world, and affect regulation capacities as well as the ability of caregivers to serve as protective shields.

Case Example

In this section we briefly present a case to illustrate the impact of cultural factors on child and family functioning. The case presented represents a composite of multiple families with whom we have worked, with elements of their treatments combined so as to illustrate key points.

Carmen, a 38-month-old Latina girl, and her mother were referred to treatment because Carmen was experiencing nightmares, separation anxiety, and temper tantrums following her parents' separation 5 months earlier. Carmen's mother immigrated to the United States from El Salvador as a teenager and was reunited with Carmen's father, whom she had dated in El Salvador. She and Carmen's father had a volatile relationship that involved verbal aggression and one incident immediately prior to the separation when Carmen's father slammed her mother against a wall and hit her face. Carmen was present for this incident, and her mother recalls her screaming "Daddy, don't hurt Mommy." Her mother called the police and filed a restraining order after this incident. Her husband refused to speak to her after this even though he has weekly visits with Carmen. His family members, who used to be very supportive, are angry with her for involving the police. Carmen's mother feels tremendous guilt for splitting up the family. She reports that in many ways the breakup has been more upsetting than the violence. Following the separation, Carmen and her mother moved in with Carmen's maternal grandmother. Her grandmother lives in a more dangerous area of the city, and Carmen has seen drug dealers and heard drive-by shootings.

During the assessment it became apparent that Carmen's grandmother played a significant role in her life and that Carmen's mother and grandmother had a highly conflicted relationship. Carmen's mother reported that when she was a child her own mother left her in El Salvador in the care of her grandmother and aunt. She stated that her mother would send money to help her grandmother care for her and her brothers and that she finally sent for them when she was a teenager. Carmen's mother reported being very rebellious as a teenager and not doing well in school. She dropped out because she had difficulty doing the classwork in English and soon became pregnant by Carmen's father.

Continuous assessment throughout the course of treatment revealed a history of multiple traumas in each generation, which were followed by numerous secondary adversities. These traumas are detailed in Figure 1.2 along with a timeline of El Salvador's recent history. It should be noted that this information was gathered over the course of treatment. As shown, Carmen's grandmother and mother lived in El Salvador during the civil war of the 1980s and early 1990s. Her grandmother was directly affected by the events in the country because a cousin she was very close to was among those who "disappeared." When the war in El Salvador was brought up, she said it was a difficult time and agreed that it made it very hard to trust others. She said that she and her husband left the country because they were worried about how dangerous it was, and they felt that life in the United States might be better. They were unsure as to what life in the United States would be like, so they left the children in the care of their grandmother and hoped to send for them as soon as they had enough money.

Carmen's mother was extremely bitter that her parents had left her and her brothers in El Salvador. She reported serious physical punishment at the hands of her grandmother. She found it hard to watch her mother take care of Carmen because she felt that her mother had never cared for her in that way. Her mother, in turn, was very disappointed that her daughter never finished school, especially after all the sacrifices she felt she had made to give her that opportunity. Carmen's mother and grandmother argued often in Carmen's presence. At times Carmen's mother would threaten to move out and not let the grandmother see Carmen.

During the assessment Carmen's mother spoke about how scared she had been when she saw her father hit her mother. She reported that although she knew a lot of families where the men hit their wives, she still felt it was wrong. She spoke with conviction and talked about how it had been hard to call the police on Carmen's father but how she wanted something different for Carmen. She discussed how his family had been especially angry because they worried that any police involvement might cause him to be deported. She brought up how losing contact with his family meant losing a significant source of support and a tie to her country. She spoke both about missing her husband and knowing that she did not want to be with someone who would hit her.

Treatment was conducted in Spanish and involved mother–child sessions and collateral meetings with the mother. The grandmother was involved in the assessment and on occasion would attend treatment sessions. Over the course of the therapy, it seemed important to address the multigenerational history of trauma and its effects on the family. The mom was able to share her anger at being abandoned as a child and talk about how she wanted something different for Carmen. In one session, which was held with just the mother and grandmother, they spoke about how the war had affected many families in their country including theirs, and each shared her feelings regarding their separation. Carmen's mother expressed anger at her mother and stated that even though she appreciated what her mother was doing for Carmen, she was still angry that she wasn't there for her earlier. They both expressed their feelings about the situation in their country and talked about how it had made it difficult to trust others. They also talked about how it was hard to be away from other family members who were still in El Salvador. The therapist highlighted how the war had broken up their family and emphasized that they were now both working together to make things better for Carmen. They agreed and were able to listen to information about how the conflict between them might be affecting Carmen, especially since she had witnessed conflict between her parents and she might worry that people go away when there is conflict.

During joint mother–child sessions Carmen used animals to play out different themes involving conflict and separation. The therapist was able to think about how these themes were salient for the mother. On one occa-

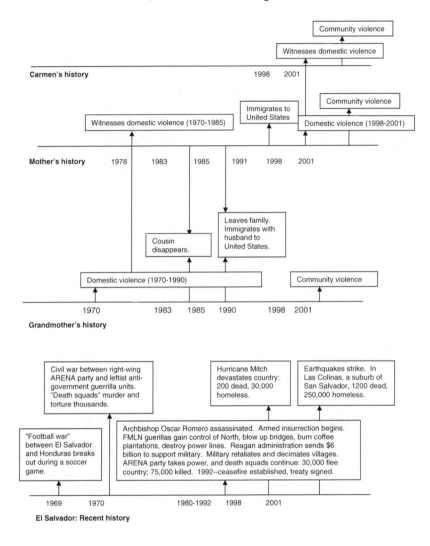

FIGURE 1.2. Case example: El Salvador historical timeline and multigenerational family history of trauma.

sion Carmen took a daddy tiger and threw him behind a chair, stating "He's not coming back." "Cry" she said to the therapist who was holding a baby tiger. The therapist made the tiger cry and talk about how she missed the daddy tiger. She then remarked to the mother that she thought Carmen was sharing how she felt about missing her daddy: "I think it's very hard for her. When she's with Daddy she misses you, and when she's with you, she misses Daddy. I think maybe you know how she feels because you also had people you missed when you were little." The mom agreed and seemed more empathic towards Carmen and more willing to help her when she was scared at night and when she had separation anxiety. She also stopped threatening to move out of the grandmother's house.

In other sessions both the mother and the grandmother expressed their wishes for Carmen. They both emphasized the importance of respect and hoped that she would be *bien educada,* meaning that she would know how to act toward others and would be loving, well mannered, and respectful. They both hoped that she would *seguir adelante,* move forward and be able to get a good education and a good profession. They were able to focus on her good qualities and to understand her temper tantrums in light of all the changes she had been through. They were also able to work together to create a more consistent caregiving routine that appeared to decrease Carmen's nightmares and separation anxiety.

Carmen's separation anxiety was also better understood during a school observation when the therapist learned that she was in a preschool class with no Spanish-speaking teachers. The only other Spanish-speaking girl in her class was older than she, and they did not get along. Carmen's mother began volunteering in the school and facilitated interactions between her and the other children. She was excited to see how Carmen was learning English, and she began thinking about taking ESL (English as a second language) classes, so she could help Carmen with her schoolwork and also could obtain a better job in the future.

DIRECTIONS FOR FUTURE RESEARCH

In a study of parent's perceptions of the degree of their children's exposure to violence, Fick, Osofsky, and Lewis (1997) found that parents typically underrated the amount of violence their child had experienced. The study was conducted with parents and children living in neighborhoods which at that time had some of the highest rates of community violence in a large urban city in the United States. The children in this same area had reported high rates of exposure to community violence. They reported violence that they witnessed, had knowledge of, and had been victim to in their neighborhoods, playgrounds, and schools. We need to know more about these discrepancies between parents' and children's reports of their experience of traumatic events.

Do parents' cultural frameworks not only mediate their emotional and behavioral practices and responses to their child but also their perception of the trauma to their child?

We need to know more about the specific roles of complicated bereavement responses, complex acculturation processes, and their interaction with ethnic identity and assimilation. We must better understand how these sociocultural processes serve as psychological foundations for the child's experience of trauma.

As noted earlier, language is the primary means of transmitting culture. Within the United States almost 20% of children speak a language other than English at home (*http://www.census.gov,2001*). Further, Spanish is the first language for nearly 70% of these children, and it is projected that by 2050 the U.S. population will be about 25% Hispanic. In 2000, foreign-born Americans made up about 11% of the U.S. population, contributing to the ongoing complexity of linguistic and cultural diversity within this country. We need to understand how developmental processes related to language and differential processes of intrafamilial acculturation and individual cultural assimilation impact parent–child relationships. The issue of language brokering by young children for their newly immigrated parents has been argued to have positive developmental outcomes, yet such brokering by youngsters also serves as a source of stress. Umaña-Taylor (2003) noted that family relations could become strained through role reversals as young children take on the responsibility of translation for their adult parents. When conveying confidential information both the child and parent may experience increased anxiety and stress. There also may be poorer educational outcomes and inhibited identity formation for children who are thrust into the position of taking on adult responsibilities as they translate English for their monolingual parents or caregivers.

Culture as a Source of Protection

We typically perceive the role of culture as a context for development. We know less about the cultural processes specifically related to attachment and the outcomes for the socioemotional domains of the relationship. An emphasis on cultural processes related to trauma and young children helps move the "blaming" aspect of the etiology of some forms of interpersonal trauma from the shoulders of biological parents. Recognizing the significance of these ecological and cultural sources of variability in children's experience of trauma underscores recent controversial positions about the declining significance of parental influences (Harris, 2003). Influences of peer group, neighborhood culture, and genetic determinants are also important to the child.

Similarly, Aptekar and Stöcklin, (1997) present compelling evidence from their extensive work with street children of Brazil that such children develop a culture of coping and survival. They argue that exposure to trauma in children can lead to positive mental health as well as social outcomes.

Culture is an underutilized resource in trauma work. Children are more than the passive recipients of cultural socialization. Their responses and needs help to shape the response of the caregiving environment. A revolutionary approach that builds on traditions in community psychology and public health might well be to view the entire group or community as a client.

Finally, we must explore further what intuitively are the most prominent social outcomes for young children, culture, and trauma—that is, the issue of social justice. In cataloging the clinical symptoms of young children exposed to various traumas, clinicians have noted the increased aggression, fearfulness, and anxiety and intense affect with triggers associated with the original trauma (Kaufman, & Henrich, 2000). Accordingly, clinical interventions and prevention efforts need to incorporate these known clinical responses in their assessment as well as intervention efforts. But does the clinical intervention with these children and their caregivers to assist with their individual experiences of grief, bereavement, and trauma impact what might be the more powerful ethnic and cultural legacies associated with the trauma? How can mental health systems best support children and their families that are vulnerable to the historical trauma of past generations? How can we build on the strengths presented by various cultural traditions, values, and beliefs that may be sources of psychic protection?

We know little about the impact of individual or group experiences of trauma on the moral development of young children. From this work, we may learn lessons in social justice and morality. In his work with the children traumatized by racial desegregation in the U.S. South, Coles (1967) notes that this cohort of children developed increased empathy and a greater sense of justice as a means of coping with the trauma of forced integration. Aptekar and Stöcklin (1997) poignantly argue for perceiving children living on the streets of Brazil not only as passive recipients of trauma but also as active agents in creating a healthy culture of cooperation and caring.

Challenge of the Complexity of Culture

Finally, we must not let the complexity of the diversity presented by a multicultural world and developmental processes dissuade us from the challenge of understanding the impact of culture on the traumatic experiences of young children (Lewis, 2000b). There are theoretical and interdisciplinary specific efforts that offer sources of hope and blueprints for what needs to be done with individual ethnic groups and families and children. Coordination of efforts, communication among disciplines, and focused resources on the intergenerational traumas of immigrant groups to the United States and existing ethnic minority groups are the next steps in advocacy and prevention. Infant mental health studies with their interdisciplinary structure and fearlessness of intense affect in children offer the ideal mechanism to address these issues.

In our work analyzing drawings of their neighborhoods done by African American children exposed to high rates of community violence, we identified a thematic element of hope. Symbols of flowers, children playing, and religious symbols were evident in these young children's drawings of violence and murder (Lewis et al., 1997). These drawings provide one source of evidence that despite the tears of trauma, children's souls are full of hope. Ultimately, the work of healing the collective traumas of cultural, ethnic, and racial groups will reverberate beyond supporting the healthy attachment in the parent–child relationship. Interrupting intergenerational legacies of trauma, pain, and tragedy will not only serve to prevent future generations of child abuse and neglect but also other forms of domestic violence in families. Our collective efforts will serve to promote the mental health and well-being of diverse young children and their families as well as social justice in the larger society.

REFERENCES

American Psychiatric Association. (1994). *Diagnostic and statistical manual of mental disorders* (4th ed.). Washington, DC: Author.

Aptekar, L., & Stöcklin, D. (1997). Children in particularly difficult circumstances. In J. W. Berry, P. R. Dasen, & T. S. Saraswathi (Eds.), *Handbook of cross-cultural psychology: Vol. 2. Basic processes and human development* (pp. 377–412). Needham Heights, MA: Allyn & Bacon.

Bagilishya, D. (2000). Mourning and recovery from trauma: In Rwanda, tears flow within. *Transcultural Psychiatry, 37*(3), 337–353.

Baker, A., & Shalhoub-Kevorkian, N. (1999). Effects of political and military traumas on children: The Palestinian case. *Clinical Psychology Review, 19*, 935–950.

Bell, C. C., & Jenkins, E. J. (1993). Community violence and children on Chicago's south side. *Psychiatry, 56*, 46–54.

Bit, S. (1991). *The warrior heritage: A psychological perspective of Cambodian trauma.* El Cerrito, CA: Author.

Bowlby, J. (1969). *Attachment and loss: Vol. 1. Attachment.* New York: Basic Books.

Bowlby, J. (1988). *A secure base.* New York: Basic Books.

Bracken, P. (2002). *Trauma: Culture, meaning and philosophy.* London: Whurr.

Brave Heart, M. Y. H. (2000). Wakiksuypi: Carrying the historical trauma of the Lakota. In M. J. Zakour (Ed.), *Disaster and traumatic stress research and intervention* (pp. 245–266). New Orleans, LA: Tulane University, School of Social Work.

Bronfenbrenner, U. (1979). *The ecology of human development.* Cambridge, MA: Harvard University Press.

Canino, I. A., & Spurlock, J. (2000). *Culturally diverse children and adolescents: Assessment, diagnosis, and treatment* (2nd ed.). New York: Guilford Press.

Chemtob, C. M., & Taylor, T. L. (2002). Treatment of traumatized children. In R. Yehuda (Ed.), *Treating trauma survivors with PTSD* (pp. 75–126). Washington, DC: American Psychiatric Press.

Coles, R. (1967). *Children of crisis: A study of courage and fear.* New York: Dell.

Danieli, Y. (1985). The treatment and prevention of long-terms effects of intergenerational transmission of victimization: A lesson from holocaust survivors and their children. In C.R. Figley (Ed.), *Trauma and its wake* (pp. 295–312). New York: Brunner/Mazel.

Deater-Deckard, K., Dodge, K. A., Bates, J. E., & Pettit, G. S. (1996). Physical discipline among African American and European American mothers: Links to children's externalizing behaviors. *Developmental Psychology, 32,* 1065–1072.

De Levita, D. (2000). Child psychotherapy as an instrument in cultural research: Treating war-traumatized children in the former Yugoslavia. In A. Robben & M. Suarez-Orozco (Eds.), *Cultures under siege: Collective violence and trauma* (pp. 131–154). New York: Cambridge University Press.

DeVries, M. W. (1996). Trauma in cultural perspective. In B. A. van der Kolk, A. C. McFarlane, & L. Weisaeth (Eds.), *Traumatic stress: The effects of overwhelming experience on mind, body, and society* (pp. 398–413). New York: Guilford Press.

Fick, A. C., Osofsky, J. D., & Lewis, M. L., (1997). Police and parents' perceptions and understanding of violence. In J. D. Osofsky (Ed.), *Children in a violent society* (pp. 261–276). New York: Guilford Press.

Garbarino, J., Dubrow, N., Kostelny, K., & Pardo, C. (1992). *Children in danger: Coping with the consequences of community violence.* San Francisco: Jossey-Bass.

Garcia Coll, C. T. (1990). Developmental outcome of minority infants: A process-oriented look into our beginnings. *Child Development, 61,* 270–289.

Goldman, R. (1997). *Circumcision, the hidden trauma: How an American cultural practice affects infants and ultimately us all.* Boston: Vanguard.

Groves, B., Zuckerman, B., Marans, S., & Cohen, D. (1993). Silent victims: Children who witness violence. *Journal of the American Medical Association, 269,* 262–264.

Harris, J. R. (2003). The outcome of parenting: What do we really know? In M. Coleman & L. Ganong (Eds.), *Points and counterpoints: Controversial relationship and family issues in the 21st century* (pp. 136–141). Los Angeles: Roxbury.

Harrison, A. O., Wilson, M. N., Pine, C. J., Chan, S. Q., & Buriel, R. (1990). Family ecologies of ethnic minority children. *Child Development, 61,* 347–362.

Harwood, R. (2002). Parenting among Latino families in the U.S. In M. Bornstein (Ed.), *Handbook of parenting: Vol. 4: Social conditions amd applied parenting* (2nd ed., pp. 21–46). Mahwah, NJ: Erlbaum.

Johnson-Powell, G. (1997). A portrait of America's children: Social, cultural, and historical context. In G. Johnson-Powell & J. Yamamoto (Eds.), *Transcultural child development: Psychological assessment and treatment* (pp. 3–33). New York: Wiley.

Kaufman, J., & Henrich, C. (2000). Exposure to violence and early childhood trauma. In C. H. Zeanah (Ed.), *Handbook of infant mental health* (2nd ed., pp. 195–208). New York: Guilford Press.

Kazdin, A. E., & Weisz, J. R. (2003). *Evidence-based psychotherapies for children and adolescents*. New York: Guilford Press.

Korbin, J. (1977). Anthropological contributions to the study of child abuse. *International Child Welfare Review, 35,* 23–31.

Lahor, N., Wolmer, L., & Cohen, D. J. (2001). Mothers' functioning and children's symptoms 5 years after a SCUD missile attack. *American Journal of Psychiatry, 158*(2), 1020–1026.

Levy-Warren, M. H. (1987). Moving to a new culture: Cultural identity, loss, and mourning. In J. Bloom-Feshbach & S. Bloom-Feshbach (Eds.), *The psychology of separation and loss: Perspectives on development, life transitions, and clinical practice* (pp. 300–315). San Francisco: Jossey-Bass.

Lewis, M. L. (1996). Trauma reverberates: Psychosocial evaluation of the caregiving environment of young children exposed to violence and traumatic loss. In J. D. Osofsky & E. Fenichel (Eds.), *Islands of safety: Assessing and treating young victims of violence* (pp. 21–28). Washington, DC: Zero to Three.

Lewis, M. L. (2000a). African American parents and their interpretations of emotions of infants. In J. D. Osofsky & H. E. Fitzgerald (Eds.) *WAIMH handbook of infant mental health* (Vol. 3, pp. 59–63). New York: Wiley.

Lewis, M. L. (2000b). The cultural context of infant mental health: The developmental niche of infant–caregiver relationships. In C. H. Zeanah (Ed.), *Handbook of infant mental health* (2nd ed., pp. 91–108). New York: Guilford Press.

Lewis, M. L., Osofsky, J. D., & Moore, M. S. (1997). Violent cities, violent streets: Children draw their neighborhoods. In J. D. Osofsky (Ed.), *Children in a violent society* (pp. 277–298). New York: Guilford Press.

Lieberman, A. F., Van Horn, P., Grandison, C. M., & Pekarsky, J. H. (1997). Mental health assessment of infants, toddlers, and preschoolers in a service program and treatment outcome research program. *Infant Mental Health Journal, 18*(2), 158–170.

Lu, F. G., Lim, R. F., & Mezzich, J. E. (1995). Issues in the assessment and diagnosis of culturally diverse individuals. In J. M. Oldham & M. Riba (Eds.), *American Psychiatric Association review of psychiatry* (Vol. 14, pp. 477–510). Washington, DC: American Psychiatric Press.

Malakoff, M. E. (1994). Refugee children and violence. In C. Chiland & G. J. Young (Eds.), *The child in the family: Vol. 11. Children and violence* (pp. 145–159). Northvale, NJ: Aronson.

McMiller, W. P., & Weisz, J. R. (1996). Help-seeking preceding mental health clinic intake among African-American, Latino, and Caucasian youths. *Journal of American Academy of Child and Adolescent Psychiatry, 35*(8), 1086–1094.

Miller, K. E. (1996). The effects of state terrorism and exile on indigenous Guatemalan refugee children: A mental health assessment and an analysis of children's narratives. *Child Development, 67,* 89–106.

Miranda, J., Azocar, F., Organista, K. C., Muñoz, R. F, & Lieberman, A. F. (1996). Recruiting and retaining low-income Latinos in psychotherapy research. *Journal of Consulting and Clinical Psychology, 64*(5), 868–874.

Munet-Vilaró, F. (1998). Grieving and death rituals of Latinos. *Oncology Nursing Forum, 25,* 1761–1763.

Okagaki, L., & Sternberg, R. J. (1993). Parental beliefs and children's school performance. *Child Development, 64,* 36–56.

Osofsky, J. D. (1995). The effects of exposure to violence on young children. *American Psychologist, 50*(9), 782–788.

Parson, E. R. (2002). Understanding children with war-zone traumatic stress exposed to the world's violent environments. *Journal of Contemporary Psychotherapy, 30*(4), 325–340.

Peddle, N., Monteiro, C., Guluma, V., Macaulay, & Thomas, E. A. (1999). Trauma, loss, and resilience in Africa: A psychosocial community based approach to culturally sensitive healing. In K. Nader (Ed.), *Honoring differences: Cultural issues in the treatment of trauma and loss* (pp. 121–149). Philadelphia: Brunner/Mazel.

Perry, B. D. (1994). Neurobiological sequelae of childhood trauma: Post-traumatic stress disorders in children. In M. Murberg (Ed.), *Catecholamines in post-traumatic stress disorder: Emerging concepts* (pp. 253–276). Washington, DC: American Psychiatric Press.

Phinney, J. S. (1996). When we talk about American ethnic groups, what do we mean? *American Psychologist, 51*, 918–927.

Pumariega, A. J. (2001). Cultural competence in treatment interventions. In H. B. Vance & A. J. Pumariega (Eds.), *Clinical assessment of child and adolescent behavior* (pp. 494–512). New York: Wiley.

Pynoos, R. S. (1994). Traumatic stress and developmental psychopathology in children and adolescents. In R. S. Pynoos (Ed.), *Posttraumatic stress disorder: A clinical review* (pp. 286–298). Lutherville, MD: Sidran Press.

Pynoos, R. S., Steinberg, A. M., & Goenjian, A. (1996). Traumatic stress in childhood and adolescence: Recent developments and current controversies. In B. A. van der Kolk, A. C. McFarlane, & L. Weisaeth (Eds.), *Traumatic stress: The effects of overwhelming experience on mind, body, and society* (pp. 331–358). New York: Guilford Press.

Pynoos, R. S., Steinberg, A. M., & Piacentini, J. C. (1999). A developmental model of childhood traumatic stress and intersection with anxiety disorders. *Biological Psychiatry, 46*, 1542–1554.

Rechtman, R. (2000). Stories of trauma and idioms of distress: From cultural narratives to clinical assessment. *Transcultural Psychiatry, 37*(3), 403–415.

Rousseau, C., Mekki-Berrada, A., & Moreau, S. (2001). Trauma and extended separation from families among Latin American and African refuges in Montreal. *Psychiatry, 64*(1), 40–68.

Ryan, C. S., & Bogart, L. M. (1997). Development of new group members' in-group and out-group stereotypes: Changes in perceived group variability and ethnocentrism. *Journal of Personality and Social Psychology, 73*, 719–732.

Salzman, M. B. (2001). Cultural trauma and recovery: Perspectives from terror management theory. *Trauma, Violence and Abuse, 2*(2), 172–191.

Scheeringa, M. S., & Gaensbauer, T. J. (2000). Posttraumatic stress disorder. In C. H. Zeanah (Ed.), *Handbook of infant mental health* (2nd ed., pp. 369–381). New York: Guilford Press.

Shalev, A. Y. (1996). Stress versus traumatic stress from acute homeostatic reactions to chronic psychopathology. In B. A. van der Kolk, A. C. McFarlane, & L. Weisaeth (Eds.), *Traumatic stress: The effects of overwhelming experience on mind, body, amd society* (pp. 77–101). New York: Guilford Press.

Sue, S., Fujino, D. C., Hu, L. T., Takeuchi, D. T., & Zane, N. W. S. (1991). Community mental health services for ethnic minority groups: A test of the cultural responsiveness hypothesis. *Journal of Consulting and Clinical Psychology, 59,* 533–540.

Super, C., & Harkness, S. (1997). The cultural structuring of child development. In J. W. Berry, P. R. Dasen, & T. S. Saraswathi (Eds.), *Handbook of cross-cultural psychology: Vol. 2. Basic processes and human development* (pp. 1–40). Needham Heights, MA: Allyn & Bacon.

Tharp, R. G. (1991). Cultural diversity and treatment of children. *Journal of Consulting and Clinical Psychology, 59*(6), 799–812.

Tolson, T. F., & Wilson, M. N. (1990). The impact of two and three generational black family structure on perceived family climate. *Child Development, 61,* 416–428.

Tully, M. A. (1999). Lifting our voices: African American cultural responses to trauma and loss. In K. Nader (Ed.), *Honoring differences: Cultural issues in the treatment of trauma and loss* (pp. 23–48). Philadelphia: Brunner/Mazel.

Umaña-Taylor, A. J. (2003). Language brokering as a stressor for immigrant children and their families. In M. Coleman & L. Ganong (Eds.), *Points and counterpoints: Controversial relationship and family issues in the 21st century* (pp. 157–159). Los Angeles: Roxbury.

Velez-Ibanez, C. G., & Parra, C. G. (1999). Trauma issues and social modalities concerning mental health concepts and practices among Mexicans of the Southwest United States with reference to other Latino groups. In K. Nader (Ed.), *Honoring differences: Cultural issues in the treatment of trauma and loss* (pp. 76–97). Philadelphia: Brunner/Mazel.

Waitzkin, H., & Magana, H. (1997). The black box in somatization: Unexplained physical symptoms, culture and narratives of trauma. *Social Science and Medicine, 45,* 811–825.

Weinhold, B. K., & Weinhold, J. B. (2000). *Conflict resolution: The partnership way.* Denver: Love.

Weisz, J. R. (1989). Culture and the development of child psychopathology: Lessons from Thailand. In D. Cicchetti (Ed.), *Rochester Symposium on Developmental Psychopathology: Vol. 1. The emergence of a discipline* (pp. 89–117). Hillsdale, NJ: Erlbaum.

Weisz, J. R., Sigman, M., Weiss, B., & Mosk, J. (1993). Parent reports of behavioral and emotional problems among children in Kenya, Thailand, and the United States. *Child Development, 64,* 98–109.

Weisz, J. R., Suwanlert, S., Chaiyasit, W., Weiss, B., Walter, B. R., & Wibulswasdi Anderson, W. (1988). Thai and American perspectives on over- and undercontrolled child behavior problems: Exploring the threshold model among parents, teachers, and psychologists. *Journal of Consulting and Clinical Psychology, 56*(4), 601–609.

Wessells, M. G. (1999). Culture, power, and community: Intercultural approaches to psychosocial assistance and healing. In K. Nader (Ed.), *Honoring differences: Cultural issues in the treatment of trauma and loss* (pp. 267–282). Philadelphia: Brunner/Mazel.

Woodcock, J. (1995). Healing rituals with families in exile. *Journal of Family Therapy, 17,* 397–409.

Yamamoto, J., Silva, J. A., Ferrari, M., & Nukariya, K. (1997). Culture and psychopathology. In G. Johnson-Powell & J. Yamamoto (Eds.), *Transcultural child de-*

velopment: Psychological assessment and treatment (pp. 34–57). New York: Wiley.

Zakour, M. J. (Ed.). (2000). *Disaster and traumatic stress research and intervention.* New Orleans, LA: Tulane University, School of Social Work.

Zayas, L. H., & Solari, F. (1994). Early childhood socialization in Hispanic families: Context, culture, and practice implications. *Professional Psychology: Research and Practice, 25*(3), 200–206.

Zea, M. C., Diehl, V. A., & Porterfield, K. S. (1997). Central American youth exposed to war violence. In J. G. Garcia & M. C. Zea (Eds.), *Psychological interventions and research with Latino populations* (pp. 39–55). Needham Heights, MA: Allyn & Bacon.

CHAPTER 2

TRAUMA AND ATTACHMENT
The Case for Disrupted Attachment Disorder

SARAH HINSHAW-FUSELIER
SHERRYL SCOTT HELLER
VICTORIA T. PARTON
LARA ROBINSON
NEIL W. BORIS

Attachment refers to a homeostatic biobehavioral system that is evident early in childhood and is operative across the lifespan. Recently, it has been argued that the study of attachment is inextricably linked to the study of emotion regulation, in that the primary attachment relationship serves as a regulatory mechanism for both positively and negatively charged affect experienced by young children (Schore, 2000). It is through interactions in the primary attachment relationship that flexible strategies for regulating emotions in the social environment are developed (Sroufe, 1989; Schore, 2001a). Increasingly, developmental research on attachment is focusing on factors associated with the organization or disorganization of the attachment system in early childhood (van IJzendoorn, Schuengel, & Bakermans-Kranenburg, 1999). Scientific advances, from narrative measures that capture how adults' own attachment experiences influence their parenting behavior to experimental paradigms that capture the processes through which experience sculpts the brain, have brought clinicians ever closer to understanding how the attachment system is organized by experience (Green & Goldwyn, 2002). Trauma has emerged as a critical factor, both in its direct impact on young children and how that impact resonates through—and alters—the developing attachment relationship.

The purpose of this chapter is to revisit an old topic: the impact of disruption in the primary attachment relationship on young children. Disruption in the early caregiving relationship has long been recognized to be traumatic, and recent research has bolstered our understanding of the negative developmental impact of trauma on attachment. Despite this knowledge, early attachment disruption is not widely recognized as a clinical issue that may require intervention. Consequently, existing diagnostic criteria for disrupted attachment disorder are not widely used to identify symptomatic children. As a result, appropriate goals for treatment may be overlooked, effective therapeutic strategies may not be employed, and desirable outcomes may be less likely to occur.

Though disentangling the general effects of early negative interactions from the specific effects of disruption in the attachment relationship is often difficult, case reports suggest that young children present with symptoms requiring intervention following disruptions in early attachment relationships, even when the disrupted caregiving environment is less than adequate (e.g., maltreated children in foster care). Our goal, then, is to demonstrate the theoretical rationale for disrupted attachment disorder (DAD) and to propose updated criteria for DAD. Attention to diagnostic criteria is important so that clinicians have a framework for understanding the etiology and symptomatic presentation of children who are adversely affected by disruptions in their primary attachment relationships. Diagnostic classification is also necessary to determine appropriate intervention goals and strategies, as well as to provide a basis for further clinical research that can refine and clarify the nature of disorders.

Though good data are limited, this chapter begins by reviewing the scope of the problem of attachment disruption in early childhood, both in the United States and in developing countries. A brief historical overview of the observational study of the impact of attachment disruption follows. This overview of past research on humans is updated by incorporating data from relevant research on animals and considering the emerging implications of recent neurobiological research. Moderators and mediators of reactions to attachment disruption are considered and a diagnostic framework for disrupted attachment disorder is presented. A longitudinal case history of a set of twins followed from infancy to the early grade school period follows, providing a springboard for the discussion of the clinical implications and possible sequelae of disrupted attachment relationships in infancy and early childhood. Consideration is given to the interplay of relationship issues and traumatic events, both for diagnosis and intervention. Finally, we emphasize the way in which clinical recognition of and experience with the problems associated with attachment disruption might shape future efforts to refine both the diagnostic nosology and intervention practices.

Before we present the history of research on attachment disruption, it is important to concede that there are perils and pitfalls of creating diagnostic categories for infant psychopathology, an issue that has been more completely addressed elsewhere (cf. Zeanah, Boris, & Scheeringa, 1997). Certainly, clinicians must weigh the risks of "labeling" an individual infant or young child when, over time, intervening biological or social factors may shift the individual toward adaptive functioning (Grossman et al., 2003). On the other hand, it is important to identify clusters of symptoms in individuals that are associated with current impairment, future developmental deviance, or both. Even if both the scientific underpinnings of diagnostic systems and the values that these systems are associated with may be challenged (Clark, Watson, & Reynolds, 1995), reliable classifications may nevertheless lead to interventions designed to restore adaptive functioning more quickly. As will be discussed later, recent neurobiological research suggests both that early experience shapes brain function and that successive symptomatic episodes may make it more likely that symptoms recur, a phenomenon known as *kindling* (Grossman et al., 2003). Though the research supporting these phenomena in humans is limited, both support the argument for early identification of "disorders," ideally coupled with effective intervention that may help mitigate the negative effects on brain development. Appropriate diagnosis and treatment may reduce the negative effects of the initial disruption by preventing successive symptomatic episodes.

SCOPE OF THE PROBLEM

The most recent survey data available document that 556,000 children are in foster care in the United States (U.S. Department of Health & Human Services, 2002). At the time of data compilation, 28% of these children were under 6 years of age and only 4% of the total number of children in care were in preadoptive homes. The Adoption and Safe Families Act of 1996 (ASFA; Children's Defense Fund, 2000) was specifically designed to decrease the amount of time young children spend in foster care, though the hoped-for effect of reducing the number of placement disruptions young children experience has yet to be widely documented. Though tracking data on reports of child maltreatment is difficult, the numbers of very young children in foster care or relative placement who are likely to be subjected to at least one additional disruption in their primary caregiving relationship appear to be increasing (Cicchetti & Toth, 1995). However, as intervention programs that address the ASFA goal are implemented, more data may become available regarding the disruptive experiences that young children have in foster care (see Malik, Crowson, Lederman, & Osofsky, 2002; Zeanah & Larrieu, 1998).

Early disruption in attachment relationships is prevalent worldwide. For example, as of 2002 an estimated 13 million children worldwide have lost one or both parents to AIDS, and that number is expected to rise to 25 million by 2010 (U.S. Agency for International Development, 2002). In Africa, where the prevalence of HIV approaches 30% of the adult population in several countries, systems of care for orphans are underdeveloped (Donahue & Williamson, 1999). For many children, substitute care will be provided by grieving caregivers who are likely to be facing economic decline. Consequently, in countries where disruptions in early relationships occur because of the death of one or both parents, disrupted attachment will be confounded by a host of other factors known to negatively impact development.

HISTORY OF THE STUDY
OF EARLY ATTACHMENT DISRUPTION

The consequences of institutionalization or prolonged hospitalization of young children are documented in the medical literature as far back as the early part of the 20th century (Chapin, 1915). However, systematic research on the consequences of separating infants and young children from their caregivers did not receive wide attention until the World Health Organization (WHO) commissioned John Bowlby to systematically review the literature following the large-scale family disruptions resulting from World War II. Bowlby (1951) concluded that disruptions in early relationships had both short- and long-term effects. In the short term, delayed physical and cognitive development had been well documented. Bowlby asserted that, in the long term, early separation from caregivers was associated with later antisocial behaviors and problematic relationships.

Bowlby's (1951) report followed the dramatic films and writings of René A. Spitz (1945, 1946), who drew attention to the plight of children exposed to institutionalized care and temporary separation from their "love object" (usually the mother). Spitz proposed a diagnostic category, "anaclitic depression," to describe the temporary change in behavior that was characterized by emotional withdrawal, immobility, weight loss, susceptibility to illness, and decrease in developmental quotient observed in these infants whose primary relationships had been disrupted.

Like Spitz, James Robertson (1953, 1958) used film to document the response to separation of young children who were placed in residential nurseries during their mothers' hospitalizations for subsequent births. Working together, Robertson and Bowlby (1952) cataloged observations of reactions to separation with the typical response following a triphasic pattern. During the initial phase of "protest," children experienced acute distress and generally displayed oppositional, tantrum-like behavior in response to bids by substitute caregivers. They were typically inconsolable and, while there were indications of a gradual decline in the intensity of distress over time, the pervasive desire for the mother's return and determined efforts to find her remained. The second phase, termed "despair," is consistent with responses of grief and mourning and is similar to Spitz's (1946) description of anaclitic depression. Finally, the third phase, termed "detachment," was characterized by extreme emotional distance and ambivalence toward the attachment figure after reunion. Children revealed a lack of pleasure and responsiveness at the initial reencounter with their mother, sometimes even appearing not to recognize her. Following reunion, the unrelenting concern of another separation remained apparent in children's anxious behavior in the face of cues that were reminiscent of the separation.

These observations, together with complementary ethological research on animals, laid the foundation for Bowlby's (1969/1982, 1973, 1980) theory of attachment. Longer-term studies of children who experienced prolonged disruption in an established caregiver–child relationship followed. For instance, researchers found that behavioral patterns of children 20 weeks following reunion included sleep difficulties, fear of losing the caregiver again, demanding behavior, alternately loving and suddenly hostile behavior with the caregiver, regression in toilet training, and sensitivity to changes in their environment (e.g., presence of a stranger; Heinicke & Westheimer, 1965). Data from retrospective studies indicated that institutionalized children and children who experienced repeated disruptions in caregiving relationships (e.g., placement in multiple foster homes or with multiple family members) continued to have distorted social and emotional relatedness, such as superficial relationships and indiscriminate friendliness, motor skill deficits, language deficits, cognitive deficits, and impulsive and delinquent behavior (Bowlby, 1944a, 1944b; Provence & Lipton, 1962).

By the early 1970s, just 20 years after Bowlby's WHO review on wartime separation of infants and young children, Rutter (1972a, 1972b) completed an updated review of the effects of "maternal deprivation," highlighting complementary emerging animal data. Shortly thereafter, Tizard and Hodges's (1978) account of the long-term developmental trajectory of children who grew up in institutions provided data on a single cohort followed over many years. Together, animal data and longitudinal follow-up of humans who had experienced institutionalization underscored the tremendous clinical implications of disrupted attachment on the developing organism.

THE PSYCHOBIOLOGICAL IMPLICATIONS OF ATTACHMENT DISRUPTION

Contributions from Animal Studies

Perhaps the greatest advance in the 20 years following Rutter's (1972b) review was the animal research highlighting the psychobiological implications of early caregiving disruptions, especially through the study of rearing in various degrees of social isolation (e.g., temporary isolation from mother; peer rearing). As Kraemer (1992) noted in his integrative review of primate studies, beginning with Harry Harlow's work in the 1970s, "it was not initially realized that isolation rearing disrupts the expression of virtually every aspect of what it means to be a social rhesus monkey, including the regulation of such basic biological functions as eating, drinking, aggression, mating and caring for offspring" (p. 496). Through careful experimental design, animal researchers have been able to isolate many mediators and moderators of the effect of social isolation on the developing organism (Hofer, 1987). A picture has emerged of the importance of caregiving interactions in the biobehavioral regulation of the developing organism. However, even with "reparative" experiences in relationships (i.e., sensitive interaction with a caregiver that helps the infant regulate negative affect), specific long-term consequences of negative experiences—or stress—have been documented (McEwen, 1999).

To help clarify the role of biology in attachment behavior, Kraemer (1992) has put forth a psychobiological theory of attachment based on animal models that is believed to be applicable to humans. Kraemer, Ebert, Schmidt, and McKinney (1991) proposed that infants' regulatory systems develop in relation to an external object. The attachment figure externally regulates the infant's behavior and physiology through behavioral and physiological responses that are attuned to the infant's cues. Through the dynamic emotional communication and regulation of the physiological states (i.e., arousal), the infant's brain adopts the regulatory characteristics of the caregiver, thereby internalizing a *caregiver icon,* a "dynamic, multimodal, temporal, and spatial sensory 'image' of the regulatory systems of the caregiver that are tuned to caregiving" (Kraemer, 1992, p. 498). This conceptualization of the caregiver icon essentially expands the established concept of an internal working model (see Bretherton & Munholland, 1999) to include the neurobiological mechanisms that are responsible for programming the infant's patterns of coping cognitively and emotionally with challenges in the social environment.

Research guided by primate social isolation studies suggests that the interactive regulation of affect, including the management of stressors, impacts the organization of the early developing right hemisphere of the brain (Schore, 2000), which is dominant for "inhibitory control" (Garavan, Ross, & Stein, 1999) and the regulation of arousal (Heilman & Van Den Abell, 1979). Additionally, the hypothalamopituitary–adrenocortical axis and the sympathetic–adrenomedullary axis, which are highly integrated into the stress response circuits, appear to play a critical role in mediating response to trauma (Schore, 2000). Right brain development, key to the increasing ability to regulate reaction to novelty and stress, is experience dependent and is embedded within the attachment relationship between the infant and the primary caregiver (Schore, 1994, 1999, 2000).

Schore's (2000) recent integrative reviews suggest that attachment-related trauma acts to inhibit the development of efficient right brain function, leaving the individual vulnerable to maladaptive stress regulation. However, specific studies of attachment disruption have not yet been conducted. Nevertheless, disturbances in basic regulatory processes such as eating, sleeping, and toileting, in addition to lowered frustration tolerance, irritability, and mood changes (e.g., sadness), have been reported in children who are separated from their attachment figures, even when an adequate or familiar substitute caregiver is provided (e.g., Robertson & Robertson, 1971, 1989; Stein & Call, 2001; Zelenko & Benham, 2002). During such a time of prolonged stress, infants would be subjected to extreme levels of arousal for a prolonged period, thereby facing the experience of having prolonged intense distress without the external regulation that should be provided by sensitive interaction with the attachment figure. Disrupted attachment likely raises levels of stress hormones, leading to biochemical alteration of the corticolimbic circuitries that are associated with the development of inefficient regulation (Schore, 1996). So, we suggest that attachment disruption may constitute a type of "relational trauma" that could interrupt the development of an efficient regulatory system that allows for adaptive regulation of social and environmental stress. However, a neuropsychobiological model specific to disrupted attachment needs to be evaluated so that a more precise understanding of the processes involved can be determined.

At the very least, it is clear that the very processes of neural development, which occur most rapidly in early childhood, are shaped by experience. The plasticity of the brain, a phenomenon more extensive and important than recognized even at the time of Kraemer's (1992) review of the psychobiology of attachment, suggests that both early recognition of children's stress responses and organized and comprehensive early intervention are important so that disturbances and disruptions in the primary attachment relationship can be addressed in an effort to reduce problematic symptomatology that could lead to social, emotional, and regulatory dysfunction.

Implications for Humans

When researchers are studying attachment disruption in humans, there is little they can do to control for moderating and mediating factors, such as preseparation relationship stability, length of separation, or number of separations. Certainly, these factors, along with ontogenic factors, will impact the course of attachment disruption for a given individual. Furthermore, children are almost never reared in isolation, and the difference between isolation and a shorter period of separation may be profound. However, given that the attachment system is thought to be similar across species, the fact that long-term social dysregulation has been noted in animals who experienced early attachment disruptions, either through postnatal separation or having been reared in isolation, strongly suggests that identifying and following children who experience early attachment disruptions is critical.

Recent observational study of children who experienced extremely deprived caregiving conditions (e.g., children adopted from institutions; maltreated children) lends support to the proposition that children who experience early caregiving disruptions should be evaluated and treated for symptoms resulting from the disruption. For example, recent research has demonstrated that children who are reared in institutions are at increased risk for behavior problems (Ames, 1997; Marcovitch et al., 1997) and disturbances and disorders of attachment (O'Connor, Bredenkamp, Rutter, & The English and Romanian Adoptees Study Team [ERA], 1999; O'Connor, Rutter, & the [ERA], 2000; Smyke, Dumitrescu, & Zeanah, 2002). Similarly, children in foster care have been reported to develop anomalous attachment behaviors that are consistent with reactive attachment disorder (RAD) and disorders of nonattachment (e.g., Albus & Dozier, 1999; Hinshaw-Fuselier, Boris, & Zeanah, 1999). When these observational findings are considered with the research regarding the neurobiology of stress, a picture emerges of the potential path from children's early disruptive caregiving experiences to long-term emotional and behavioral vulnerabilities. Children who are exposed to disrupted caregiving are at risk for continued difficulty in emotion regulation and deficits in what has been called social cognitive processing. (Price & Landsverk, 1998).

A first goal, then, is to reliably identify children who experience attachment disruptions. Symptomatology needs to be assessed according to diagnostic criteria for disrupted attachment disorder. As greater numbers of children are identified and followed over time, criteria can be refined according to the picture that emerges regarding the etiology and course of the disorder. As a clearer picture emerges regarding the symptoms and potential sequelae of disrupted attachment, the efficacy of intervention practices can be assessed and treatment practices can be tailored to the specific needs of young children whose primary caregiving relationship is disrupted.

TOWARD REFINED CRITERIA FOR DIFFERENTIAL DIAGNOSIS OF DISRUPTED ATTACHMENT DISORDER

There is clearly overlap between criteria for disrupted attachment disorder (DAD) and criteria for other disorders that may occur in early childhood. Shared symptomatology is a problem in current conceptualizations of psychopathology, as is comorbidity (Clark et al., 1995). Given the dearth of research on infant psychopathology, it is difficult to hierarchically organize classifications and decide whether each category represents an etiologically distinct disorder. A first step in refining nosologies is to establish the clinical phenomenology of each proposed disorder through careful case studies (Cantwell, 1996). Following the section on differential diagnosis is a case example that both highlights the kinds of early symptoms that may be evident around the time of an attachment disruption and the difficulties in sorting out which symptoms are the result of the disruption and which symptoms might have been preexisting.

Disrupted Attachment Disorder

The currently proposed DAD criteria (see Table 2.1) include behaviors characteristic of the triphasic syndrome of protest, despair, and detachment that Robertson and Bowlby (1952) outlined. These include searching for the absent parent figure, emotional withdrawal, disruptions in regulatory functions, and either indifference to reminders of the caregiver or extreme sensitivity to such reminders or to themes connected to separation or loss (e.g., playing hide-and-seek; Lieberman & Zeanah, 1995). While not all of these symptoms listed in Table 2.1 need to be present for DAD to be considered, the clinical picture should include a grouping of the aforementioned symptoms that *occur at the time of a separation from or loss of a primary attachment figure* and impair young children's ability to participate adaptively in their social environment.

Case examples illustrate that symptoms of DAD may evolve over time, even if children have transferred the attachment bond to another caregiver or have been reunited with their parent figure. However, published case examples often involve children in foster care who are not reunited with the caregiver, rather than temporary separation from an established caregiver. In fact, other than Robertson's observational data, there are no available data on the prevalence of significant symptoms following brief separations in the context of stable relationships in low-risk families. In high-risk cases, fear of abandonment and vulnerability to loss may persist (Lieberman & Zeanah, 1995). In some cases, ongoing anxiety may be expressed as excessive clinginess or extreme distress upon separation from the caregiver (Lieberman & Zeanah, 1995). Furthermore, anxiety in the young child is sometimes accompanied by contradictory restrictions in direct expression of affection with the caregiver (Gaensbauer, Chatoor, Drell, Siegel, & Zeanah, 1995), extended sadness and apathy (Stein & Call, 2001; Zelenko & Benham, 2002), and frequent or severe angry outbursts (Lieberman & Zeanah, 1995; Zelenko & Benham, 2002). Children's play may also be impacted, such as in the case of a little girl who obsessively hid little toys after being transferred to an adoptive home from a foster home where she had lived for 14 months (Lieberman & Zeanah, 1995).

TABLE 2.1. Diagnostic Criteria for Disrupted Attachment Disorder

A. The child has experienced a sudden separation from or loss of the attachment figure.

B. Symptoms include one or more of the following:
   1. Irritability and angry protest
   2. Search behavior for the missing caregiver
   3. Clinginess to the replacement caregiver
   4. Angry protest toward or withdrawal from reminders of the caregiver

C. Accompanying symptoms include one or more of the following:
   1. Lack of interest in age-appropriate activities (e.g., positive affective involvement in play)
   2. Diminished appetite or food stuffing or hoarding (usually late features)
   3. Disrupted sleep patterns
   4. Flat or sad affect
   5. Emotional withdrawal
   6. Lethargy

D. The disturbances in the child's affect and/or behavior impair social interaction.

Note. Adapted from Zeanah, Boris, Bakshi, and Lieberman (2000). Copyright 2000 by John Wiley & Sons. Adapted by permission of John Wiley & Sons.

Differential Diagnosis

Posttraumatic Stress Disorder and Disrupted Attachment Disorder

Some symptoms, such as anxious avoidance, may be seen with both PTSD and DAD. When death (or other loss) of a caregiver is involved, intrusive thoughts of the caregiver, avoidance of reminders of the caregiver, restricted range of affect, loss of interest in age-appropriate activities, difficulty concentrating, and sleep difficulties may herald either disorder. The distinguishing features of PTSD in such circumstances would be fearfulness, vigilance, and anxiety (Scheeringa & Gaensbauer, 2000), rather than emotional withdrawal combined with the anomalous attachment behaviors that would characterize DAD.

Reactive Attachment Disorder—Inhibited Subtype and Disrupted Attachment Disorder

A complicating factor in the differential diagnosis of DAD is that some children who meet the criteria for DAD may have had such inadequate preseparation relationship experiences that they met the criteria for RAD-inhibited at the time of separation. It may be very difficult to establish whether symptomatic neglected or maltreated children who experience a prolonged separation from their caregiver should be diagnosed with RAD-inhibited or DAD. The most salient overlapping symptoms between RAD-inhibited and DAD are emotional withdrawal and disinterest in social interaction (e.g., refusal to accept comfort from others and/or lack of comfort seeking, even in times of acute distress). Inhibited children, like those with DAD, may exhibit a lack of age-appropriate interest in activities. However, inhibited children are likely to show fear responses, especially with their primary caregivers, and would not be expected to be clingy. In some cases, there may be evidence that the withdrawal symptoms increase significantly at the time of prolonged separation, which would support a DAD diagnosis.

As opposed to children who meet criteria for RAD, children with adequate preseparation attachment relationships will likely have engaged in some degree of preferred attachment behaviors (e.g., preferential comfort seeking in times of distress; reference to the caregiver in novel situations) with their caregivers prior to the disruption in the relationship. For these children, DAD should be considered if the observed symptoms arise in response to a sudden separation from or loss of a particular caregiver *and* if the observed perturbations in attachment behaviors represent a sudden change in an established pattern.

Depression and Disrupted Attachment Disorder

Unlike depressive symptomatology (see Luby, 2000), DAD criteria require deviations in attachment-relevant behaviors as well as problems with mood. If depressive symptomatology (e.g., restricted affect; decreased interest in activities; sadness) accompanies changes in attachment behaviors and a prolonged separation from or loss of the primary caregiver has occurred, DAD should be considered.

CASE EXAMPLE

This case involves a set of fraternal twins born at 36 weeks gestation into a family who had an extensive history of involvement with Child Protective Services (CPS). In fact, before the twins were born, four older children from the family had been placed in foster care. The four siblings were followed for more than 2 years by a clinical intervention project, the Infant Team (IT), which served young maltreated children (see Zeanah & Larrieu, 1998, for a program description). At birth, the children's mother, Mrs. Clark, had a positive toxicology screen for cocaine. Just after the twins' birth, the biological parents voluntarily transferred custody of the twins (Lynn and Charlie) to a relative, their mother's stepmother, who was also their godmother.

The biological parents had very limited caregiving responsibility for the twins; thus, the majority of this case history will focus on the twins' relationship with their two primary caregivers, Mrs. Step, the maternal stepgrandmother, and Mrs. King, the foster mother. The twins' history, developmental status, and symptomatology will be presented in the order the evaluations were administered. Follow-up information collected from two research projects, spanning 5 years following the twins' initial clinical evaluation, will also be presented.

The Clark Family's Social History

The Clarks were initially referred to the IT when their four oldest children were placed in foster care for neglect and abandonment. After 2 years of intensive multimodal treatment, their parental rights for the four older children were terminated. The Clarks had been unable to maintain stable housing, demonstrated extremely poor decision-making and problem-solving skills, exhibited limited ability to empathize with or understand their children's perspectives, and reported a volatile relationship with each other, including serial separations and reconciliations.

Mr. Clark reported a childhood history fraught with abuse and emotional neglect. He was parented by an erratic mother and an alcoholic father. Mrs. Clark reported being abandoned by her mother and physically abused by her maternal grandmother, who raised her. She alleged that she was gang raped at the age of 12, after which she began experimenting with drugs and alcohol. She screened positive for cocaine on several toxicology screens throughout her evaluation and treatment.

The Twins' History

Little is known about the twins' development in their first 9 months, though it is believed that Mrs. Step had primary responsibility for them. When they entered foster care at 9 months of age they were unable to sit unsupported, crawl, or pull up into a standing position. Their foster mother reported that the twins' primary caregiver told her that Charlie was deaf, developmentally delayed, and asthmatic. In his new foster home, Charlie regularly needed comforting at night, banged his head when frustrated/angry, and frequently exhibited brief trance-like states. His foster mother also noted that Charlie appeared to be responsive to sound, and subsequent evaluation revealed that his hearing was normal. Mrs. King reported that Lynn came to her with a severe diaper rash, gastroesophageal reflux, and little capacity for self-soothing nor any interest in actively seeking comfort.

The foster mother was interviewed several months later (as part of a research study) about the twins' symptoms at placement. The interview included specific questions about their attachment-related behaviors. The foster mother described both children as showing signs of a "significant emotional disturbance" following separation from the maternal stepgrandmother at 9 months of age. However, the pattern of their behavior was different. Charlie's affect was described as being very flat ("no animation"). He was emotionally withdrawn and appeared lethargic, showing little interest in toys. His sleep patterns were disrupted, but primarily because he woke to eat frequently. At times, he even stuffed food in his mouth and cried pitifully when a jar of food was empty. At other times, when stressed, he "stared off" and was quite unresponsive—even to the point of not orienting to sound or touch. He was otherwise not irritable, showed little search behavior for his previous caregiver, and, for the first 4–6 weeks of placement, did not show a reaction when separated from his new caregiver.

Lynn was described as irritable: "She could really get herself into a tizzy." Her affect was also flat much of the time, though she was more reactive than Charlie and she was immediately clingy with her new caregiver. Her sleep was disrupted, and she frequently "[awoke] with a high-pitched scream." At these times, she was difficult to console and she even resisted comforting. Her appetite was normal. She showed some interest in toys and was less withdrawn and lethargic than her brother. She protested separation from her foster mother vigorously immediately after being placed with her, though she did not search for her previous caregiver.

Within 6 weeks of placement in foster care, both children were able sit unassisted, crawl, and pull up into a standing position. Two weeks later the Bayley Developmental Assessment was administered to both twins. They scored at the 7-month level, which placed them both in the significantly delayed range of development, though Lynn's mild noncompliance during the exam may have interfered with obtaining an accurate testing of her developmental level. Nevertheless, both twins had made rapid developmental strides in their foster home. However, their biological parents' wish to have the children returned to Mrs. Step, deemed by the state a viable relative placement, necessitated an evaluation to determine the most appropriate placement for the children.

Infant Team Placement Evaluation

When the twins were 19 months of age (in care for 10 months) they completed a comprehensive relationship-based clinical evaluation with Mrs. King and Mrs. Step. The twins' birth parents, despite initial cooperation with visitation, had withdrawn their petition to care for their children, retracted their accusations that the twins had been neglected in Mrs. Step's care, and repeatedly expressed their desire to have the state name her as guardian. The evaluation included structured caregiver–child interactions with each child. When observed with Mrs. Step, Charlie appeared wary, anxious, and avoidant. For example, he rarely interacted with Mrs. Step, instead wandering about the room watching her from a distance. He even attempted to exit the room several times on his own. Although Lynn did not appear avoidant of Mrs. Step, she also did not exhibit much affection toward her. Mrs. Step exhibited low-to-moderate levels of emotional and instrumental support toward both children; however, she was very inconsistent in displaying this support. In particular, she had exceptional difficulty providing emotional support to Charlie. For example, Mrs. Step was unable to anticipate Charlie's frustration, despite its frequent occurrence. Moreover, she was unable to calm or soothe him when he became frustrated with a toy.

In contrast, the assessment with their foster mother was quite positive. Both Charlie and Lynn were clearly able to seek and be comforted by their foster mother when they needed her. When either child became frustrated or lost interest in the task, Mrs. King was able to support them in a positive and calm manner, thus helping to regulate their stress. When the twins were 21 months, their foster family volunteered to participate in a research project that included an in-home observation. At this point in time, the twins exhibited a healthy and positive attachment relationship with their foster mother. Both children sought and were able to use their foster mother as a source of comfort when they were distressed, they referenced their mother when wary or unsure, and they appeared to genuinely enjoy interacting with their foster mother. The twins' foster mother was exceptionally sensitive to their cues, able to help them to regulate both positive and negative emotions, exhibited developmentally appropriate support, and clearly delighted in the children as individuals.

Follow-Up

The Clarks lost their parental rights when the twins were 25 months of age. The twins remained in the care of the Kings throughout the adoption process. When the twins were 5 years old, the adoption by the Kings was finalized.

When the twins were 6 years old, they were reevaluated as part of another research study. This evaluation included measures to assess the child's current cognitive abilities, peer interactions, family relationships, school behavior, and psychiatric symptomatology. The children, their adoptive mother, and their teacher reported on their current functioning. The children were interviewed using the Berkeley Puppet Interview (Ablow & Measelle, 1993). This interview, created specifically for use with young children, uses puppets to interview young children about their perception of various aspects of their lives. Data suggest that child report from the Berkeley Puppet Interview correlates well with parent report (gleaned from a standardized measure that uses the same framework as the interview; Ablow et al., 1999).

Both children participated in cognitive testing using the Kaufman Brief Intelligence Test (K-BIT) and the Peabody Picture Vocabulary Test (PPVT).

Both Lynn and Charlie scored within the normal range on vocabulary and matrices subtests. Both Charlie and his adoptive mother reported that he had more difficulty than his peers paying attention and being impulsive. Both of them also endorsed items indicating that Charlie exhibited more oppositional and defiant behaviors than his peers. Charlie endorsed items that reflect a higher level of anxiety and a lower level of prosocial behavior than his peers. He also endorsed items reflecting less paternal warmth and marital harmony than his peers. Charlie's teacher described him as a sweet child who "for the most part is liked by other children." She described him as lacking confidence and indicated that he exhibited a need to seek out and receive her approval.

Lynn, her teacher, and her adoptive mother all endorsed items indicating that Lynn exhibited more oppositional/defiant and less prosocial behaviors than her peers. Both Lynn's adoptive mother and her teacher endorsed items that indicate that Lynn was more aggressive and had more attention problems than her peers. The items Lynn and her teacher endorsed indicated that Lynn was bullied by her peers more often than her age-mates, yet they also reported that she had a higher level of academic engagement and competence than her peers. Lynn indicated that her adoptive parents exhibited a higher level of marital conflict than her peers' parents; however, she also reported higher levels of marital affection and resolution. Lynn's teacher reported that Lynn had a problem soiling her pants at the beginning of the school year, which led her to being ostracized by her classmates. The teacher described Lynn as a "very sweet and loving child" and that it "broke her heart" to see Lynn being treated in this manner. She also reported that Lynn spent the first 2 months of the school year crying every morning and that the other students became "tired of hearing this."

DISCUSSION

Diagnosing psychopathology in infancy and early childhood is difficult. In particular, traumatic experiences that impact the attachment relationship may be reflected in the ways infants and young children interact with their caregivers. Unfortunately, often limited or unreliable history is available at the time of presentation, even when observed behavior is of clinical concern.

In the case presented here, the children's developmental delays at the time of foster care placement, followed by their rapid developmental gains while in the care of their foster family, can be taken as indicators that their initial caregiving environment was less than adequate and that they were likely neglected. While both twins experienced neglect, each presented with a different collection of symptoms, neither of which is captured by any single diagnostic category. For example, Charlie was lethargic and exhibited a lack of interest in age-appropriate activities, symptoms that are associated with depression. His wariness with his first primary caregiver and his lack of interest in his foster mother and lack of comfort seeking with her are evidence of a disorder of attachment. However, it is debatable whether his symptoms are best captured by the inhibited subtype of RAD or by DAD. In addition, he had a sleep disturbance and exhibited food stuffing, a symptom reported in cases of neglect but not captured in the nosology (Hinshaw-Fuselier et al., 1999).

Though Lynn displayed more mild withdrawal than Charlie (e.g., moderate interest in her environment), she had more severe regulatory problems (e.g., marked sleep disturbance). Like Charlie, Lynn displayed anomalous attachment behaviors that may be found with RAD-inhibited children, though the pattern was different than Charlie's (e.g., seemingly incompatible behaviors, such as her excessive clinginess and her distress upon separation and refusal of comfort when extremely distressed at night). Her attachment behavior suggests that she was attached to her primary caregiver prior to placement in foster care, though the relationship was likely not consistent and sensitive enough for Lynn to develop a secure attachment relationship with her. Lynn's extreme sensitivity to separation was notable and may have been related to the disruption she suffered in her first primary attachment relationship. Therefore, her symptoms may be best captured by a diagnosis of DAD.

Though it may be difficult to arrive at the best diagnosis in cases such as these, in which good information about the preseparation relationship isn't available and symptoms cross diagnostic categories, it is nonetheless important to do so, as diagnosis shapes treatment. The first intervention imperative for the twins was to be placed in a stable environment with a sensitive and consistent caregiver with whom they could develop an organized attachment relationship. Whether a diagnosis of RAD-inhibited or DAD is deemed best, the most essential piece of treatment in a case involving preseparation relationship difficulties and relationship disruption is to provide the opportunity for children to develop a stable and organized attachment relationship. Through repeated interactions with the children over time, a sensitive caregiver who is attuned to children's cues can provide the external regulation that the children need to regulate their stress, particularly in response to separation. Thus, the sensitive caregiver makes available a reparative environment in which children whose attachment relationship has been disrupted may be able to internalize more efficient regulatory patterns over time. It is possible that when this occurs early and effectively, when the neuroplasticity of the brain is at its greatest, problematic brain development patterns may be interrupted. However, it remains unclear whether reparative experiences are sufficient to preempt future difficulties that may be related to early attachment-related trauma.

Another factor for consideration is that diagnosis and treatment of disrupted attachment is complicated by characteristics of the pre- and post-separation attachment relationship(s). In this case, it appears that neither of the twins had a secure attachment relationship with their primary caregiver prior to the disruption. In fact, Charlie may not have had an established attachment relationship at all, while Lynn may have had an insecure and possibly disorganized primary attachment relationship. The suspected difference in the twins' preseparation relationship experience may explain the differences in their postseparation symptomatology. These types of relationship differences have implications for treatment as well. Given the adequacy of the foster mother's caregiving, little intervention was provided, aside from marginal support services (e.g., ongoing involvement of CPS). However, had problematic relationship patterns been observed with the foster mother or had the twins been reunited with Mrs. Step, for example, their treatment might have varied. Foster parents may be offered auxiliary services for their children, such as occupational therapy, speech therapy, or individual therapy with a mental health professional, which may help offset problematic behaviors that children bring into the relationship. In addition, foster parents may benefit from participation in interactive group therapy with their young foster children or a more individually tailored intervention to help them learn to manage the particular difficult behaviors in which their foster children engage (see Heller, Smyke, & Boris, 2002, for an in-depth discussion of clinical intervention with foster families). When relationship problems precede disruption or complicate a reunion with biological parents or placement with relatives or foster parents, a gentle approach to treatment is advisable. Favorable results may be obtained by reaching out to the family using a nonthreatening technique such as *interaction guidance* (McDonough, 2000), in which families' strengths are the focus of intervention. This may be an effective way of building a therapeutic relationship that can be used to promote a sensitive and consistent caregiving relationship for young children with their primary caregiver, which is the heart of intervention in cases of disrupted or disturbed attachment.

Despite the provision of a stable and sensitive caregiving relationship, the longer-term clinical picture of the twins presented here is similar to that reported in descriptive studies of nonhuman primates whose early caregiving was disrupted. As with primates reared in isolation, the twins had long-term clinical symptoms years after their initial presentation, despite what was thought to be effective intervention following their early trauma. A comprehensive battery of standardized tests from multiple reporters at age 6 confirmed that both children had difficulty in peer relationships and both had disruptive behavior problems (e.g., inattention; impulsive and/or oppositional behavior). While current family conditions and other intervening factors cannot be ruled out as contributing to these long-term social and regulatory difficulties, the twins' symptoms at age 6 are nonetheless clinically significant. We suggest, as others have, that the neurobiological responses to stress that shape neural pathways early in childhood predisposed these twins to experience social and regulatory problems later in childhood (Schore, 1996, 2001b) despite their apparent development of an organized and probably eventually secure attachment relationship with their adoptive mother.

Clearly, much research is needed to address the lack of information pertaining to the diagnosis and treatment of disrupted attachment, the diagnostic category of DAD should be reviewed to help determine its accuracy and relevance to the clinical syndrome(s) associated with attachment disruptions. It would be beneficial to follow a large sample of children who experience attachment disruption to document both the immediate trauma and the long-term sequelae associated with early relationship disruption. Diagnostic criteria need to be refined based on common symptoms across large groups of children. For example, as the foregoing case study indicates, nonshared factors preceding the disruption (e.g., relationship characteristics) may result in symptoms that are different enough to support disorder subtypes. Once diagnostic reliability is established, it should be possible to study intervening factors that mediate or moderate children's response to attachment disruption. In this way, effective intervention following diagnosis can be identified. In the meantime, currently used intervention techniques should be systematically studied with children who experience disruptions and are reunited with their attachment figures and with children who experience disruption and are placed with alternate caregivers. Particular attention should be given to children in foster care who experience repeated disruption, to determine the effects of multiple disruptions and the efficacy of relationship-based treatment efforts in mitigating those effects.

Refining diagnostic criteria through the study of disruptions in attachment relationships will also shed light on how various kinds of traumatic experiences impact attachment. Given the hundreds of thousands of children who undoubtedly will experience relationship disruptions in the foster care system in addition to the millions of children worldwide who will experience the sudden loss of their primary caregivers as the AIDS pandemic runs its course, the need to both identify symptomatic children early and intervene effectively is clear.

REFERENCES

Ablow, J. C., & Measelle, J. R. (1993). *Berkeley puppet interview: Administration and Scoring System Manuals*. Berkeley: University of California.

Ablow, J. C., Measelle, J. R., Kraemer, H. C., Harrington, R., Luby, J., Smider, N., Dierker, L., Clark, V., Dubicka, B., Heffelfinger, A., Essex, M. J., & Kupfer, D. J. (1999). The MacArthur three-city outcome study: Evaluating multi-informant measures of young children's symptomatology. *Journal of the American Academy of Child and Adolescent Psychiatry, 38*(12), 1580–1590.

Albus, K. E., & Dozier, M. (1999). Indiscriminate friendliness and terror of strangers in infancy: Contributions from the study of infants in foster care. *Infant Mental Health Journal, 20*(1), 30–41.

Ames, E. L. (1997). *The development of Romanian orphanage children adopted to Canada.* Vancouver, British Columbia, Canada: Simon Fraser University.

Bowlby, J. (1944a). Forty-four juvenile thieves: Their characters and home-life. *International Journal of Psycho-Analysis, 25,* 19–53.

Bowlby, J. (1944b). Forty-four juvenile thieves: Their characters and home-life (II). *International Journal of Psycho-Analysis, 25,* 107–128.

Bowlby, J. (1951). *Maternal care and mental health.* New York: Columbia University Press.

Bowlby, J. (1973). *Attachment and loss: Vol. 2. Separation.* New York: Basic Books.

Bowlby, J. (1980). *Attachment and loss: Vol. 3. Loss.* New York: Basic Books.

Bowlby, J. (1982). *Attachment and loss: Vol. 1. Attachment* (2nd ed.). New York: Basic Books. (Original work published 1969)

Bretherton, I., & Munholland, K. A. (1999). Internal working models in attachment relationships: A construct revisited. In J. Cassidy & P. R. Shaver (Eds.), *Handbook of attachment: Theory, research, and clinical applications* (pp. 520–554). New York: Guilford Press.

Cantwell, D. P. (1996). Classification of child and adolescent psychopathology. *Journal of Child Psychology and Psychiatry, 37,* 3–12.

Chapin, H. D. (1915). Are institutions for infants necessary? *Journal of the American Medical Association, 64,* 1–3.

Children's Defense Fund (2000). Adoption and Safe Families Act (ASFA) basics. Retrieved March 31, 2003, from the World Wide Web: *http://www.childrens defense.org/ss_asfa_basics.php*

Cicchetti, D., & Toth, S. L. (1995). A developmental psychopathology perspective on child abuse and neglect. *Journal of the American Academy of Child and Adolescent Psychiatry, 34,* 541–565.

Clark, L. A., Watson D., & Reynolds S. (1995). Diagnosis and classification of psychopathology: Challenges to the current system and future directions. *Annual Review of Psychology, 46,* 121–153.

Donahue, J., & Williamson, J. (1999). *Community mobilization to mitigate the impacts of HIV/AIDS.* Washington, DC: Displaced Children & Orphans Fund.

Gaensbauer, T., Chatoor, I., Drell, M., Siegel, D., & Zeanah, C. H. (1995). Traumatic loss in a one-year-old girl. *Journal of the American Academy of Child and Adolescent Psychiatry, 34,* 94–102.

Garavan, H., Ross, T. J., & Stein, E. A. (1999). Right hemisphere dominance of inhibitory control: An event-related functional MRI study. *Proceedings of the National Academy of Sciences, USA, 96,* 8301–8306.

Green, J., & Goldwyn, R. (2002). Annotation: Attachment disorganization and psychopathology: New findings in attachment research and their potential implications for developmental psychopathology in childhood. *Journal of Child Psychology and Psychiatry, 43,* 835–846.

Grossman, A. W., Churchill J. D., McKinney B. C., Kodish I. M., Otte S. L., & Greenough, W. T. (2003). Experience effects on brain development: Possible contributions to psychopathology. *Journal of Child Psychiatry, Psychology, and Allied Disciplines, 44,* 33–63.

Heilman, K. M., & Van Den Abell, T. (1979). Right hemispheric dominance for mediating cerebral activation. *Neuropsychologia, 17,* 315–321.

Heinicke, C. M., & Westheimer, I. (1965). *Brief separations:* New York: International Universities Press.

Heller, S. S., Smyke, A. T., & Boris, N. W. (2002). Very young foster children and foster families: Clinical challenges and interventions. *Infant Mental Health Journal, 23*(5), 555–575.

Hinshaw-Fuselier, S., Boris, N., & Zeanah, C. H. (1999). Reactive attachment disorder in maltreated twins. *Infant Mental Health Journal, 20*(1), 42–59.

Hofer, M. A. (1987). Early social relationships: A psychologists's view. *Child Development, 58,* 633–647.

Kraemer, G. W. (1992). A psychobiological theory of attachment. *Behavioral and Brain Sciences, 15,* 493–541.

Kraemer, G. W., Ebert, M. H., Schmidt, D. E., & McKinney, W. T. (1991). Strangers in a strange land: A psychobiological study of infant monkeys before and after separation from real or inanimate mothers. *Child Development, 62,* 548–566.

Lieberman, A., & Zeanah, C. H. (1995). Disorders of attachment in infancy. In *Child and Adolescent Psychiatric Clinics of North America, 4*(3), 571–588.

Luby, J. L. (2000). Depression. In C. H. Zeanah (Ed.), *Handbook of infant mental health* (2nd ed., pp. 382–396). New York: Guilford Press.

Malik, N. M., Crowson, M. M., Lederman, C. S., & Osofsky, J. D. (2002). Evaluating maltreated infants, toddlers, and preschoolers in dependency court. *Infant Mental Health Journal, 23*(5), 576–592.

Marcovitch, S., Goldberg, S., Gold, A., Washington, J., Wasson, C., Krekewich, K., & Handley-Derry (1997). Determinants of behavioral problems in Romanian children adopted into Toronto. *International Journal of Behavioral Development, 20,* 17–31.

McDonough, S. C. (2000). Interaction guidance: An approach for difficult-to-engage families. In C. H. Zeanah (Ed.), *Handbook of infant mental health* (2nd ed., pp. 485–493). New York: Guilford Press.

McEwen, B. S. (1999). Stress and hippocampal placticity. *Annual Review of Neuroscience, 22,* 105–122.

O'Connor, T. G., Bredenkamp, D., Rutter, M., & the English and Romanian Adoptees Study Team [ERA]. (1999). Attachment disturbances and disorders in children exposed to early severe deprivation. *Infant Mental Health Journal, 20*(1), 10–29.

O'Connor, T. G., Rutter, M., & the English and Romanian Adoptees Study Team [ERA]. (2000). Attachment disorder behavior following early severe deprivation: Extension and longitudinal follow-up. *Journal of the American Academy of Child and Adolescent Psychiatry, 39*(6), 703–712.

Price, J. M., & Landsverk, J. (1998). Social information-processing patterns as predictors of social adaptation and behavior problems among maltreated children in foster care. *Child Abuse and Neglect, 22*(9), 845–858.

Provence, S., & Lipton, R. C. (1962). *Infants in institutions.* New York: International Universities Press.

Robertson, J. (Director). (1953). *A two-year old goes to hospital* [Film: 16mm, 40 minutes, in English and French]. (Available from Concord Video and Film Council, Rosehill Centre, 22 Hines Road, Ipswich, Suffolk, 1P3 9BG England)

Robertson, J. (Director). (1958). *Going to hospital with mother.* [Film: 16mm, 40 minutes, in English and French]. (Available from Concord Video and Film Council, Rosehill Centre, 22 Hines Road, Ipswich, Suffolk, 1P3 9BG England)

Robertson, J., & Bowlby, J. (1952). Responses of young children to separation from their mothers. *Courrier du Centre Internationale d'Enfance, 2,* 131–142.

Robertson, J., & Robertson, J. (1971). Young children in brief separation: A fresh look. *Psychoanalytic Study of the Child, 26,* 264–315.

Robertson, J., & Robertson, J. (1989). *Separation and the very young child.* London: Free Association Books.

Rutter, M. (1972a). Maternal deprivation reassessed. *Journal of Psychosomatic Research, 16,* 241–250.

Rutter, M. (1972b). *Maternal deprivation reassessed.* Baltimore: Penguin.

Scheeringa, M. S., & Gaensbauer, T. J. (2000). Posttraumatic stress disorder. In C. H. Zeanah (Ed.), *Handbook of infant mental health* (2nd ed., pp. 369–381). New York: Guilford Press.

Schore, A. N. (1994). *Affect regulation and the origin of the self: The neurobiology of emotional development.* Hillsdale, NJ: Erlbaum.

Schore, A. N. (1996). The experience-dependent maturation of a regulatory system in the orbital prefrontal cortex and the origin of developmental psychopathology. *Development and Psychopathology, 8,* 59–87.

Schore, A. N. (1999, December). *Parent–infant communication and the neurobiology of emotional development.* Paper presented at the Zero to Three 14th Annual Training Conference, Los Angeles, CA.

Schore, A. N. (2000). Attachment and the regulation of the right brain. *Attachment and Human Development, 2*(1), 23–47.

Schore, A. N. (2001a). The effects of a secure attachment relationship on right brain development, affect regulation, and infant mental health. *Infant Mental Health Journal, 22*(1–2), 7–66.

Schore, A. N. (2001b). The effects of early relational trauma on right brain development, affect regulation, and infant mental health. *Infant Mental Health Journal, 22*(1–2), 201–269.

Smyke, A. T., Dumitrescu, A., & Zeanah, C. H. (2002). Attachment disturbances in young children: I. The continuum of caretaking casualty. *Journal of the American Academy of Child and Adolescent Psychiatry, 41*(8), 972–982.

Spitz, R. A. (1945). Hospitalism: An enquiry into the genesis of psychiatric conditions in early childhood. *Psychoanalytic Study of the Child, 1,* 53–74.

Spitz, R. A. (1946). Anaclitic depression: An enquiry into the genesis of psychiatric conditions in early childhood. II. *Psychoanalytic Study of the Child, 2,* 131–342.

Sroufe, L. A. (1989). Relationships, self, and individual adaptation. In A. J. Sameroff & R. N. Emde (Eds.), *Relationship disturbances in early childhood* (pp. 70–94). New York: Basic Books.

Stein, M. T., & Call, J. D. (2001). Extraordinary changes in behavior in an infant after a brief separation. *Journal of Developmental and Behavioral Pediatrics. 22*(2, Suppl.), S11–S15.

Tizard, B., & Hodges, J. (1978). The effect of early institutional rearing on the development of eight-year-old children. *Journal of Child Psychology and Psychiatry, 19,* 99–118.

U.S. Agency for International Development (2002). *Children on the brink 2002: A joint report on orphan estimates and program strategies* (Contract No. HRN-C-00-99-00005-00). Washington, DC: TvT Associates.

U.S. Department of Health & Human Services. (2002). *Adoption and foster care analysis and reporting system report.* Rockville, MD: Administration for Children & Families, Children's Bureau.

van IJzendoorn, M. H., Schuengel, C., & Bakermans-Kranenburg, M. J. (1999). Disorganized attachment in early childhood: Meta-analysis of precursors, concomitants, and sequelae. *Development and Psychopathology, 11,* 225–249.

Zeanah, C. H., Boris N. W., Bakshi, S., & Lieberman, A. F. (2000). Attachment disorders of infancy. In J. D. Osofsky & H. E. Fitzgerald (Eds.), *WAIMH handbook of infant mental health* (Vol. 4, pp. 93–122). New York: Wiley.

Zeanah, C. H., Boris, N. W., & Scheeringa, M. S. (1997). Psychopathology in infancy. *Journal of Child Psychiatry, Psychology, and Allied Disciplines, 38,* 81–99.

Zeanah, C. H., & Larrieu, J. A. (1998). Intensive intervention for maltreated infants and toddlers in foster care. *Child and Adolescent Psychiatric Clinics of North America, 7*(2), 357–371.

Zelenko, M. A., & Benham, A. (2002). Attachment theory, loss, and trauma: A case study. *Clinical Child Psychology and Psychiatry, 7*(2), 199–209.

CHAPTER 3

"HIDDEN TRAUMA" IN INFANCY

Attachment, Fearful Arousal, and Early
Dysfunction of the Stress Response System

MICHELLE R. SCHUDER
KARLEN LYONS-RUTH

The traditional perspective on trauma views trauma from the perspective of the traumatic event and its characteristics. How life threatening was the event? How unanticipated? How often repeated? Who was the perpetrator? The psychological sequellae of trauma are thus most often viewed as following from the characteristics of the event. Characteristics of the child experiencing the trauma, as well as his or her social context, have received less attention except that a consensus exists that large individual differences do exist in how traumatic events are experienced.

In this chapter we do not focus on characteristics of traumatic events or trauma responses. Instead, we argue here that the impact of trauma on the developing child cannot be understood apart from the social and psychological resources available to buffer the effects of fearful arousal on the child's psychobiological functioning. In early childhood the primary attachment relationship serves that function. Therefore, physiological and psychological responses to threatening events in early childhood can be understood fully only in reference to the quality of psychobiological regulation available within primary attachment relationships.

We intend to elaborate the view here that trauma in infancy has special characteristics and must be defined differently than trauma at later ages. According to the fourth edition of the *Diagnostic and Statistical Manual of*

Mental Disorders (DSM-IV) a traumatic event involves threat to the physical integrity of oneself or another person (American Psychiatric Association, 1994). In human infancy, however, experienced threat is closely related to the caregiver's affects and availability rather than to the actual degree of physical or survival threat inherent in the event itself. Equipped with limited behavioral and cognitive coping capacities, the very young infant is dependent on external regulation to avoid overwhelming levels of physiological arousal that exceed available coping capacities.

Thus, the relevant traumas of infancy most often result from the "hidden traumas" of caregiver unavailability and interactive dysregulation. These hidden traumas are woven into the fabric of interaction between the caregiver and the infant and do not necessarily stand out as salient events to the observer. However, the physiological evidence reviewed below indicates that these more subtle traumatic events of infancy engender similar physiological consequences in stress response systems during the infancy period as do the more obvious threat events salient to older children and adults.

Finally, new evidence suggests that the infant does not come equipped with a particular level of stress tolerance at birth that continues into the preschool and school years. Instead, the expression of the infant's genetic predisposition appears to be substantially under the influence of caregiver regulation. The sensitively attuned caregiver, able to navigate the pathway from heightened states of arousal to homeostatic recovery, shapes the infant's psychobiological response to environmental stressors, creating an infant who is able to tolerate challenges to his or her internal psychobiological milieu. Conversely, insensitive caregiver response to heightened infant arousal may promote dysregulated response to stress in the infant, characterized by under- or overactivity in the stress response system. Sensitively attuned caregiver regulation effectively resets the infant's propensity to react to stressors with more enduring states of arousal. Therefore, these subtle regulatory events of early infancy shape the subsequent functioning of neuroendocrine stress response systems in enduring ways. Specifically, these hidden traumas of infancy contribute to the early hyper- or hyporegulation of stress responses mediated through the hypothalamic–pituitary–adrenocortical (HPA) axis.

In developing a view of the regulatory processes in the caregiver–infant system that contribute to dysregulation, we integrate insights from the literature on early brain development and early dysfunction of the HPA axis with an intersubjective and bioregulatory model of the early functioning of the attachment system. We recontextualize the functioning of the attachment relationship over the first year within a revised evolutionary framework. This framework anticipates dual-level mechanisms embedded in the infant–caregiver relationship governing the regulation of fearful arousal in infancy, including both direct physiological mechanisms and intersubjective processes.

ATTACHMENT RELATIONSHIPS
AND REGULATION OF FEARFUL AROUSAL

In this chapter we integrate various strands of the developmental literature to advance a model of the likely mechanisms through which caregiver behavior impacts the stress response system in human infancy. The literature most central to such a model is the literature on the development of the attachment relationship. The infant's attachment behavioral system is viewed as the set of infant behaviors that mediates felt security, or reductions in fearful arousal, by maintaining proximity or contact with the caregiver. In-depth reviews of this literature are available elsewhere (Cassidy & Shaver, 1999; Lyons-Ruth & Jacobvitz, 1999). Here we reference this literature selectively in regard to the interface of attachment behavior and the regulation or dysregulation of the stress response system, as evidenced by activity in the HPA system.

The caregiving system has received considerable attention from attachment theorists over the past 40 years. John Bowlby put forth the critical concept of an attachment motivational system that functions to promote the infant's proximity to the caregiver and thereby to regulate both the infant's actual safety and the infant's sense of "felt security" in the environment. He asserted that infants are biologically predisposed to become attached to their caregivers and that early disturbances in primary attachment relationships could lead to emotional insecurity and later disturbances in the development of meaningful relationships (Bowlby, 1969, 1973, 1980).

Ainsworth, Blehar, Waters, and Wall (1978) developed a means of classifying the quality of a child's attachment to a caregiver, referred to as the "Strange Situation" procedure. Twelve- to 18-month-old infants' responses to brief separations from and reunions with the caregiver allow the researcher to classify the infant's attachment organization as *secure, avoidant,* or *resistant/ambivalent.* The mother's sensitivity to the infant's signals and communications in the home predicted secure organization, whereas maternal rejection and unpredictability predicted detached avoidance and overtly anxious resistance/ambivalence, respectively (Main, 2000).

Mary Main and Judith Solomon subsequently developed a fourth category of infant strange situation behavior, called *disorganized/disoriented.* These infants exhibited an array of odd, disoriented, and overtly conflicted behaviors in the presence of a parent. Main and Hesse (1990) hypothesized that for these infants the caregiver was both the source of comfort and a source of alarm, so that these infants experienced a simultaneous need to approach and to flee their parent. Lyons-Ruth, Bronfman, and Atwood (1999) have noted that absence of caregiver regulation also leads to infant disorganization, so that absence of regulation rather than fear of the caregiver per se may be the more general mechanism related to disorganization. Consistent with these hypotheses regarding caregiver behavior, studies have indicated that 83% of abused or neglected infants display disorganized attachment behaviors toward the parent (V. Carlson, Cicchetti, Barnett, & Braumwald, 1989). However, it is likely that caregiver behaviors less extreme than overt maltreatment are involved as well. Approximately 15% of infants in low-risk samples demonstrate disorganized attachment patterns (van IJzendoorn, Schuengel, & Bakermans-Kranenburg, 1999). While a subset of these infants may have been maltreated, Hesse and Main (2000) have speculated that other parents may demonstrate anomalous forms of threatening, fearful, and/or dissociative behavior related to unresolved trauma in their own histories.

A large body of research on fearful arousal has documented the range of individual coping responses to fear displayed by different individuals when they are exposed to severe stressors. These have been captured by the summary label "fight or flight." In addition, Seligman (1975) and others have described "freezing" and "learned helplessness" as responses occurring when more active coping responses are unavailable or ineffective. More recently, Taylor and colleagues (2000) have advanced a "tend-or-befriend" hypothesis regarding primary responses to threat among social primates, arguing that "fight or flight" may be more relevant to the stress responses of males while various forms of affiliative responses may be more common stress responses of females.

This entire array of coping or defensive responses appears in some form in the infant behaviors that are part of the disorganized spectrum. For example, freezing, huddling on the floor, and other depressed behaviors are part of the coding criteria for disorganized behaviors, as are contradictory approach–avoidance behaviors that often mix angry resistance with avoidant behaviors such as running away or hiding under a chair. Not surprisingly, infants exhibiting disorganized attachment strategies often demonstrate atypical physiological responses to stressors, as detailed in a later section.

As is evident from these descriptions, disorganized infants can look very different from one another. Within this broad array of behaviors there are at least two distinct subgroups. Disorganized attachment behaviors may occur in concert with other insecure behaviors that are part of an avoidant or ambivalent attachment strategy, resulting in a primary classification of disorganized attachment and a secondary classification of avoidant or ambivalent (referred to hereafter as D-insecure). However, disorganized behaviors may also be displayed in the context of behaviors that are usually part of a secure strategy, such as protesting separation, seeking contact with mother at reunion, and ceasing distress after being picked up, as shown in Table 3.1. This disorganized subgroup is given a secondary classification of secure (referred to hereafter as D-secure). In the National Institute of Child Health and Human Development child care study (K. McCartney, personal communication, April, 1993), D-Secure infants made up 52% of the disorganized group.

There are parallel differences in the maternal behaviors associated with infant disorganization. Mothers of D-insecure infants have displayed significantly higher rates of role confusion, negative-intrusive behavior, and frightening behavior than mothers of D-secure infants. In contrast, mothers of D-secure infants have exhibited significantly higher rates of withdrawal than mothers of D-insecure infants (Lyons-Ruth, Bronfman, & Atwood, 1999). These two profiles of maternal behavior have been referred to as "hostile–self-referential" and "helpless–fearful." The behaviors contributing to these profiles are described in more detail in Lyons-Ruth, Bronfman, and Atwood (1999).

The subtle nature of the helpless–fearful profile of maternal behavior is important to note, as is the subtlety of many of the disorganized behaviors of D-secure infants. The more hostile–self-referential maternal behaviors and the more avoidant and ambivalent disorganized infant behaviors are much easier to identify as maladaptive, yet recent data indicate that these behaviors characterize less than half of mothers and infants who experience disorganized attachment relationships.

Another form of atypical attachment behavior that is likely to be predictive of long-term impairment in social behavior is the indiscriminate attachment behavior seen among infants reared in institutional settings with very poor care and with no selective attachment figure available (O'Connor, Rutter, & the English and Romanian Adoptees Study Team [ERA], 2000). However, a lack of selectivity in attachment behavior is also noted clinically among high-risk home-reared infants and can be observed in the standard attachment assessment in the infant's tendency to accept comfort from an unfamiliar lab assistant even though actively distressed.

From this body of attachment research, we understand trauma in a 12- to 18-month-old infant to be related both to the directly traumatic experience of maltreatment as well as to effects of parental behaviors that are frightening, frightened, withdrawing, role reversed, or otherwise atypical.

TABLE 3.1. Subgroups of Disorganized Attachment in Infancy

Disorganized–secure ("pseudo-secure")	Disorganized–insecure ("avoidant–resistant [A/C]")
• Disorganized behaviors	• Disorganized behaviors
• Little avoidance or resistance	• Avoidance, resistance, or both
• Distress to separation	• Often appears quite conflicted
• Calms in parent's presence	• May combine marked separation distress with marked avoidance at reunion
• Some proximity seeking	
• May appear passive, depressed, aimless, hesitant, or apprehensive	

Unlike mildly rejected or inconsistently treated infants, who demonstrate inadequate stress-reducing behavioral strategies, the infant whose caregiver has been unable to provide basic regulation around fearful arousal fails to develop any coherent behavioral attachment strategies for retaining organization and reducing physiological arousal in the face of moderate stress.

While these data have been compelling in establishing a relational basis for the infant's regulation of fearful arousal by the end of the first year, this literature has two limitations. First, attachment security cannot be assessed prior to the end of the first year of life because the standard assessment depends on the infant's display of particular types of behavioral organization not available to younger infants. Second, while the assessment of attachment security claims to index "felt security," we have had little in the way of converging physiological indicators of the infant's states or "felt" experience. Instead, those experiences have had to be inferred primarily from how the infant organizes his or her emotional displays and behavioral responses. However, contemporary research (Spangler & Schieche, 1998; Nachmias, Gunnar, Mangelsdorf, Parritz, & Buss, 1996) suggests that observed behavioral and emotional responses are not always reliably associated with underlying physiological indicators of felt security or fearful arousal, as reviewed below. Measures of infant physiological states provide opportunity to assess internal psychobiological states more directly, regardless of displayed behavior or changes in behavioral capacities, during the first year of life.

How might we elaborate our model of attachment and trauma during the first year of life to incorporate the caregiver's earliest environmental contributions to fundamental biological and behavioral systems in the infant? The caregiving environment impacts the infant's development much earlier and in a more physiological manner than the pioneer attachment theorists were able to demonstrate. As our neuroscientific tools accumulate, we can begin to elaborate a model of attachment and trauma during the first years of life that is more sensitive to very early psychobiological and developmental processes, as well as to distinguish that model from the models that are more reflective of processes at later ages.

THE ENVIRONMENT'S ROLE
IN REGULATION OF GENE EXPRESSION

Findings from a decade of developmental neuroscience indicate that experience shapes neuronal function and brain architecture (Kandel, 1992; LeDoux, 2002; Greenough & Black, 1992). We no longer believe that brain anatomy matures on a fixed ontogenetic calendar. Instead, we recognize environmental experience to be critical to the differentiation of brain tissue itself. We now view the infant brain as an open, nonlinear dynamic system in which an initial set of genetic predispositions serve as a constraint on an open system that takes its organization partially from the organization of the surrounding environment of care. During the prenatal period and first months of life, the primary caregiver essentially defines the environment for the altricial human infant.

Research indicates considerable plasticity in neuronal development in infancy. Mechanisms mediating such experience-expectant change in neuronal development include sensitive periods, behavioral induction, synaptic overproduction, and subsequent pruning (Greenough & Black, 1992; Huttenlocher, 1994; Nelson, 1999). Plasticity may involve not only the creation of new synaptic connections among neurons but also growth of new neurons across the lifespan (Ericksson et al., 1998).

Recently, a number of studies using animal models have generated compelling data that the quality of early caregiving can alter infant physiology, including basic gene expression (Francis, Diorio, Liu, & Meaney, 1999; Liu et al., 1997; Caldji et al., 1998). For example, rat pups separated from their mothers in the first 2 weeks of life incurred a permanent increase in the expression of genes controlling the secretion of corticotropin-releasing factor (CRF), a factor related to effective stress response (Plotsky & Meaney, 1993). In addition, among nonseparated pups, dams who showed increased care of their pups by licking and grooming them during nursing seemed to provide them with a life-long protection from stress, whether or not the pup and dam were genetically related. This latter process appeared to be mediated through the enhanced expression of genes regulating glucocorticoid receptors and the consequent suppression of genes regulating CRF synthesis (Liu et al., 1997). Similar effects of maternal care on offspring CRF have been reported in primates (Coplan et al., 1996).

John Bowlby himself presaged the last decade's findings concerning a socially constructed brain some 40 years ago when he called for a deeper understanding of the ways that an immature organism is critically shaped by its primordial relationship with a mature, adult member of its species. He suggested that the infant's emerging social, psychological, and biological capacities could not be understood apart from its relationship with the mother. More specifically, Bowlby (1958) inquired into the mechanisms by which the infant forms a secure bond characterized by emotional communication with the mother and how this early socioemotional learning is then internalized in the form of an enduring capacity to regulate states of emotional security.

STRESS AND THE HYPOTHALAMIC–PITUITARY–ADRENOCORTICAL SYSTEM

Bowlby (1969) also noted more than 30 years ago that the attachment relationship directly influenced the infant's capacity to cope with stress through the maturation of a control system in the infant's brain that comes to regulate the attachment behavioral system. This behavioral control system is now understood to have complex feedback relations with the hypothalamic–pituitary–adrenocortical (HPA) system, which takes a central role in managing perceived threats to well-being.

Stress describes both the subjective experience induced by a novel, potentially threatening or distressing situation and the behavioral and/or neurochemical reactions to it (Weinstock, 1997). The stress response involves a cascade of biochemical and hormonal events that has evolved to restore homeostasis and promote survival. While successful adaptation often requires the integrated action of most of the regulatory systems of the body, including the autonomic nervous system, the immune system, the neuroendocrine system, and behavioral coping systems, the main systems of the stress response are the norepinephrine-sympathetic adrenomedullary (NE-SAM) system and the hypothalamic–pituitary–adrenocortical (HPA) system. These two systems work together to restore the well-being of the organism by increasing energy resources through increasing heart rate; metabolizing fat and protein stores; and inhibiting digestion, the immune system, and the growth system.

Although both systems are vital to restoring internal homeostasis (Chrousos & Gold, 1992; Stratakis & Gold, 1995), the HPA system has been widely studied in children because its end product, cortisol, provides a marker of the stress response to a perceived homeostatic disruption that can be measured nonintrusively in samples of saliva. Exposure to traumatic events in later childhood and adulthood has been clearly related to alterations in the functioning of the HPA axis, including alterations toward both hypo- and hyperresponsive functioning (Gunnar & Donzella, 2001). Accordingly, in this chapter, we focus on the HPA axis and develop a model of the events associated with its dysregulation in infancy.

Corticotropin-Releasing Hormone and the Hypothalamic–Pituitary–Adrenocortical Axis

Corticotropin-releasing hormone (CRH) is the principal hypothalamic regulator of the pituitary–adrenocortical axis. Produced in the paraventricular nucleus (PVN) of the hypothalamus, CRH, together with the synergistic actions of vasopressin (VP), stimulates the secretion of adrenocorticotropic hormone (ACTH) and endorphins by the anterior pituitary (Chrousos, 1997). Cells on the cortex of the adrenal gland respond to ACTH leading to the release of glucocorticoids. In primates, cortisol is the primary glucocorticoid. In nonprimates, corticosterone is the primary glucocorticoid released. Circulating glucocorticoids complete a negative feedback loop to shut off the current HPA axis activity and to modulate HPA axis activation through their actions at glucocorticoid receptors distributed at different levels of the HPA axis, including the pituitary, hypothalamus, hippocampus, and frontal cortex.

Glucocorticoids

Normally, glucocorticoids are responsible for restraining the stress response by inhibiting HPA axis activation. Glucocorticoids prevent the consequences of prolonged or excessive stress response. At basal or resting levels, glucocorticoids tend to restore or permit processes that support homeostatic defense mechanisms (Munck & Naray-Fejes-Toth, 1994; Gunnar, 2000). Glucocorticoid increases in this basal range generally promote mental and physical health and development (Gunnar, 2000; deKloet, Rots, van den Berg, & Oitzl, 1994). Higher, stress-related elevations in glucocorticoids have suppressive and potentially destructive effects (Sapolsky, 1997; Gunnar, 2000). The regulatory effects of higher glucocorticoid levels may be necessary to prevent overreaction of other body systems, which, if unchecked, lead to injury (Munck & Naray-Fejes-Toth, 1994). These opposing permissive versus suppressive effects appear to operate in part through different receptor systems (Sapolsky, 1997), mineralocorticoid receptors (MRs) and glucocorticoid receptors (GRs).

MRs are largely occupied when glucocorticoids are low and mediate many of the protective functions of the hormone. Basal levels of cortisol follow a daily rhythm mediated in part through the activity of MRs in the hippocampus (Gunnar, 2000). Response to stress, which provokes elevations in cortisol over baseline daily levels, is contained in part through GRs. GRs are highly responsive to increasing levels of glucocorticoids, and their binding is related to termination of CRH production by the PVN of the hypothalamus, reduction of ACTH from the pituitary, and consequently the termination of glucocorticoid production (Liu et al., 1997). The differential properties of MRs and GRs suggest that a balance between the occupation of the MRs and GRs is important to the functioning of the HPA system (DeKloet, Vreugdenhil, Citel, & Joek, 1998).

Assessment of Cortisol Secretion as a Marker of Stress Response Functioning

In humans, the final product of the HPA system is the adrenocortical steroid hormone cortisol. Although cortisol secretion provides only a partial understanding of the activity of the neuroendocrine system, its regulation appears to bear importantly on human growth and development (Gunnar & Donzella, 2001).

Studies of the HPA system in young children require the use of noninvasive measures. CRH has never been assessed in children because it involves sampling cerebrospinal fluid. Similarly, assessment of ACTH requires blood sampling (Dahl et al., 1991). Measurement of salivary cortisol, conversely, offers a noninvasive and relatively simple method for assessing cortisol production in young children (Schwartz, Granger, Susman, Gunnar, & Laird, 1998; Gunnar & Donzella, 2001). Reliance on salivary cortisol measures imposes limitations on our understanding of the regulation and dysregulation of the HPA system in children. The HPA, for example, often maintains normal cortisol levels in response to chronic stressors, while pituitary levels of ACTH often reveal significant effects of chronic stress (Heim, Ehlert, & Hellhammer, 2000). Nevertheless, a considerable literature on the social regulation of cortisol activity has emerged over the past 15 years, during which the assessment of salivary cortisol has entered into common use (Gunnar & Donzella, 2001).

There are two important features of cortisol secretion that typically are considered in the assessment of this hormone. First, cortisol exhibits a typical daily secretion that is unrelated to a stressful challenge, whereby cortisol levels are highest on awakening and lowest at the end of the daily activity phase (Bailey & Heitkemper, 1991). Second, cortisol secretion is activated when a stressful environmental challenge is identified.

First, we examine typical daily cortisol production. As with other hormones in the body, cortisol has a circadian rhythm that is unrelated to stressful challenge. Under typical conditions, mature cortisol levels peak in the morning, are at half of morning levels by late afternoon, and are negligible by midnight (Bailey & Heitkemper, 1991; Knutsson et al., 1997; Sikes, 1992). Cortisol levels should be close to zero in the evening at the end of the activity cycle. Failure to bring cortisol concentrations to low levels at this time of day is believed to reflect a fundamental dysregulation of the stress physiology system. Indeed, elevations in evening levels have been found in some children evidencing psychological disorder (Brent, Ryan, Dahl, & Boris, 1995; De Bellis et al., 1999).

Notably, young children do not evidence a fully adult pattern of basal cortisol production. Newborns exhibit two peaks 12 hours apart that are not correlated with time of day (Sippell, Becker, Versmold, Bidlingmaier, & Knorr, 1978). Typically, the single early morning peak in cortisol is reliably established by 3 months of age (Price, Close, & Fielding, 1983), although Larson, White, Cochran, Donzella, and Gunnar (1998) report an early morning peak in cortisol production as early as 6 weeks of age when group averages are taken. A reliable decrease in cortisol from morning to afternoon is evident by about 4 years of age, reflecting the development of mature sleep–wake patterns by this age (Gunnar & Donzella, 2001).

In contrast to its generally stable daily secretion pattern, cortisol levels generally increase in response to a stressor (although we later discuss a number of exceptions evidenced in recent investigations). Adaptive response to stress typically involves a number of behavioral and physiological responses dedicated to the provision of energy necessary to overcome an identified challenge. A brisk elevation in cortisol production is viewed as one aspect of the organism's adaptive effort to reestablish homeostasis in the face of challenge. Notably, the ability to appropriately regulate the stress response may be as important as the ability to initiate it. Containment of the stress response is crucial to avoid the behavioral and physical consequences of the mobilization of behaviors and resources (Johnson, Kamilaris, Chrousos, & Gold, 1992).

An efficient HPA system is thought to be one that expresses moderate basal glucocorticoid levels, elevated glucocorticoid response when stressors arise, and quick response termination when stressors subside. The development of this efficient HPA system is highly dependent on a healthy GR system (DeKloet, 1991; DeKloet & Reul, 1987). GRs have a low affinity for glucocorticoids and are primarily responsible for reactive negative feedback following an acute stressor. Suppressive, potentially destructive effects of glucocorticoids become more pronounced when GRs are occupied for longer periods of time (Sapolsky, 1997). An inverted U-function has been found for many effects of glucocorticoids. Small increases in the hormone, or brief elevations even to high levels, often enhance behavioral performance and support health-promoting physiological processes. Larger increases, particularly if they result in prolonged occupation of GRs, lead to impairments and threats to health (Gunnar, 2000).

Caregiving and Neuroendocrine Regulation in Nonhuman Mammals

A large body of rodent research has shown that separation of the pup from the dam for prolonged periods, particularly when such separation disrupts maternal behavior, leads to heightened responsivity and poorer regulation of the HPA axis into the adulthood of the animal (Caldji et al., 1998; Levine, 1994; Plotsky & Meaney, 1993). When rat pups are separated from the dam on a daily basis for 3-hour periods, the separation produces hyperstress reactivity (Plotsky & Meaney, 1993). Rats subjected to this paradigm demonstrate reduced GR numbers, increased CRH activity, and larger and longer glucocorticoid responses to restraint stress and novel environments (Liu et al., 1997). Moreover, as noted above, pups reared by mothers who engage in less licking and grooming show larger HPA axis responses to restraint stress, heightened fear, and reduced GR-mediated negative feedback containment of the glucocorticoid stress response (Caldji et al., 1998).

Early experiences in nonhuman primates also appear to affect the development of reactivity and regulation of the HPA axis. Rhesus monkeys raised under conditions of deprivation on cloth surrogates or raised only with peers exhibit larger and more prolonged elevations in cortisol to stressful stimulation (Higley, Suomi, & Linnoila, 1992). Similarly, the presence of the rhesus mother provides a powerful buffer against cortisol reactivity to stressors like capture, separation, and handling—even if the infant cannot physically contact her (Bayart, Hayashi, Faull, Barchas, & Levine, 1990). Disturbing mother–infant interaction by making maternal food supply unpredictable has also been shown to lead to increases in CRH levels measured when the offspring are adults (Coplan et al., 1996). Although mother–infant separations produce striking increases in HPA activity in nonhuman primates, a discontinuity has been noted between hormonal and behavioral manifestations of stress following the initial separation and after multiple separations. Hennessy (1986) found that young monkeys continue to respond to separation hormonally but not vocally, even after having been separated 80 times before. Behavior then, particularly vocalization, may be a less sensitive index of the distress caused by long-term maternal deprivation than endocrine reactivity.

Human Caregiving and Regulation of the Neuroendocrine Stress Response System

While the evidence that early experiences have long-term effects on the HPA axis comes largely from animal research, other research with human infants also suggests that events embedded in daily typical interactions between the caregiver and the infant affect the development of the HPA system. A growing body of literature suggests that HPA axis activity in infants and young children varies with characteristics of the caregiving environment and the quality of the child's relationships with the caregiver (Spangler & Schieche, 1998; Nachmias et al., 1996; Ashman, Dawson, Panagiotides, Yamadar, & Wilkinson, 2002; Gunnar, Mangelsdorf, Larson, & Hertsgaard, 1989).

Caregiver-Regulated Stress Hyporesponsivity

While the human newborn demonstrates a highly reactive adrenocortical response to stressors (Gunnar, 1992), there is evidence that reactivity of the HPA system gradually dampens over the first year of life as a function of quality caregiving (Gunnar & Donzella, 2001). Indeed, attempts to elicit elevations in cortisol to psychosocial stressors in the second year of life have often met with failure (Gunnar et al., 1989; Gunnar & Nelson, 1994; Spangler & Grossmann, 1993). Sensitivity, responsiveness, and attention from primary caregivers appears crucial to sustaining low cortisol activity during this period (Gunnar & Donzella, 2001). As with the infant rat, which also exhibits a period of relative stress hyporesponsivity between postnatal days 4 and 14 (Rosenfeld, Suchecki, & Levine, 1992), the absence of an available and sensitive caregiver may lead to significant elevations in glucocorticoid levels, larger than those observed in older children and adults (Gunnar & Donzella, 2001).

Attachment Quality and the Hypothalamic–Pituitary–Adrenocortical Axis

As noted by Spangler and Schieche (1998), research on adrenocortical function in the Strange Situation suggests, when taken together, that infants classified as securely attached do not demonstrate elevations in cortisol levels (Spangler & Grossmann, 1993). Indeed, the pattern typically observed is one of decreasing cortisol levels from the beginning to 30 minutes after the end of the procedure. In contrast, studies examining disorganized patterns of attachment behavior have found that these children produce larger increases in cortisol than do children classified as securely or insecurely attached (Spangler & Grossmann, 1993; Hertsgaard, Gunnar, Erickson, & Nachmias, 1995). Children classified as insecurely attached exhibited more equivocal and complicated results. The findings suggest an interplay between attachment and temperamental factors. Infants with low behavioral inhibition, both secure and insecure, did not exhibit adrenocortical responses. Adrenocortical activation was observed in behaviorally inhibited infants with an insecure attachment, both ambivalent and avoidant, but not in those with secure relationships. These findings suggest that secure attachment relationship may function as a social buffer against less adaptive temperamental dispositions.

Normal Disjunction between Behavioral and Physiological Responses in Early Development

Spangler and Schieche's (1998) own research suggests that emotional distress and adrenocortical activity are unrelated in secure infants. However, high distress is associated with adrenocortical activation in ambivalent, avoidant, and disorganized infants. Unlike emotional expression in securely attached children, it appears that emotional expression in children with insecure and disorganized attachment patterns does not fulfill its social function as a means to manage fearful arousal through the help of a caregiver.

Similarly, Nachmias and colleagues (1996) found that 18-month-olds who responded fearfully to a series of strange, novel events were likely to show elevations in cortisol only if they were insecurely attached to the parent who accompanied them and helped them to manage their emotional responses to events. No differences in fearful or wary behavior were noted as a function of attachment security. These data tend to be more consistent with the view that secure relationships buffer the HPA axis in early childhood, rather than the view that temperamental differences in fearfulness or inhibition produce the differences in attachment classification and/or elevations in cortisol to strange and potentially threatening events.

Thus, as with nonhuman primate data, it appears that a sensitive and responsive caregiving system can provide a HPA axis buffer for the human infant and toddler. When this system functions correctly, the young child appears to be able to experience conditions that elicit behavioral distress and that produce inhibition of approach or fearfulness without producing increases in glucocorticoids. This point is elaborated by Spangler and Grossmann (1999), who argue that securely attached infants possess appropriate stress-reducing behavioral strategies and therefore exhibit negligible increases in cortisol levels when aroused. Insecurely attached infants who demonstrate inadequate behavioral strategies and disorganized infants who demonstrate no coherent strategies must both rely on physiological response to arousal in the wake of inadequate behavioral response.

Dozier and colleagues (2001) also report disjunction in the opposite direction between overt affective/behavioral expression and underlying physiological responses in a group of maltreated children beginning relationships with new foster mothers. These children evidence secure-appearing behavioral responses to separations and reunions while still evidencing extremely aberrant hyper- or hyporesponsive HPA functioning.

Hypercortisolism in Early Childhood

Ashman and colleagues (2002) presented evidence that a mother's depression in the first 2 years of the child's life is the best predictor of cortisol elevations at age 7 years. Similarly, in a study of 282 children 4.5 years old, Essex, Klein, Eunsuk, and Kalin (2002) reported that maternal depression beginning in infancy was the most potent predictor of children's cortisol levels at 4.5 years of age. Other research indicates that when a depressed mother interacts with her infant, she typically expresses less positive and more negative affect, sometimes in intrusive behavioral patterns and sometimes in more withdrawn patterns (Cohn, Matias, Tronick, Connell, & Lyons-Ruth, 1986; Lyons-Ruth, Zoll, Connell, & Grunebaum, 1986). A depressed mother is also likely to respond less contingently to her infant's emotional responses (Dawson & Ashman, 2000; Lyons-Ruth et al., 1986). Ashman and colleagues (2002) hypothesize that early exposure to the more negative and unpredictable caretaking of a depressed mother sensitizes the neural pathways that mediate the stress response and increases vulnerability to depression. This explanation is consistent with the animal models of effects associated with disturbed caregiving described earlier.

Hypocortisolism

Despite the central tenet that stress is associated with elevated levels of cortisol production, accumulating evidence suggests that some children demonstrate blunted cortisol responses to challenge. As recently reviewed by Gunnar and Vasquez (2001), some highly stressed children and adults evidence a hyporesponsive rather than hyperresponsive cortisol pattern, in which baseline cortisol levels can be low and fail to increase in response to acute stressors. In addition, a flattening of the usual daytime rhythm of cortisol release also appears to occur in these groups. These flatter daily patterns are due largely to lower early morning cortisol values as opposed to higher or elevated values at the nadir of the cycle. As Gunnar and Vasquez (2001) also note, such responses are sometimes, but not always, found in children or adults who have experienced more severe acute or chronic adverse life histories. The occurrence of these hyporesponsive patterns is frequent enough that more work is needed to understand their psychosocial, genetic, and biomolecular etiological contributors.

Hypothalamic–Pituitary–Adrenocortical Axis Functioning among Orphanage-Reared Children

Children reared in orphanages in Romania have been the focus of several studies of the relation between environmental regulation and HPA axis activity. Ten years ago, Romanian orphanages were described as grossly depriving, that is, lacking in social stimulation, physical stimulation, and opportunities for attachment relationships (Ames, 1990). M. Carlson and her colleagues (Carlson et al., 1995a, 1995b; Carlson & Earls, 1997) assessed salivary cortisol levels among toddlers in Romanian orphanages over several days at wakeup, noon, and late afternoon/evening in a group of 2-year-olds who had lived in the orphanage for most of their lives. Compared to home-reared 2-year-old Romanian children, the orphanage-reared children showed no evidence of the expectable daily rhythm in cortisol levels (a peak in the morning, at half of morning levels by late afternoon, and negligible levels by midnight) over the daytime hours. Moreover, cortisol levels of the orphanage-reared children were not clearly elevated over those of family-reared children. Instead, many of the orphanage-reared children appeared to have lower than expected morning levels of cortisol.

In a different study, Romanian children reared in orphanages and then adopted into homes in British Columbia were studied 6.5 years after adoption (Gunnar, Morison, Chisholm, & Schuder, 2001). All of the children had lived in orphanages for over 8 months prior to adoption and most were under 3 years of age when adopted. Parents collected saliva samples at wakeup, noon, and before bed for 3 days. Averaging over days, the orphanage-adopted children showed the expected daily rhythm, or slope, in cortisol production but had higher morning, afternoon, and evening levels than both Romanian children adopted near birth ("early-adopted") and Canadian-born children reared in their families of origin. Additionally, orphanage stay was positively associated with cortisol level, so that the length of time that the orphanage-adopted Romanian children had lived in orphanages prior to adoption predicted their levels of cortisol 6.5 years later.

Unfortunately, we have no information as to whether children who continue to live in orphanages begin to show elevated cortisol levels as they get older or whether a more typical daily rhythm of cortisol production emerges. Nor can we be certain whether there is a causal relation between immersion in an enriched family environment and the emergence of a normal daily rhythm in cortisol production. However, as reported by Gunnar et al. (2001), Russian children under the age of 4 years living in orphanage settings evidence a similarly absent daily rhythm is cortisol production (Kroupina, Gunnar, & Johnson, 1997). In contrast, Bruce, Kroupina, Parker, and Gunnar (2000) found lower bedtime than wakeup cortisol levels in a small group of infants and toddlers who had been adopted after some 4–18 months of orphanage care and had been living in their adoptive families for approximately 2 months. Taken together, these findings suggest that orphanage rearing fails to support the development of a normal daily rhythm in cortisol production in young children whereas adoption into a family may promote the emergence of an expected daily rhythm. This hypothesis awaits further investigation, as most of the information presented above is based on small samples and/or pilot data.

These findings from orphanage rearing studies, however, are consistent with reports of daytime cortisol patterns for neglected infants reared in their families of origin (Gilles, Berntson, Zipf, & Gunnar, 2000) and a foster care intervention study with preschool-age children (Fisher, Gunnar, Chamberlain, & Reid, 2000). Gilles and colleagues investigated daytime cortisol levels in family-reared children who were characterized either as high-risk infants (i.e., risk factors for neglect but not meeting criteria for neglect), low-risk infants, or neglected. Salivary cortisol was assessed in the morning, at noon, and in the evening. Both the neglected and high-risk groups had a flatter and lower pattern of daytime cortisol production than did the low-risk infants. Neglected infants demonstrated the lowest early morning levels and also had the flattest pattern of daytime cortisol production. Fisher and colleagues found that preschool-age children placed in foster care exhibited a less marked daytime rhythm in cortisol production than did home-reared children, but this rhythm became more typical in children who had been placed with foster families specifically trained to work with behaviorally and emotionally disturbed children.

BRIDGING NORMAL AND ABNORMAL DEVELOPMENT: HIDDEN REGULATORS AND "TIPPING POINTS"

The data reviewed thus far clearly point to a role for caregiver regulation in the normal development of HPA axis function. Attachment research and associated studies of mutual regulatory processes between parents and infants have provided a very general model of how parental sensitive responsiveness leads to the development in the infant of organized coping strategies in the face of stress and to confidence in the caregiver's availability.

However, the existing data do not yet allow for a detailed specification of how sensitive and responsive caregiving acts at the physiological level to facilitate normal HPA axis development. In addition, while sensitive parenting and its correlates have been extensively studied, little is known about the "tipping points" where inadequate regulation precipitates qualitatively different forms of physiological organization in the developing infant. These tipping points would be the points where less adequate caregiving regulation crosses the line to become a hidden trauma of infancy, in that the infant's developing stress response system would be reset in a negative and enduring way.

Identification of developmental tipping points in human infancy is complicated both by the difficulty of conducting experimental studies and by the complexity of the human caregiving process. The concept of sensitive responsiveness itself has shown only a limited, though quite consistent, ability to explain infant outcomes, probably due in part to its very general definition and operationalization in attachment research (van IJzendoorn, 1995). At the other extreme, researchers have investigated abusive or neglecting caregiving and, again, consistent results emerge. However, these extreme family environments conflate many sources of adverse care and can go only a limited way toward identifying the tipping points that precipitate alternative forms of physiological function in the infant.

Since it is increasingly clear that critical parameters of HPA functioning are being set during the first year of life, a more detailed account of the regulation of fearful arousal through the attachment relationship is critical to a model of what constitutes trauma during the vulnerable period of infancy. Two levels of mechanisms for the regulation of fearful arousal are likely to be embedded in the early infant–caregiver relationship: direct physiological regulators and intersubjective regulators. We next address each of these in turn.

Direct Physiological Mechanisms as Hidden Regulators of Attachment and Fearful Arousal

The findings regarding early regulation of the HPA axis by the primary caregiver reviewed above are consistent with Myron Hofer's (1995) contention that the evolutionary survival value of proximity to the caregiver goes well beyond protection (Bowlby, 1969) or felt security (Sroufe & Fleeson, 1986). Hofer's central thesis is that different specific aspects of the experience of proximity to or separation from the caregiver affect different specific features of an infant's response to separation from the caregiver. These physiological regulatory processes are hidden within the more overt transactions between the mother and the infant. He proposes that the attachment relationship provides an opportunity for the mother to shape both the developing physiology and the behavior of her infant through discrete regulatory pathways that he refers to as "hidden regulators of attachment" (Hofer, 1995).

Hofer conceptualizes attachment first as a biological event. He reminds us that attachment has an evolutionary history among social mammals as a physiological process long before humans evolved the capacity to communicate intersubjectively and to cognitively represent the attachment experience. The point is particularly relevant when we consider the underdeveloped cognitive systems of very young infants. The absence of sophisticated cognitive awareness means that the young infant is constrained to deal with the vicissitudes of the attachment relationship at an affective and physiological level. As noted earlier, the very young infant has extremely limited coping strategies, whether behavioral or cognitive. A few examples will illustrate Hofer's contention.

While studying the development of autonomic cardiovascular regulation in rats, Hofer (1973b) reported that a dam escaped from the maternity cage overnight and the next morning the cardiac rates of her 2-week-old pups were 40% below the norm for their age. The pups were slowed and hyporesponsive, and appeared to be experiencing the "conservation withdrawal" phase of response to loss.

Suspecting that the slow heart rates could be due to cooling of the cardiac pacemaker cells, Hofer heated the cage floor, maintaining the core temperature of the separated pups throughout a 24-hour separation period. Cardiac rates remained the same; however, the rat pups became hyperactive. Thus, a period of 24 hours of separation could result in either depressed or overreactive behavior, depending on whether one aspect of maternal care, warmth, was available to the pups (Hofer, 1975).

Curious as to what aspects, if any, of maternal care might regulate cardiac rate, Hofer conducted a series of further experiments, ultimately revealing that a supply of milk prevented the pups' cardiac response to separation but had no effect on behavioral hyperactivity. Instead, the pups' hyperactivity was found to be prevented by the presence of a nonlactating foster mother who failed to influence the pups' reduced cardiac rates (Hofer, 1973a, 1973c).

These results led Hofer to conclude that different aspects of the separation experience affected different features of the pups' bioregulatory systems. The pups' behavioral activity was regulated by the amount of warmth supplied by their mother. Their cardiac rates could be "set" anywhere from normal to 40% below normal by adjusting the rate at which milk was infused to the separated pups through a gastric canula.

Rather than responding to a single cue or signal of the dam's absence with an integrated behavioral and physiological response, then, it appeared that different systems in the separated pups responded to different signals of the mother's absence. As with primates, loss of all regulators at once produced a complex web of responses in different systems, their direction, timing, and magnitude varying with the characteristics of individual systems (Kraemer, 1992). The pups' response to separation then could be viewed as an assemblage of different processes reflecting the withdrawal or loss of a number of different regulatory processes that had been hidden within the pups' relationship with their mother.

Maternal Regulators of Hyporesponsiveness to Stress

There are also discrete hidden mechanisms embedded within the attachment relationship that regulate stress hyporesponsiveness at the beginning of life. As noted previously, many species of animals, including humans, demonstrate a period of hyporesponsiveness to stress. This period is characterized by little or no response to stressors, as evidenced by the level of corticosterone in nonhuman animals and by the levels of cortisol in humans. Newborn rats typically show vigorous corticosterone response to mild and severe stress from 0 to 4 days after birth but then demonstrate very little response to such stressors from 4 to 14 days after birth—the stress hyporesponsive period.

However, researchers have demonstrated that 7- to 14-day-old maternally separated pups show a vigorous corticosterone response rather than the typical hyporesponsiveness demonstrated in nonseparated pups. Two different regulators, maternal milk and tactile interaction, were discovered to be responsible for the loss of the pups' hyporesponsive period. Maternal milk delivery acted at the level of the adrenal cortex, and tactile stimulation acted at the hypothalamic and/or pituitary level. Two different regulators, then, maternal milk and touch, hidden within the normal mother–infant interaction, act individually on different levels of the HPA axis to ensure a hyporesponsive period to stress in the young pup (Hofer, 1995).

Maternal Regulators of Stereotyped Rocking Behavior

Another example of the hidden regulators concept comes from research with a group of maternally deprived rhesus monkeys. Many kinds of monkeys, whether raised alone or with inanimate artificial mothers, develop a distinctive stereotyped pattern of body rocking (Mason & Berkson, 1975). Mason and Berkson hypothesized that the body rocking was the consequence of release from a particular maternal regulator, in this case a mobile mother. These researchers decided to raise a group of rhesus monkeys for a year without any maternal interaction. Instead, half of the monkeys were given a standard terry cloth surrogate and the other half were given the same surrogate except that the surrogate was suspended on a rope a few inches off the floor so the surrogate would swing if jumped on or pushed.

Results of the investigation indicated that although both groups of monkeys looked identical on a number of behaviors typical of maternal deprivation, the "surrogate on a rope" group failed to demonstrate any of the stereotypical rocking behavior typically evidenced by deprived monkeys (and humans).

Peer Rearing of Nonhuman Primates

Several prospective longitudinal studies have found that peer-reared monkeys consistently exhibit more extreme behavioral, adrenocortical, and noradrenergic reactions to social separations than do their mother-reared cohorts, even after living in the same social group for extended periods (Higley & Suomi, 1989). Peer-only-reared monkeys, for example, exhibit larger cortisol responses to psychosocial stressors as adults than do mother-reared infants (Higley & Suomi, 1989). Similarly, research attempting to identify neurochemical substrates that may be regulated by the primate caregiver suggests that maternal separation may produce cytoarchitechtural changes in dopamine (DA), norepinephrine (NE), and serotonin (5-HT)—collectively referred to as the biogenic amine systems—that result in functional dysregulation of these systems (Kraemer & Clarke, 1990). Kraemer, Ebert, Schmidt, and McKinney (1989) conducted a longitudinal study examining the levels of cerebrospinal fluid (CSF) NE in rhesus monkeys reared in three different rearing conditions (mother-deprived, mother-reared/peer-reared, and mother-reared/peer-deprived settings) up to 22 months of age. Mother rearing after birth produced an increase in CSF NE in all infants by comparison to infants that did not have a mother. Peer-reared monkeys also consistently show lower CSF concentrations of 5-hydroxyindoleacetic acid (5-HIAA), the primary central serotonin metabolite (Champoux, Higley, & Suomi, 1997) than their mother-reared counterparts. Serotonin is a prominent inhibitory neurotransmitter implicated in ubiquitous aspects of metabolic, regulatory, and emotional functioning.

Taken together, the research reviewed above concurs with Hofer's contention that regulation should not be conceived of strictly in terms of affects but also in terms of discrete regulating mechanisms that act directly on developing physiological systems. The first function of the infant–caregiver system is that of the physiological regulation of both members of the dyad. At the most basic level, the infant's sense of security may result from adequate homeostatic regulation within the caregiving relationship, with the earliest form of secure attachment encoded physiologically in the experience of nondisruptive and need-satisfying regulation of early physiological systems. Attachment, then, is not an end in itself but rather a system adapted by evolution to fulfill key ontogenetic physiological and psychological tasks. Because of the obstacles to conducting controlled experiments with human infants, there is little information on how these physiological mechanisms related to body warmth, milk supply, tactile stimulation, and movement might impact the developing stress response system. However, given their importance in other primates, it is likely that similar mechanisms play a role in fostering the emergence of normal organization in the HPA system over the first year of life.

Intersubjective Processes as Hidden Regulators of Attachment and Fearful Arousal

Hofer (1994a, 1994b, 1995) confines his point concerning "hidden regulators" of attachment to the domain of direct physiological mechanisms. In addition, the elaborated human capacity for intersubjective sharing of affective signals is another likely regulator of early infant attachment and stress responsivity. However, at the time Bowlby (1969) was writing, the knowledge bases regarding both developmental neuroscience and the intersubjective capacities of the infant were limited. Therefore, in discussing the attachment behavioral system during the first year of life, Bowlby (1958) located the human attachment system within the context of primate evolution and identified the human attachment behaviors shared with other primates, such as clinging, following, sucking, smiling, and crying, as the critical mediators of the attachment relationship during the first year. Ainsworth et al. (1978) then emphasized much more clearly the role of the mother's sensitivity to infant cues over the first year in fostering open emotional communication and felt security in the infant. However, the standard attachment assessment focuses on infant behaviors that mature at the end of the first year, so that the attachment security or disorganization of the infant cannot currently be assessed at earlier ages.

Since Bowlby's early writing, however, numerous studies using diverse methodologies have demonstrated that human infants are equipped with much more elaborate capacities than other primates have for sharing both affective signals and intersubjective states with others (e.g., Jaffe, Beebe, Feldstein, Crown, & Jasnow, 2001; Tomasello, 1999). Tomasello has argued that only humans have an awareness of others' minds as being like their own and that this capacity is clearly seen by the end of the first year. Human infants then use this awareness to coordinate behavior with others and to learn from others.

Others have observed that a specifically human coordination of intersubjective information between the mother and the human infant begins much earlier than the end of the first year. Trevarthen (2001) has noted that from birth the infant organizes his or her behavior toward people and objects differently. In face-to-face interaction with people, 2- to 4-month-old infants display preadapted behavior patterns that appear to be organized around the intention to communicate, with focused attention on the face, rhythmic cycling of legs and arms, lip and tongue movements, cooing vocalizations, and responsiveness to the partner's expressions. In addition, young infants display turn taking in communicative acts and disruption in behavior to incomprehensible or mistimed partner behavior (Murray & Trevarthen, 1985). Murray and Trevarthen concluded that there is a preadapted intention toward cooperative communication and a preadapted capacity for coordination of subjectivities; in their words, "the forms and communicative values of human emotions are innately formulated" (1985, p. 194). This more developed intersubjective capacity of the human infant partially displaces the human attachment system from its primate base and recontextualizes attachment within particularly human forms of inter-subjective relatedness from the beginning of life. Therefore, to understand the relations among the attachment system and the hidden traumas that produce dysregulation of the HPA axis during the first year, it is necessary to elucidate how attachment processes during the first year are embedded within a matrix of intersubjective communication. Little attention has been paid to delineating the pathways toward disorganized attachment strategies across the first year of life. Consequently, little is understood about how the caregiving deviations associated with disorganization by the end of the first year impact the infant's first year of development and, more specifically, how those same caregiving deviations affect the HPA system.

Primary Intersubjective Communication

As just reviewed, contemporary biologists have reconceptualized the capacity to regulate states of emotional security as a developmental process that begins with the dyadic regulation of the infant's earliest physiological homeostasis. The caregiver facilitates the infant's capacity to maintain internal homeostasis by adjusting the mode, amount, timing, and variability of her relational stimulation to the infant's signals.

A well-controlled study of caregiver contribution to very early physiological regulation was conducted by Sander, Julia, Stechler, and Burns (1972). Sander and colleagues randomly assigned newborn infants who were waiting to be given into foster care either to the regular hospital routine for the first 10 days or to a rooming-in relationship with a single nurse who cared for and fed the infant on demand. The regular hospital routine consisted of care in the newborn nursery by a rotating series of nurses who fed the infant on a preset schedule. The two intermediate conditions of demand feeding in the nursery and scheduled feedings by a rooming-in nurse were also evaluated. Regardless of rooming-in status, demand feeding during the first 10 days promoted earlier differentiation of day–night sleep cycles in the first days of life and greater individual stability in feeding behavior and sleep–wake cycles—stability that persisted over the first 2 months of life. Infants who had rooming-in caregivers during the first 10 days had longer awake periods and longer sleep periods by the second 10 days of life.

This careful study indicated that caregiving inputs that were timed to respond to cues from the infant had maximum regulatory impact, enhancing the infant's emergent self-organizing capacities, whereas caregiver inputs that were not contingent on infant cues were less effective in contributing to infant physiological regulation. The timing and fittedness of caregiver responses in relation to infant cues is likely to be fundamental to adequate early development.

The human infant also appears uniquely well equipped at birth to exchange affective signals with a caregiver. Ekman and Oster (1979) identified 24 distinct facial action patterns evident in early infancy, and emotions such as sadness, anger, disgust, fear, joy, and interest can be identified reliably from the facial displays of infants 1–9 months of age. The resulting subtlety of this capacity for exchanging affective signals in face-to-face communication by 2–3 months of age has been described in detail in time series analyses (e.g., Jaffe et al., 2001). In this earliest expression of intersubjective communication, the "topic" or referent of the shared affective "comment" is simply the hedonic quality of the relationship itself. There is a primary affective communication of "We make pleasure or displeasure together," with no reference to outside objects or events.

Very little research has examined as yet the relations among disorganized attachment strategies at 1 year of age, the characteristics of infant–mother affective communication, and infant stress responsiveness in the first 6 months of life. While it is clear that interaction is necessary for adequate development (Spitz, 1949), it is not known what aspects of early interaction are critical to the damping down of the HPA axis over the early months. In addition, it is likely that there are different developmental consequences to the HPA axis of parental withdrawal and of parental insensitive intrusiveness—or, in their most extreme form, of parental loss or neglect and of parental abuse. Jaffe and colleagues (2001) found that in a face-to-face interaction, "hypervigilant" tight vocal rhythm tracking by both the mother and the baby at 4 months of age, combined with the baby's postural and visual avoidance, was a predictor of disorganization of attachment strategies at 12 months of age. Jaffe et al. (2001) also found that babies who became disorganized showed more vocal and facial distress at age 4 months. A range of other early dysregulated interactive patterns are also likely to predict infant disorganization, but it is not clear where the tipping points are located along the spectrum of nonoptimal caregiving behaviors. It is also unclear what relative roles are played by such aspects of early interaction as physical touch, movement, soothing of distress, sharing of positive affects, quantity of interaction, or timing and fittedness of responses in the emergence of organized attachment strategies and normative HPA axis functioning. However, Thompson et al. (2003) have reported that cortisol response to a mildly stressful event occurs in the same direction for the mother and the baby by 6 months of age, and, as noted earlier, Ashman et al. (2002) have found cortisol elevations among infants of depressed mothers. Additional work is needed to elaborate our understanding of this critical early period in the formation of disorganized attachment relationships and dysregulated stress responses.

Secondary Intersubjective Communication

As infants approach 9 months of age, they increasingly look to their familiar social partners for affective cues to guide responses to objects and events outside the relationship itself, a process referred to as "social referencing." This capacity has been related to other indicators of a broad capacity for mutual sharing of subjective states, or affective comments toward other objects and events, that emerges during the last quarter of the first year and that Tomasello (1999) has described as uniquely human (for a review, see Lyons-Ruth & Zeanah, 1993). As an infant becomes more mobile, social referencing of the parent serves as an anticipatory affective guide to inform the infant about sources of danger or pleasure and serves to regulate the infant's affect and behavior from a distance. The sense of shared emotional states and mutually regulated affective displays underlying this behavior probably emerges from the earlier processes of affective communication in face-to-face play observed during the first 6 months of life.

However, little is known about what happens to subsequent intersubjective capacities if early affective communication with the caregiver is highly distorted. The literature on social referencing and secondary intersubjectivity has not yet been extended to infants at social risk, nor has it been related theoretically to attachment processes. However, we hypothesize that it is precisely this emergent capacity for using parental affective signals as cues to safety in the larger environment that promotes the shift from security mediation by close physical holding to the goal-corrected behavioral organization of attachment strategies at 12 months of age, in which security is partially mediated by maintaining proximity within visual/affective signaling distance. In a slightly different but related speculation, the developmental onset of 9-month-old infants' wariness with strangers may also stem from the increased intersubjective sharing capacity of 9- to 12-month-old infants, a capacity that makes the stranger's unknown affective communicative repertoire a source of uncertainty and potential lack of safety.

Clinical description of the absence of cautious behavior among children who have experienced early deprivation and neglect point to potential disruptions in the development of normal social referencing behavior among some groups of high-risk infants and toddlers. The indiscriminate friendliness evidenced by young children from severely depriving institutional settings also may rest on a disruption in normal social referencing capacities and suggests the fruitfulness of further explorations of the links between developing forms of intersubjective communication and risk-related deviations in attachment and HPA axis functioning (O'Connor, Rutter, & the English and Romanian Adoptees Study Team [ERA], 2000).

The emergence of elevated cortisol levels to stressful events among disorganized infants has not been studied over the first year, nor has disorganization been studied in relation to disrupted or hypervigilant social referencing behavior. There are also few data to relate particular profiles of atypical caregiver behavior to particular alterations in infant stress physiology, including hyper- or hyporesponsiveness or circadian rhythm disturbances, so it remains unclear whether there are tipping points in caregiver behavior that produce these shifts in infant functioning. However, given the diversity of atypical caregiver behaviors associated with infant disorganization, it is likely that helpless or withdrawing caregiving and hostile or intrusive caregiving produce different infant intersubjective regulatory strategies and different infant physiological correlates over time.

It is also unclear how circadian rhythm disturbances in infancy relate to hyper- or hyporesponsiveness of the HPA axis to stressors. Orphanage rearing is related to both elevated cortisol levels and shifts in circadian rhythms by the end of the first year of life (M. Carlson et al., 1995a, 1995b), but it is not clear whether the two forms of disturbance are related to one another or to the same aspects of caregiving. However, it is clear that disturbances in daily rhythm of cortisol release may occur under much more apparently benign conditions than orphanage rearing. For example, two recent studies have documented that circadian rhythm changes can occur under conditions of high-quality infant–toddler day care (Dettling, Gunnar, & Donzella, 1999; Dettling, Parker, Lane, Sebane, & Gunnar, 2000). Therefore, the tipping points for infant physiology may be much less extreme than the current emphasis on abuse or neglect would anticipate.

Collaborative Communication as Hypothalamic–Pituitary–Adrenocortical Axis Regulator

Multiple lines of evidence, then, indicate that a sensitive and responsive caregiving system can provide an HPA axis buffer for the human infant and toddler. When this system functions effectively, the young child appears to be able to experience conditions that elicit behavioral distress and that produce inhibition of approach or fearfulness without producing increases in glucocorticoids. The finding is consistent with Bowlby's (1973) assertion that securely attached infants need not rely on physiological adaptation within the "inner ring of life-maintaining systems" because regulation can be established through behavioral interaction with the caregiver in the "outer, or socially mediated ring" of homeostasis.

This socially mediated homeostasis is critically dependent on the shared intersubjectivities of the mother and the infant due to the prolonged helplessness and lack of mobility characteristic of human infancy and, we would propose, to the critical role of attuned and responsive social communication as a hidden regulator of HPA axis activity in human life. This proposal finds support in the work of Sethre-Hofstad, Stansbury, and Rice (2002), who examined attunement in adrenocortical response between the mother and the child as a function of maternal sensitivity. Sixty-four mother–child pairs with biological children age 24–51 months participated. Adrenocortical responsiveness was found to be highly correlated in sensitive mothers and their children, whereas responses in less sensitive mothers and their children were not significantly related. Because of the apparent role of the caregiver environment in fostering the adequate development of the infant's stress response system, primary trauma, or what we have referred to as hidden trauma, impacts the initial structuring of the system itself.

SUMMING UP

In this chapter, we have emphasized first the unique nature of trauma in infancy. Unlike many of the more observable discrete traumatic experiences that characterize later childhood, the traumas of infancy are woven into the moment-to-moment regulatory transactions experienced in the infant–caregiver system and are consequently nonevident. Frame-by-frame analysis (Beebe & Lachmann, 2002) has revealed a subtle dialogue involving synchronous rapid movements and fast changes in affective expressions. We suggest that trauma occurs within this "split second world of the mother and infant" (Stern, 1977) through varieties of caregiver unavailability and interactive dysregulation. These hidden traumas of early dysregulation appear to have the capacity to reset the infant's stress response system and therefore to influence the infant's and young child's responses to later stress or trauma. In one notable finding, infant disorganization and caregiver emotional unavailability in the first 2 years of life were shown to be stronger predictors than abuse experiences of dissociative symptoms in early adulthood (Ogawa, Sroufe, Weinfield, Carlson, & Egeland, 1997).

The interactive regulation provided in the context of the earliest caregiver–infant interactions appears critical to the development of adaptive psychobiological functioning. Indeed, contemporary thinkers have reconceptualized the capacity to regulate states of emotional arousal as a developmental process that begins with the regulation of the infant's physiological homeostasis or equilibrium in the earliest transactions between the caregiver and the infant (Sander, 1962; Sander et al., 1972; Sroufe, 1996; Trevarthen, 2001). The attuned caregiver, who is able to monitor her own internal signals and differentiate her own affective state, is able to facilitate the infant's capacity to maintain internal homeostasis by adjusting the mode, amount, timing, and variability of the onset and offset of environmental stimulation. The mother and infant experience repeated state transitions, as they move together from low arousal to heightened arousal to restored equilibrium. The attuned caregiver matches her activity level to her infant's during periods of playful engagement, allows the infant to recover quietly when the child prefers disengagement, and sensitively responds to bids for reengagement after a period of decelerated arousal (Beebe, Jaffe, and Lachmann, 1994; Beebe & Lachmann, 2002; Shore, 2003). A dyadic regulatory system evolves where the infant's moment-to-moment state changes are understood and responded to by the caregiver, thereby achieving their regulation.

The caregiver who is unable to provide consistent affective attunement and containment of the infant's psychobiological responses during transitions from heightened arousal to homeostatic return contributes to heightened and enduring states of psychobiological arousal in the infant. The limited behavioral and cognitive resources of early infancy are insufficient to the task of regulation when the infant is aroused. Instead, psychobiological regulation during early infancy is dependent on external regulation by a caregiver to avoid overwhelming levels of physiological arousal that exceed available coping capacities. These uncontained and enduring states of overwhelming psychobiological arousal engender physiological consequences in the stress response system of the infant that are similar to the physiological consequences observed subsequent to the more salient traumatic events of childhood.

The considerable evidence across rodent, nonhuman primate, and human primate literatures presented above supports the contention that response to emotional arousal, as evidenced in the development of the stress physiology system, is regulated in part by nongenomic relational transactions with the caregiver from the earliest months of life. This conclusion perforce causes us to reconceptualize our model of attachment as not merely an end in and of itself but rather a system adapted by evolution to fulfill key ontogenetic physiological and psychological tasks. As Hofer asserts, a series of discrete regulatory mechanisms exist within the attachment relationship. We suggest that the development of an efficient stress response system in the infant results in part from adequate homeostatic regulation within the caregiving relationship, with the earliest form of secure attachment encoded physiologically in the experience of nondisruptive and need-satisfying regulation of early physiological systems, specifically the stress response system.

Bowlby suggests that inadequate attachment creates vulnerability to later stressors primarily through the development of maladaptive inner working models. Our revised view of attachment complements this perspective by suggesting that there are two mechanisms by which the hidden traumas of infancy can leave individuals vulnerable to adverse outcomes.

One is related to the maintenance of internal neurophysiological homeostasis, as described above. The provision of insensitive, inadequate caregiver regulation shapes the atypical development of the stress physiology system. The other mechanism is related to the development of intersubjectivity. Researchers have observed that the specifically human coordination of intersubjective information between the mother and the human infant begins much earlier than the end of the first year. Infants traumatized during the first year, then, may fail to develop fully their capacity for social communication. The relationship between disturbance in facility with intersubjectivity in infancy and the development of atypical stress physiology and subsequent psychopathology requires further investigation. Indeed, Claussen, Mundy, Mallik, and Willoughby (2002) recently reported a relationship between disorganized attachment status and a diminished capacity to initiate bids for joint attention in a group of 56 high-risk toddlers. No group differences in the capacity to respond to bids were observed. The findings suggest that infants with a disorganized attachment style may develop a diminished capacity for joint attention and other subsequent aspects of intersubjectivity. The capacity to initiate bids for joint attention in the second year of life has been linked to language, cognitive, and behavioral development in several studies (Mundy & Gomes, 1998). To understand the relations, then, among the attachment system and the hidden traumas that produce dysregulation in the HPA axis during the first year, we must expand our understanding of how attachment processes during the first year are embedded within a matrix of intersubjective communication.

Increasingly, we understand that the parameters of HPA functioning and the capacity for intersubjectivity are being set during the first year of life. Consequently, a more detailed account of the regulation of fearful arousal through the attachment relationship is critical to a model of what constitutes trauma during infancy. Different kinds of caregiver unavailability and interactive dysregulation may initiate unique physiological and intersubjective mechanisms that lead to distinct developmental outcomes. The proposed psychobiological dysregulation, evidenced in the HPA axis, consequent to inadequate, insensitive caregiving during infancy, may predispose young children to physical and psychological disorder, but the tipping points, the mechanisms leading to atypical stress physiology functioning, are no doubt complex, nonlinear, and permeable to environmental variables. Future research is needed to investigate aspects of caregiver availability that are most critical to adaptive psychobiological functioning in infancy. A few of the numerous factors that merit consideration include the following: the mediating influence of developing intersubjectivity; the importance of contingency and periodicity in caregiver responsiveness; the developmental timing of certain "regulatory actions"; the potential for sensitive periods in the first year, during which neural development may be more vulnerable to caregiver inadequacies; and the effects of subtle variations in the frequency and severity of interactive dysregulation.

We might ask as well whether the vulnerabilities incurred as a consequence of caregiver unavailability and interactive dysregulation may be reconceptualized as protective factors in certain contexts or with respect to certain developmental tasks or developmental phases. Some aspects of altered stress physiology functioning may be protective rather than harmful. While the literature reveals clear associations between atypical HPA axis functioning and problematic emotional and behavioral outcomes, we should not lose sight of the fact that early vulnerabilities transact with their environment across development. Depending on the context and developmental period, vulnerability may be recast as strength.

REFERENCES

Ainsworth, M. D. S., Blehar, M., Waters, E., & Wall, S. (1978). *Patterns of attachment*. Hillsdale, NJ: Erlbaum.

American Psychiatric Association. (1994). *Diagnostic and statistical manual of mental disorders* (4th ed.). Washington, DC: Author.

Ames, E. W. (1990). Spitz revisited: A trip to Romanian "orphanages." *CPA Section on Developmental Psychology Newsletter, 9*(2).

Ashman, S. B., Dawson, G., Panagiotides, H., Yamada, E., & Wilkinson, C. W. (2002). Stress hormone levels of children of depressed mothers. *Developmental Psychopathology, 14,* 333–349.

Bailey, S. L., & Heitkemper, M. M. (1991). Morningness–eveningness and early-morning salivary cortisol levels. *Biological Psychiatry, 32,* 181–192.

Bayart, F., Hayashi, K. T., Faull, K. F., Barchas, J. D., & Levine, S. (1990). Influence of maternal proximity on behavioral and psychological responses to separation in infant rhesus monkeys (*Macaca mulatta*). *Behavioral Neuroscience, 104,* 98–107.

Beebe, B., Jaffe, J., & Lachmann, F. (1994). A dyadic systems model of mother–infant mutual regulation: Implications for the origins of representations and therapeutic action. *Psychologist Psychoanalyst, 14,* 27–33.

Beebe, B., & Lachmann, F. (2002). *Infant research and adult treatment*. Hillsdale, NJ: Analytic Press.

Benes, F. M. (1998). Developmental changes in stress adaptation in relation to psychopathology. *Development and Psychopathology, 6,* 723–739.

Bowlby, J. (1958). The nature of the child's tie to his mother. *International Journal of Psycho-Analysis, 39,* 1–24.

Bowlby, J. (1969). *Attachment and loss: Vol. 1. Attachment*. London: Hogarth Press & Institute of Psychoanalysis.

Bowlby, J. (1973). *Attachment and loss: Vol. 2. Separation—Anxiety and anger*. London: Hogarth Press.

Bowlby, J. (1980). *Loss: Vol. 3. Attachment*. New York: Basic Books.

Brent, D. A., Ryan, N., Dahl, R., & Boris, B. (1995). Early-onset mood disorder. In F.

Bloom & D. Kupfer (Eds.), *Psychopharmacology: The fourth generation of progress* (pp. 1631–1642). New York: Raven Press.

Bruce, J., Kroupina, M., Parker, S., & Gunnar, M. R. (2000, July). *The relationship between cortisol patterns, growth retardation, and developmental delay in postinstitutionalized children.* Paper presented at the International Conference on Infant Studies, Brighton, England.

Caldji, C., Tannenbaum, B., Sharma, S., Francis, D., Plotsky, P. M., & Meaney, M. J. (1998). Maternal care during infancy regulates the development of neural systems mediating the expression of fearfulness in the rat. *Proceedings of the National Academy of Sciences, USA, 95,* 5445–5340.

Carlson, M., Dragomir, C., Earls, F., Farrell, M., Macovei, O., Nystrom, P., & Sparling, J. (1995a). Cortisol regulation in home-reared and institutionalized Romanian children. *Society of Neuroscience Abstracts, 698,* 1.

Carlson, M., Dragomir, C., Earls, F., Farrell, M., Macovei, O., Nystrom, P., & Sparling, J. (1995b). Effects of social deprivation on cortisol regulation in institutionalized Romanian infants. *Society of Neuroscience Abstracts, 218,* 12.

Carlson, M., & Earls, F. (1997). Psychological and neuroendocrinological sequelae of early social deprivation in institutionalized children in Romania. *Annals of the New York Academy of Sciences, 807,* 419–428.

Carlson, V., Cicchetti, D., Barnett, D., & Braunwald, K. (1989). Disorganized/disoriented attachment relationships in maltreated infants. *Developmental Psychology, 25,* 525–531.

Cassidy, J., & Shaver, P. (Eds.). (1999). *Handbook of attachment: Theory, research, and clinical implications.* New York: Guilford Press.

Champoux, M., Higley, J. D., & Suomi, S. J. (1997). Behavioral and physiological characteristics of Indian and Chinese-Indian hybrid rhesus macaque infants. *Developmental Psychobiology, 31,* 49–63.

Chrousos, G. P. (1997). Stressors, stress and neuroendocrine integration of the adaptive response. *Annals of the New York Academy of Sciences, 816,* 311–335.

Chrousos, G. P., & Gold, P. W. (1992). The concepts of stress and stress system disorders: Overview of physical and behavioral homeostasis. *Journal of the American Medical Association, 267*(9), 1244–1252.

Claussen, A. H., Mundy, P. C., Mallik, S. A., & Willoughby, J. C. (2002). Joint attention and disorganized attachment status in infants at risk. *Development and Psychopathology, 14,* 279–291.

Cohn, J. F., Matias, R., Tronick, E. Z., Connell, D., & Lyons-Ruth, K. (1986). Face-to-face interactions of depressed mothers and their infants. In E. Z. Tronick & T. Field (Eds.), *Maternal depression and infant disturbance* (pp. 31–45). San Francisco: Jossey-Bass.

Coplan, J. D., Andrews, M. W., Owens, M. J., Friedman, S., Gorman, J. M., & Nemeroff, C. B. (1996). Persistent elevations of cerebrospinal fluid concentrations of corticotropin-releasing factor in adult nonhuman primates exposed to early-life stressors: Implications for the pathophysiology of mood and anxiety disorders. *Proceedings of the National Academy of Sciences, USA, 93,* 1619–1623.

Dahl, R., Ryan, N., Puig-Antich, J., Nguyen, N., Al-Shabbout, M., Meyer, V., & Perel, J. (1991). 24-hour cortisol measures in adolescents with major depression: A controlled study. *Biological Psychiatry, 30,* 25–36.

Dawson, G., & Ashman, S. B. (2000). On the origins of a vulnerability to depression:

The influence of the early social environment on the depression of psychobiological systems related to risk for affective disorder. In C. Nelson (Ed.), *Minnesota Symposium on Child Psychology: Vol. 31. The effects of early adversity on neurobehavioral development* (pp. 245–279). Mahwah, NJ: Erlbaum.

De Bellis, M. D., Baum, A. S., Birmaher, B., Keshavan, M. S., Eccard, C. H., Boring, A. M., Jenkins, F. M., & Ryan, N. D. (1999). Developmental traumatology: Part 1. Biological stress systems. *Biological Psychiatry, 45*(10), 1259–1270.

DeKloet, E. R. (1991). Brain corticosteroid receptor balance and homeostatic control. *Frontiers in Neuroendocrinology, 12*(2), 95–164.

DeKloet, E. R., & Reul, J. M. (1987). Feedback action and tonic influence of corticosteroids on brain function: A concept arising from the heterogeniety of brain receptor systems. *Psychoneuroendocrinology, 12*(2), 83–105.

DeKloet, E. R., Rots, N. Y., van den Berg, D. T., & Oitzl, M. S. (1994). Brain mineralocorticoid receptor function. *Annals of the New York Academy of Sciences, 746*, 8–20.

DeKloet, E. R., Vreugdenhil, E., Oitel, M. S., & Joek, A. (1998). Brian corticosteroid receptor balance in health and disease. *Endocrine Reviews, 19*, 269–301.

Dettling, A. C., Gunnar, M. R., & Donzella, B. (1999). Cortisol levels of young children in full-day childcare centers: Relations with age and temperament. *Psychoneuroendocrinology, 24*(5), 519–536.

Dettling, A. C., Parker, S. W., Lane, S., Sebanc, A., & Gunnar, M. R. (2000). Quality of care and termperament determine changes in cortisol concentrations over the day for young children in childcare. *Psychoendocrinology, 25*(8), 819–836.

Dozier, M., Levine, S., Gordon, K., Manni, M., Gunnar, M. R., Fisher, P. R., & Stovall-McClough, K. C. (2001). *Atypical daytime patterns of cortisol production among young children who entered foster care in infancy.* Paper presented at the biennial meeting of the Society for Research in Child Development, Minneapolis, MN.

Ekman, P., & Oster, H. (1979). Facial expressions of emotion. *Annual Review of Psychology, 30*, 527–554.

Eriksson, P. S., Perfilieva, E., Bjork-Eriksson, T., Alborn, A.-M., Nordborg, C., Peterson, D. A., & Gage, F. H. (1998). Neurogenesis in the adult human hippocampus. *Nature Medicine, 11*, 1313–1317.

Essex, M., Klein, M., Eunsuk, C., & Kalin, N. (2002). Maternal stress beginning in infancy may sensitize children to later stress exposure: Effects on cortisol and behavior. *Biological Psychiatry, 52*(8), 776–784.

Fisher, P. A., Gunnar, M. R., Chamberlain, P., & Reid, J. B. (2000). Specialized foster care for maltreated preschoolers: Impact on children's behavior, neuroendocrine activity, and foster parent functioning following placement in a new foster home. *Journal of the American Academy of Child and Adolescent Psychiatry, 39*(11), 1356–1364..

Francis, D., Diorio, J., Liu, D., & Meaney, M. (1999). Nongenomic transmission across generations of maternal behavior and stress responses in the rat. *Science, 286*, 1155–1158.

Gilles, E. E., Berntson, G. G., Zipf, W. B., & Gunnar, M. R. (2000, July). *Neglect is associated with a blunting of behavioral and biological stress responses in human infants.* Paper presented at the International Conference of Infant Studies, Brighton, England.

Greenough, W., & Black, J. E. (1992). Induction of brain structure by experience: Substrates for cognitive development. In M. R. Gunnar & C. A. Nelson (Eds.), *Minnesota Symposium on Child Psychology: Vol. 24. Developmental behavioral neuroscience* (pp. 155–200). Mahwah, NJ: Erlbaum.

Gunnar, M. R. (1992). Reactivity of the hypothalamic pituitary adrenocortical system to stressors in normal infants and children. *Pediatrics, 90,* 491–497.

Gunnar, M. R. (2000). Early adversity and the development of stress reactivity and regulation. In C. A. Nelson (Ed.), *Minnesota Symposia on Child Psychology: Vol. 31. The effects of early adversity on neurobehavioral development* (pp. 113–162). Mahwah, NJ: Erlbaum.

Gunnar, M. R., & Donzella, B. (2001). Social regulation of the cortisol levels in early human development. *Psychoneuroendocrinology, 27*(1–2), 199–220.

Gunnar, M. R., Mangelsdorf, S., Larson, M., & Hertsgaard, L. (1989). Attachment, temperament and adrenocortical activity in infancy: A study of psychoendocrine regulation. *Developmental Psychology, 25,* 355–363.

Gunnar, M. R., Morison, S., Chisholm, K., & Schuder, M. (2001). Salivary cortisol levels in children adopted from Romanian orphanages. *Developmental Psychopathology, 13,* 611–628.

Gunnar, M. R., & Nelson, C. (1994). Event-related potentials in year-old infants: Relations with emotionality and cortisol. *Child Development, 65,* 80–94.

Gunnar, M. R., & Vasquez, D. (2001). Low cortisol and a flattening of expected daytime rhythm: Potential indices of risk in human development. *Development and Psychopathology, 13,* 515–538.

Heim, C., Ehlert, U., & Hellhammer, D. H. (2000). The potential role of hypocortisolism in the pathophysiology of stress-related bodily disorders. *Psychoneuroendocrinology, 25*(1), 1–35.

Hennessy, M. B. (1986). Multiple, brief maternal separations in the squirrel monkey: Changes in hormonal and behavioral responsiveness. *Physiology and Behavior, 36*(2), 245–250.

Hertsgaard, L., Gunnar, M. R., Erickson, M. F., & Nachmias, M. (1995). Adrenocortical responses to the strange situation in infants with disorganized/disoriented attachment relationships. *Child Development, 66*(4), 1100–1106.

Hesse, E., & Main, M. (2000). Disorganized infant, child, and adult attachment: Collapse in behavioral and attentional strategies. *Journal of the American Psychoanalytic Association, 48,* 1097–1127; discussion, 1175–1187.

Higley, J. D., & Suomi, S. J. (1989). Temperamental reactivity in non-human primates. In G. A. Kohnstamm, J. E. Bates, & M. K. Rothbart (Eds.), *Temperament in childhood* (pp. 153–167). New York: Wiley.

Higley, J. D., Suomi, S. J., & Linnoila, M. (1992). A longitudinal study of CSF monoamine metabolite and plasma cortisol concentrations in young rhesus monkeys: Effects of early experience, age, sex, and stress on continuity of individual differences. *Biological Psychiatry, 32,* 127–145.

Hofer, M. A. (1973a). Maternal separation affects infant rats' behavior. *Behavioral Biology, 9*(5), 629–633.

Hofer, M. A. (1973b). The effects of brief maternal separations on behavior and heart rate of two week old rat pups. *Physiology and Behavior, 10*(3), 423–427.

Hofer, M. A. (1973c). The role of nutrition in the physiological and behavioral effects of early maternal separation on infant rats. *Psychosomatic Medicine, 35*(4), 350–359.

Hofer, M. A. (1975). Studies on how early maternal separation produces behavioral change in young rats. *Psychosomatic Medicine, 37*(3), 245–264.

Hofer, M. A. (1994a). Early relationships as regulators of infant physiology and behavior. *Acta Paediatrica Scandinavica Supplement 397*, 9–18.

Hofer, M. A. (1994b). Hidden regulators mediating early attachment, separation and loss. In N. A. Fox (Ed.), The development of emotion regulation. *Monographs of the Society for Research in Child Development, 59*(2–3, Serial No. 2040), 192–207.

Hofer, M. A. (1995). Hidden regulators: Implications for a new understanding of attachment, separation, and loss. In S. Goldberg & R. Muir (Eds.), *Attachment theory: Social, developmental, and clinical perspectives* (pp. 203–230). Hillsdale, NJ: Analytic Press.

Huttenlocher, P. R. (1994). Synaptogenesis, synapse elimination, and neural plasticity in human cerebral cortex. In C. A. Nelson (Ed.), *Minnesota Symposium on Child Psychology: Vol. 27. Threats to optimal development: Integration biological, psychological, and social risk factors* (pp. 35–54). Mahwah, NJ: Erlbaum.

Jaffe, J., Beebe, B., Feldstein, S., Crown, C., & Jasnow, M. (2001). Rhythms of dialogue in infancy. *Monographs of the Society for Research in Child Development, 66*(2), 1–132.

Johnson, E. O., Kamilaris, T. C., Chrousos, G. P., & Gold, P. W. (1992). Mechanisms of stress: A dynamic overview of hormonal and behavioral homeostasis. *Neuroscience and Biobehavioral Reviews, 16*, 115–130.

Kandel, E. R. (1992). Early experience, critical periods, and developmental fine tuning of brain architecture. In E. R. Kandel, J. H. Schwartz, & T. Jessell (Eds.), *Principles of neural science* (2nd ed., pp. 757–770). New York: Elsevier.

Knutsson, U., Dahlgren, J., Marcus, C., Rosberg, S., Bronnegard, M., Stierna, P., & Albertsson-Wikland, K. (1997). Circadian cortisol rhythms in healthy boys and girls: Relationship with age, growth, body composition, and pubertal development. *Journal of Clinical Endocrinology and Metabolism, 82*, 536–540.

Kraemer, G. W. (1992) A psychobiological theory of attachment. *Brain and Behavioral Sciences, 15*, 493–541.

Kraemer, G. W., & Clarke, S. A. (1990). The behavioral neurobiology of self-injurious behavior in rhesus monkeys. *Progress in Neuro-Psychopharmacology and Biological Psychiatry, 14*(Suppl.), S141–S168.

Kraemer, G. W., Ebert, M. H., Schmidt, D. E., & McKinney, W. T. (1989). A longitudinal study of the effects of different rearing environments on cerebospinal fluid norepinephrine and biogenic amine metabolites in rhesus monkeys. *Neuropsychopharmacology, 2*, 175–189.

Kroupina, M., Gunnar, M. R., & Johnson, D. E. (1997). *Report on salivary cortisol levels in a Russian baby home*. Minneapolis: University of Minnesota, Institute of Child Development.

Larson, M., White, B. P., Cochran, A., Donzella, B., & Gunnar, M. R. (1998). Dampening of the cortisol response to handling at 3–months in human infants and its relation to sleep, circadian cortisol activity, and behavioral distress. *Developmental Psychobiology, 33*, 327–337.

LeDoux, J. (2002). *Synaptic self: How are brains become who we are*. New York: Penguin.

Levine, S. (1994). The ontogeny of the hypothalamic–pituitary–adrenal axis: The influence of maternal factors. *Annals of the New York Academy of Sciences, 746,* 275–288.

Liu, D., Diorio, J., Tannenbaum, B., Caldji, C., Francis, D., Freedman, A., Sharma, S., Pearson, D., Plotsky, P. M., & Meaney, M. J. (1997). Maternal care, hippocampal glucocorticoid receptors, and hypothalamic–pituitary–adrenal responses to stress. *Science, 277,* 1659–1662.

Lyons-Ruth, K., Bronfman, E., & Atwood, G. (1999). A relational diathesis model of hostile–helpless states of mind: Expressions in mother–infant interactions. In J. Solomon & C. George (Eds.), *Attachment disorganization* (pp. 33–70). New York: Guilford Press.

Lyons-Ruth, K., Bronfman, E., & Parsons, E. (1999). Maternal disrupted affective communication, maternal frightened or frightening behavior, and disorganized infant attachment strategies. In J. Vondra & D. Barnett (Eds.), Atypical patterns of infant attachment: Theory, research and current directions. *Monographs of the Society for Research in Child Development, 64*(Serial No. 258), 67–96.

Lyons-Ruth, K., & Jacobvitz, D. (1999). Attachment disorganization: Unresolved loss, relational violence, and lapses in behavioral and attentional strategies. In J. Cassidy & P. Shaver (Eds.), *Handbook of attachment: Theory, research, and clinical implications* (pp. 520–554). New York: Guilford Press.

Lyons-Ruth, K., & Zeanah, C. (1993). The family context of infant mental health: Part I. Affective development in the primary caregiving relationship. In C. Zeanah (Ed.), *Handbook of infant mental health* (pp. 14–26). New York: Guilford Press.

Lyons-Ruth, K., Zoll, D., Connell, D., & Grunebaum, H. (1986). The depressed mother and her one-year-old infant: Environmental context, mother–infant interaction and attachment, and infant development. In E. Tronick & T. Field (Eds.), *Maternal depression and infant disturbance* (pp. 61–82). San Francisco: Jossey-Bass.

Main, M. (2000). The organized categories of infant, child, and adult attachment: flexible vs. inflexible attention under attachment-related stress. *Journal of the American Psychoanalytic Association, 48,* 1055–1096; discussion 1175–1187.

Main, M., & Hesse, E. (1990). Parents' unresolved traumatic experiences are related to infant disorganized attachment status: Is frightened and/or frightening parental behavior the linking mechanism? In M. Greenberg, D. Cicchetti, & E. M. Cummings (Eds.), *Attachment in the preschool years: Theory, research and intervention* (pp. 161–184). Chicago: University of Chicago Press.

Mason, W. A., & Berkson, G. (1975). Effects of maternal mobility on the development of rocking and other behaviors in the rhesus monkeys: A study with artificial mothers. *Developmental Psychobiology, 8,* 197–211.

Munck, A., & Naray-Fejes-Toth, A. (1994). Glucocorticoids and stress: Permissive and supressive actions. *Annals of the New York Academy of Sciences, 746,* 115–130.

Mundy, P. A., & Gomes, A. (1998). Individual differences in joint attention skill development in the second year. *Infant Behavior and Development, 21,* 469–482.

Murray, L., & Trevarthen, C. (1985). Emotional regulation of interactions between two-month olds and their mothers. In T. M. Field & N. A. Fox (Eds.), *Social perception in infants* (pp. 177–197). Norwood, NJ: Ablex.

Nachmias, M., Gunnar, M. R., Mangelsdorf, S., Parritz, R. H., & Buss, K. (1996).

Behavioral inhibition and stress reactivity: the moderating role of attachment security. *Child Development, 67*(2), 508–522.

Nelson, C. (1999). Change and continuity in neurobehavioral development: Lessons from the study of neurobiology and neural plasticity. *Infant Behavior and Development, 22*(4), 415–429.

O'Connor, T. G., Rutter, M., & the English and Romanian Adoptees Study Team [ERA]. (2000). Attachment disorder behavior following early severe deprivation: Extension and longitudinal follow-up. *Journal of the American Academy of Child and Adolescent. Psychiatry, 39*(6), 703–712.

Ogawa, J. R., Sroufe, L. A., Weinfield, N. S., Carlson, E. A., & Egeland, B. (1997). Development and the fragmented self: Longitudinal study of dissociative symptomatology in a nonclinical sample. *Development and Psychopathology, 9*(4), 855–879.

Plotsky, P. M., & Meaney, M. J. (1993). Early, postnatal experience alters hypothalamic corticotropin-releasing factor (CRF) mRNA, median eminence CRF content and stress-induced release in adult rats. *Molecular Brain Research, 18,* 195–200.

Price, D. A., Close, G. C., & Fielding, B. A. (1983). Age of appearance of circadian rhythms in salivary cortisol values in infancy. *Archives of Disease in Children, 58,* 454–456.

Rosenfield, P., Suchecki, D., & Levine, S. (1992). Multifactorial regulation of the hypothalamic–pituitary–adrenal axis during development. *Neuroscience and Biobehavioral Review, 16,* 553–568.

Sander, L. W. (1962). Issues in early mother–child interaction. *Journal of the American Academy of Child Psychiatry, 1,* 141–166.

Sander, L. W., Julia, H. L., Stechler, G., & Burns, P. (1972). Continuous 24-hour interactional monitoring in infants reared in two caretaking environments. *Psychosomatic Medicine, 34*(3), 270–282.

Sapolsky, R. M. (1997). The physiological relevance of glucocorticoid endangerment of the hippocampus. *Annals of the New York Academy of Sciences, 746,* 294–307.

Schwartz, D. B., Granger, D. A., Susman, E. J., Gunnar, M. R., & Laird, B. (1998). Assessing salivary cortisol in studies of child development. *Child Development, 69,* 1503–1513.

Seligman, M. E. D. (1975). *Helplessness: On depression, development and death.* San Francisco: Freeman.

Sethre-Hofstad, L., Stansbury, K., & Rice, M. (2002). Attunement of maternal and child adrenocortical response to child challenge. *Psychoneuroendocrinology, 27*(6), 731–748.

Shore, A. N. (2003). *Affect regulation and the repair of the self.* New York: Norton.

Sikes, P. J. (1992). Endocrine responses to the stress of critical illness. *AACN Clinical Issues, 3,* 397–391.

Sippell, W. G., Becker, H., Versmold, H. T., Bidlingmaier, F., & Knorr, D. (1978). Longitudinal studies of plasma aldosterone, corticosterone, deoxycosterone, progesterone 17-hydroxyprogesterone, cortisol, and cortisone determined simultaneously in mother and child at birth and during the early neonatal period. *Journal of Clinical Endocrinology and Metabolism, 46,* 971–985.

Spangler, G., & Grossmann, K. E. (1993). Biobehavioral organization in securely and insecurely attached infants. *Child Development, 64,* 1439–1450.

Spangler, G., & Grossmann, K. (1999). Individual and physiological correlates of attachment disorganization in infancy. In J. Solomon & C. George (Eds.), *Attachment disorganization* (pp. 95–124). New York: Guilford Press.

Spangler, G., & Schieche, M. (1998). Emotional and adrenocortical responses of infants to the strange situation: The differential function of emotional expression. *International Journal of Behavioral Development, 22,* 681–706.

Spitz, R. A. (1949). The role of ecological factors in emotional development in infancy. *Child Development, 20,* 145–156.

Sroufe, L. A. (1996). *Cambridge studies in social and emotional development.* New York: Cambridge University Press.

Sroufe, L. A., & Fleeson, J. (1986). Attachment and the construction of relationships. In W. Hartup & Z. Rubin (Eds.), *Relationships and development* (pp. 51–71). Hillsdale, NJ: Erlbaum.

Stern, D. (1977). *The first relationship.* Cambridge, MA: Harvard University Press.

Stratakis, C. A., & Gold, G. P. (1995). Neuroendocrinology and pathophysiology of the stress system. *Annals of the New York Academy of Sciences, 771,* 1–18.

Taylor, S. E., Klein, L. C., Lewis, B. P., Gruenewald, T. L., Gurung, R. A., & Updegraff, J. A. (2000). Biobehavioral responses to stress in females: Tend-and-befriend, not fight-or-flight. *Psychological Review, 107,* 411–429.

Thompson, L. A., Trevathan, W. R., Diaz, L. E., Licon, D. B., Fields, L. L., Villarreal, R., & Silva, K. (2003). *Mother/infant synchrony in cortisol and behavior: Relations with learning in 6-month-old infants.* Poster presented at the biennial meeting of the Society of Research in Child Development, Tampa, FL.

Tomasello, M. (1999). *The cultural origins of human cognition* (chap. 6). Cambridge, MA: Harvard University Press.

Trevarthen, C. (2001). Intrinsic motive for companionship in understanding: Their origin, development, and significance for infant mental health. *Infant Mental Health Journal, 22*(1–2), 95–131.

van IJzendoorn, M. H. (1995). Adult attachment representations, parental responsiveness, and infant attachment: A meta-analysis on the predictive validity of the Adult Attachment Interview. *Psychological Bulletin, 117,* 387–403.

van IJzendoorn, M. H., Schuengel, C., & Bakermans-Kranenburg, M. J. (1999). Disorganized attachment in early childhood: Meta-analysis of precursors, concomitants, and sequelae. *Development and Psychopathology, 11,* 225–249.

Weinstock, M. (1997). Does prenatal stress impair coping and regulation of the hypothalamic–pituitary–adrenal axis? *Neuroscience and Biobehavioral Review, 21*(1), 1–10.

PART II

ASSESSMENT, DIAGNOSIS, AND TREATMENT

WHAT ARE WE ASSESSING FOR, AND WHY?

In 1997, Robert J. Harmon and I edited a special issue of the *Infant Mental Health Journal* on *Evaluating Infants and Toddlers for Treatment*. At that time, we referred to René Spitz's classic work from 1945 and 1946 describing two psychiatric syndromes, hospitalism and anaclitic depression, for which he suggested their etiology and offered recommendations for treatment. In 1997, we agreed that while the field of *infant mental health* has expanded greatly since the time that Spitz made these then revolutionary observations and diagnoses, issues of what kind of nosology or diagnostic classification systems to use, what type of evaluations to do, and what treatment approaches are most effective continue to be issues for the field. In 1997, we concluded that there do not seem to be any agreed upon "standards" for the field of the best evaluation and treatment strategies, but rather a number of shared principles and practices that are central to most clinical infant mental health evaluation and treatment programs. In the past 6 years, we have made considerable progress in expanding training, evaluation, and treatment programs in infant mental health. The DC: 0–3 Diagnostic Classification System has been used widely in the past 6 years, with a 2003 special issue of the *Infant Mental Health Journal* reviewing international as well as U.S.-based work with the system. Generally accepted evaluation and treatment strategies have been put in place in many centers, and studies of their effectiveness are ongoing (with some of these reports being included in this book). In Part II, different strategies for assessing and treating young children and families in various settings and with diverse types of trauma are presented.

Alicia F. Lieberman and Patricia Van Horn focus in Chapter 4 on treatment of children exposed to domestic violence. They propose that the assessment of young children requires a multidimensional approach, where areas of competence and vulnerability are evaluated in overlapping biological, emotional, social, and cognitive domains, and where the child's individual functioning is considered in the context of the child's relationships and the family's ecological niche, including socioeconomic circumstances and childrearing values (Shonkoff & Phillips, 2000; Zero to Three/National Center for Clinical Infant Programs, 1994; Cicchetti & Cohen, 1995). Lieberman and Van Horn also propose that such a multidimensional approach is particularly relevant to the assessment of traumatized children because a child's response to trauma is influenced by his or her overall functioning and by the environmental supports available for recovery.

In Chapter 5, Stacy A. Klapper, Nancy S. Plummer, and Robert J. Harmon present their perspective on diagnostic and treatment issues focusing on the ways that children with different temperaments, personalities, and psychological resources react to trauma, especially severe abuse and neglect. They discuss assessment and treatment strategies in working with chronically abused and neglected children, a far too common form of trauma perpetrated on unsuspecting and defenseless children. Many of the assessment and treatment plans discussed are applicable to children who have experienced any type of traumatic experience, including accidents of various types, automobile accidents, dog bites, etc. In their chapter, the authors share their experience of having treated abused and neglected children in a therapeutic preschool setting for more than 10 years.

Julie A. Larrieu and Shana M. Bellow in Chapter 6 also focus on the problematic behaviors, perceptions, and relationship disruptions typically manifested by maltreating parents and their young children. They describe a comprehensive assessment procedure and common themes uncovered in the work of their team with maltreating parents and their children, ages birth to 47 months. The initial task of the Infant Team is to conduct a thorough assessment of each child and family (who have generally experienced multiple challenges and stressors) in order to make recommendations about permanency planning for Child Protective Services (CPS) and the Juvenile Court. The assessment procedure is designed to cast light on the relationship experiences of the parent and the child that brought them to abuse and neglect as an answer to life's stressors. In Chapter 7, Betsy McAlister Groves and Marilyn Augustyn take a departure from the traditional mental health settings to introduce the reader to an important nontraditional site for identification, assessment, and treatment of traumatized children—the pediatric clinic. The authors emphasize that despite the growing awareness of this need, there are many young children who have histories of trauma that may not be adequately identified within the current pediatric health system. Groves and Augustyn address the importance of screening for trauma in pediatric settings, describe the role of the health provider in identification of children, and propose a strategy for screening young children and their parents.

In Chapter 8, concluding Part II, Theodore J. Gaensbauer illustrates the ways in which our understanding of early trauma, as discussed in previous chapters, can be translated into actual practice. He begins with a general overview of the processes of evaluation and treatment as experienced by him in his work with traumatized young children and their families, followed by the description of a clinical case exemplifying his approach to therapy. Gaensbauer's work in a private practice setting tends to focus on traumas that are more circumscribed in nature, generally involving unintentional injuries such as those caused by medical illnesses and/or treatments or accidents of various types. Where abuse or violence has occurred, the perpetrator is likely to have been someone outside the nuclear family rather than the parents. Family settings are generally stable, and parents are able to provide relatively uncomplicated support around the trauma. The types of trauma Gaensbauer treats in his clinical practice contrast with situations of parental abuse where work with the parents is complicated by their direct responsibility for the child's trauma and where the child's loss of trust in adults has been doubly damaged by the knowledge that the trauma was intentionally inflicted on him or her by those who were supposed to nurture the youngster.

REFERENCES

Cicchetti, D., & Cohen, D. J. (Eds.). (1995). *Developmental psychopathology: Vol. 2. Risk, disorder, and adaptation.* New York: Wiley.

Shonkoff, J., & Phillips, D. (2000). *From neurons to neighborhoods: The study of early childhood development.* Washington, DC: National Academy Press.

Zero to Three/National Center for Clinical Infant Programs. (1994). *Diagnostic classification of mental health and developmental disorders of infancy and early childhood.* Arlington, VA: Author.

CHAPTER 4

ASSESSMENT AND TREATMENT OF YOUNG CHILDREN EXPOSED TO TRAUMATIC EVENTS

ALICIA F. LIEBERMAN
PATRICIA VAN HORN

The impact of traumatic events on infants, toddlers, and preschoolers is only beginning to be systematically documented and understood. This dearth of information about young children's responses to violence, accidents, natural disasters, and other traumatic events is perhaps the result of a pervasive wish to think of infancy and early childhood as a time of safety and well-being, when adult protection buffers children from the experience of pain. Even a cursory look at young children's experience shows that this is far from the case. As just one example, abuse is the leading cause of death in the first year of life after the perinatal period (National Center on Child Abuse and Neglect, 1995), and a high percentage of the children placed in foster care as a result of abuse are under 5 years of age (U.S. Department of Health and Human Services, 1994). Abuse has been empirically associated with disturbances of emotional regulation and social relatedness (Erickson, Egeland & Pianta, 1989; Main & George, 1985), disorganization of attachment (Cichetti & Barnett, 1991), and impairments of communication in infants and toddlers (Beeghly & Cicchetti, 1987, 1994). There is increasing evidence that trauma in infancy and early childhood can derail the course of normative development (Osofsky, 1997a, 1997b; Pynoos, 1990).

In the first years of life, the experience of trauma represents for children a loss of the developmentally appropriate expectation that their parents will protect them from harm. Young children rely on their parents for the consolidation of their sense of self, which is established through regulation of body rhythms, modulation of emotion, formation and socialization of interpersonal relationships, and learning from exploration of the environment. Each of these processes is disrupted when a child suffers a traumatic event or lives in chronic circumstances of traumatic stress. The child cannot then develop a mental representation of the parent as a reliable protector, and the interplay between this lack of trust and the child's traumatic responses can have pervasive negative effects on the course of development.

Children respond to trauma in ways that reflect the particular developmental tasks and challenges they are attempting to master (Marans & Adelman, 1997; Pynoos, Steinberg, & Wraith, 1995). Infants in the first year of life show a disruption of the developmentally salient processes of establishing neurophysiological regulation and forming secure attachments with the parents and other primary caregivers. Such disruptions may be manifested in eating and sleeping difficulties, problems with digestion and elimination, inconsolable crying, difficulty being soothed, intense separation anxiety, head banging or other self-injurious behaviors, unmodulated affect, and lack of consistent behavioral strategies to derive a sense of safety from the attachment figure. Toddlers may engage in similar dysregulated behaviors as those described for infants in the first year of life, while also experiencing age-specific difficulties in attaining an emotionally satisfying balance between attachment and autonomy. The resulting distortions of secure base behavior may be manifested in recklessness or inhibition of exploration, intractable temper tantrums, aggression toward caregivers, peers, and animals, and angry noncompliance. Preschoolers also show the symptoms described for infants and toddlers, with additional disturbances of age-specific issues such as distortions and constrictions of symbolic play, excessive preoccupation with body integrity, sibling rivalry, and the polarities of power versus submission and dominance versus victimization.

The overlap of symptoms across the first 5 years of life is an indication that, although specific developmental tasks may be more salient at particular ages, all of these tasks continue to be active in the course of development. In this sense, "clinical issues are issues for the life span, not phases of life" (Stern, 1985, p. 23). Responses to early trauma need to be understood as the initial manifestations of long-term risks to the child's unfolding development. This chapter describes assessment strategies designed to identify traumatic responses in a developmental and contextual framework, and presents forms of intervention aimed at alleviating traumatic responses in the present and at preventing the consolidation of these responses into chronic patterns of emotional, social, and cognitive dysfunction.

ASSESSMENT OF TRAUMATIZED INFANTS, TODDLERS, AND PRESCHOOLERS

The assessment of young children requires a multidimensional approach, where areas of competence and vulnerability are assessed in overlapping biological, emotional, social, and cognitive domains, and where the child's individual functioning is considered in the context of the child's relationships and the family's ecological niche, including socioeconomic circumstances and childrearing values (Shonkoff & Phillips, 2000; Zero to Three/ National Center for Clinical Infant Programs, 1994; Cicchetti & Cohen, 1995; Cicchetti & Howes, 1991). This multidimensional approach is particularly relevant to the assessment of traumatized children because the child's response to trauma is influenced by the child's overall functioning and by the environmental supports available for recovery.

Parents and caregivers are essential providers of information about the specific features of the trauma and the child's functioning before and after the traumatic event because young children's cognitive immaturity and language limitations restrict their ability to provide comprehensive and reliable self-reports. The assessor needs to create a collaborative stance with the parents in order to elicit accurate information about the child's trauma experience. A focus on building this collaboration is particularly relevant when the parents might be consciously or unconsciously motivated to withhold or alter information, for example, if they might be implicated in the child's trauma either through direct actions or through failure to protect the child. The assessor may choose to address the parents' experience as the initial course of action whenever the parents' reliability as reporters is compromised by intense emotions, including fear for the child's physical and emotional health, guilt, anger at the perpetrator or authority figures involved, or concern about possible legal ramifications such as criminal prosecution or foster care placement of the child. A supportive stance on the assessor's part, even when the parents' role in the trauma is ambiguous or suspect, can elicit parental cooperation and enhance the quality of the information obtained.

A "best practices" approach includes approximately three to five 45-minute assessment sessions (Zero to Three/National Center for Clinical Infant Programs, 1994). The assessment should include a history of the child's development before and after the traumatic events, observation of the child–parent interaction, and the child's narrative of the traumatic experience through the use of toys, drawing, storytelling, or other evocative materials. Additional sources of information may include observing the child in the child-care setting, interviews with child-care providers, and standardized assessment procedures. Optimally, the assessment will yield a comprehensive picture of the child's neurophysiological regulation, sensorimotor functioning, quality of the relationship with the parents and other important figures, language skills, level of symbolic play, expression and modulation of affect, areas of strength and vulnerability, and symptoms preceding and following the traumatic events.

Although a good assessment is ideally the basis for treatment, the goal of assessing the child should not preclude immediate therapeutic interventions in crisis situations. When a child is referred for services soon after a traumatic event, "psychological first aid" can be provided for immediate emotional relief by identifying specific age-related responses and administering developmentally appropriate interventions (Pynoos & Nader, 1993). These immediate therapeutic interventions can do double duty as assessment strategies because they help to elucidate the child's and family's initial responses to the trauma as well as their areas of resilience and vulnerability and ability to collaborate in the treatment. Optimally, assessment is an ongoing process that continues throughout treatment and involves continued monitoring of the child's functioning in response to new developmental skills and challenges, environmental changes, and the influence of treatment.

Assessment Domains

The assessment needs to incorporate a sustained focus on a variety of domains that influence the child's functioning. These domains are described below.

Briefing about the Circumstances and Sequence of the Trauma

Accurate information about the traumatic events is the factual foundation for a solid understanding of the child's responses. This information includes the circumstances of the trauma, participants, sequence of events, nature of the child's involvement, availability of the parents or other attachment figures, and aftermath of the traumatic event. Traumatic events are sudden and unpredictable and tend to occur very quickly, so that different participants may have different recollections and perceptions of what happened. The adults may overlook the experience of a small child as they mobilize to respond to the immediate threat. Whenever possible, a reconstruction of what the child might have seen or heard should be confirmed through reports from police, Child Protective Services (CPS), eye witnesses, or media coverage.

Child's Emotional, Social, and Cognitive Functioning

The assessment should include an evaluation of the child's functioning both before and after the traumatic event in order to determine its impact on the child's developmental progress. The child's constitutional characteristics and temperamental style may contribute to the nature of the child's traumatic response. For example, temperamentally reserved children may tend to respond to the trauma with internalizing behaviors such as affective numbing, social withdrawal, constricted exploration, separation anxiety, and new fears. In contrast, very active and outgoing children may be more prone to respond with externalizing behaviors such as recklessness, temper tantrums, defiance, and aggression. Young children are also likely to show a high co-occurrence of externalizing and internalizing symptoms, and may alternate periods of clingy and fearful behavior with episodes of anger and defiance. Because externalizing behaviors tend to be more frequently reported than symptoms of anxiety and depression, assessors should probe systematically for internalizing behaviors when the parents or other informants highlight the child's aggression, defiance, or noncompliance during the referral and assessment process.

The level of social and emotional functioning is manifested in the child's quality of attachment to the parents, the affective range of relatedness to others, and the ability to cope with age-appropriate expectations and stresses. There are broad cultural variations in the value that parents give to children's autonomous functioning, such as self-feeding or sleeping alone. Within these cultural variations, there are also normative trends in children's use of the parents as a secure base and in their ability to tolerate everyday frustration. The "goodness of fit" between the parent and the child in these areas, assessed through parental report and direct observation, is a useful gauge of the age appropriateness of the child's social and emotional behavior in the context of the family's cultural values and expectations.

Young children's cognitive development is intricately connected with their social and emotional functioning. Traumatic experiences can derail the child's readiness to learn, either temporarily or for the long term, through such mechanisms as hypervigilance, constriction of exploration, misattribution of hostile intention to others, preemptive and self-protective aggression, generalized fears, and preoccupation with internal processes so that attention is deployed to the self rather than to the environment. The child's negative affect may in turn generate ambivalence, rejection, anger, and emotional withdrawal in the parents and caregivers, confirming the child's mistrust in others and reinforcing a psychological stance that interferes with the learning of healthier forms of adaptation.

Cognitive functioning is buttressed by the child's capacity to remember. Contrary to the widespread popular belief that infants and toddlers cannot recall events, there is increasing empirical evidence that they are able to encode and retrieve early experiences. Two types of memory are generally described in the literature: implicit or nondeclarative memory, and explicit or declarative memory (Schachter, 1987). Implicit memory involves parts of the brain that are fully mature at birth, including the amygdala and other limbic areas associated with emotion; it is nonverbal, exists largely outside of awareness, and has been demonstrated experimentally in conditioning studies with newborns and infants in the first months of life. Explicit memory, usually expressed through verbal recall, requires focal attention for encoding and a subjective sense of recollection for retrieval. There is debate about the existence of explicit memory in the first year of life, although there is suggestive evidence supporting this possibility (Fivush, 1994).

A key question in determining whether infants and toddlers have long-term recall of a situation is the *memorability* of the event (Nelson, 1994). This concept refers to events that are worth remembering over time, given the quick developmental progression and changing interests and skills of the first few years of life. Assessing what constitutes a memorable event from the perspective of a young child is a pivotal issue in early memory research. From a clinical perspective, there is little doubt that a traumatic event can be considered memorable because it is unique, dramatic, and elicits intense emotion. The question here is whether young children are able to consciously remember and describe traumatic events that they experienced before acquiring language. Several clinical reports converge in concluding that, once they acquire language, children are able to narrate traumatic events that occurred while they were preverbal, and that they produce accurate behavioral reenactments even in the absence of verbal narrative (Gaensbauer, 1995; Sugar, 1992; Terr, 1988). This does not mean that everything children say and reenact about a traumatic experience is factually accurate. Distortions and omissions may be introduced by a variety of factors, including the child's misunderstanding of the purpose of certain actions. For example, an infant or toddler may misinterpret an intrusive medical procedure as an angry attack and respond with intense fear to the sight of the physician long after the procedure has been completed. Nevertheless, children's verbal and nonverbal communications should be considered as meaningful expressions of the child's mental representation of the traumatic experience and should be incorporated as integral elements of the treatment plan (Gaensbauer, 1995).

The child's sensorimotor, emotional, social, and cognitive functioning can be interpreted in the context of a brain–mind model of behavior. There is growing evidence that neurobiological alterations may occur when the child's adaptive responses are overwhelmed by the traumatic experience, particularly when it is in the form of maltreatment (see Cohen, Perel, DeBellis, Friedman, & Putnam, 2002, for a review). These neurobiological alterations may involve changes in brain structure and functioning, including hyperresponsiveness of the amygdala, which is involved in the expression and modulation of emotions and emotional memory processing; disruptions in the hypothalamic–pituitary–adrenocortical (HPA) axis, which mediates the stress response; and underreactivity of the medial prefrontal cortex, which normally releases neurotransmitters such as dopamine, norepinephrine, and serotonin, and which is involved in planned behaviors, working memory, motivation, and the ability to differentiate between internal and external models of the world. These changes in central nervous system functioning can leave a traumatized child feeling perpetually anxious and on edge, or psychologically numb. They can lead to the child's experiencing persistent and overgeneralized fears. Although there are not yet empirical findings to link particular central nervous system dysregulation to behavior, a careful assessment and treatment plan ought to take the risk for dysregulation into account and incorporate interventions designed to help the child regain physiological homeostasis. Such interventions should aim to restore the child's trust in the predictability of the world and relationships, restore the child's trust in her bodily sensations, and help her realistically assess threat.

Quality of Relationship with the Parents

Traumatic events can have an alienating impact on the child–parent relationship. Young children have a developmentally appropriate expectation that their parents will protect them in all circumstances, and they perceive the traumatic experience as an indication of the parent's anger, indifference, or incompetence in keeping them safe. The child's trust in the parent as a source of safety and protection can suffer long-lasting and perhaps irreversible damage, manifested in loss of intimacy and affectionate behavior and in increases in angry, rejecting, controlling, or punitive behavior directed to the parent. The child may show signs of preferring one parent to the other, and this favoritism may create tension between the spouses and compound the mutual recriminations that are frequent by-products of a traumatic event.

Most parents suffer intensely when their children are traumatized. When the trauma was the result of an accident, guilt and self-recrimination can have the paradoxical effect of creating parental self-absorption and diminishing attunement to the child's needs. Defensive processes may involve denial, isolation of affect, overidentification with the child, or other mechanisms that interfere with the parent's emotional availability. When the trauma was inflicted by the parents, for example, through physical abuse or exposure to severe domestic violence, the effect of the specific event may be compounded by the cumulative influence of stresses caused by longstanding psychological disorders, family conflicts, and disturbances in parenting. The relationship between the parent and the child may also be aggravated by the negative impact of external circumstances, such as the involvement of the legal system and the child's placement in foster care. These patterns need to be carefully evaluated in order to build into the treatment plan interventions aimed at addressing the impact of the trauma on the quality of the parent–child relationship.

Traumatic Reminders

The child's behavior may be strongly influenced by stimuli that act as triggers for memories of the traumatic experience, flooding the child with intrusive images and other proprioceptive and sensory experiences. Traumatic reminders tend to remain unidentified when they operate outside of the child's conscious awareness or when the child cannot use language to describe what is happening. Sensory stimuli may also act as triggers for traumatic stress responses when they are associated with secondary stresses that followed the trauma. For example, the siren of an ambulance or police car, the sight of a policeman, or walking into the lobby of the hospital where the child was taken for emergency care may acquire the qualities of traumatic reminders. Seemingly irrational fears, or efforts on the child's part to avoid ostensibly benign people or situations, can be signs that the child is associating the stimulus with some aspect of the traumatic event. When these inexplicable behaviors are reported, systematic efforts to understand their possible association with a traumatic reminder may yield valuable information about the child's experience.

The parent may have been exposed to the same traumatic situation as the child and may respond to similar or different traumatic reminders. An evaluation of the parent's traumatic experience, quality of coping, and sources of support are important elements of the assessment because this information will enable the assessor to determine the parent's capacity to cooperate in implementing the treatment plan.

Continuity versus Disruption of Daily Routines

A traumatic event often has a disruptive effect on family life. Well-established routines may be altered, including mealtimes and bedtime rituals that anchor the child's sense of predictability. These disruptions may act as secondary stresses that amplify the immediate effects of the traumatic event by introducing additional elements of uncertainty (Pynoos, Steinberg, & Piacentini, 1999). The assessment provides an opportunity to gather information about daily routines and their disruption following the trauma, and to discuss strategies that will enable the parents to build or restore a reassuring structure to everyday life.

Family Circumstances

The ecological context of the family helps to determine areas of resilience and vulnerability in recovering from trauma. The traumatic event may consist of a discrete episode that, although damaging in itself, can be relatively contained in its ramifications because the child is surrounded by well-functioning adults who are able to provide the material and emotional resources needed to support the child's recovery. Alternatively, the traumatic event may occur as part of a continuum of stressful circumstances that overwhelm both the child and the family. Poverty, unemployment, lack of education, and lack of acculturation in immigrant families provide the backdrop for lack of access to needed resources, ranging from safe neighborhoods and reliable transportation to prompt medical and psychological services and quality child care. In very severe circumstances, the trauma befalling the child may be a reflection of chaotic or dangerous patterns of family life, including excessive substance use, untreated mental illness and chronic child neglect or abuse. A careful evaluation of the family circumstances is the foundation for assessing the protective and risk factors in the child's recovery process and for drawing and implementing an effective treatment plan.

Family Belief Systems and Cultural Values

Trauma often serves as a catalyst for strong family beliefs and traditions, often rooted in cultural values, about ways of helping the child through the recovery process. The family may use rituals such as prayer, invocations, exorcisms, and body-based interventions. These practices are often embedded in belief systems about child development and childrearing values. The assessor's active efforts to learn about the family's understanding of trauma and recovery can lead to a fruitful integration of traditional healing and modern interventions on behalf of the child (Kleinman, 1980).

Making a Clinical Diagnosis

The information gathered during the assessment period helps the assessor to determine whether the child has a diagnosable clinical condition. Making a psychiatric diagnosis in the first 5 years of life is fraught with ethical and conceptual dilemmas because of concerns about labeling the child, the rapid pace of early development, the organizing roles of emotional relationships and quality of caregiving in the child's functioning, and the quick changes in emotional, social, and cognitive performance that may occur in response to situational factors and changed circumstances (Emde, Bingham, & Harmon, 1993). Young children have a relatively limited behavioral repertoire, and different diagnostic pictures may be expressed through similar behavioral configurations. For example, irritability and aggressive behavior in a toddler may signal depression, anxiety, or a traumatic stress reaction, depending on the circumstances. Comorbidity is prevalent not only among adults but in children as well, complicating efforts to arrive at a clear-cut diagnosis.

There are clinical as well as practical reasons to support the desirability of a diagnosis in spite of these difficulties. An accurate diagnostic picture provides a clear rationale for an effective treatment plan. It facilitates communication among different professionals by providing a common vocabulary of concepts and terms. Making a diagnosis can also help to obtain reimbursement for services from insurance companies and from federal and state programs, including funds for victims of crime.

Two diagnostic manuals provide classifications of mental health disorders for young children: the fourth edition of the *Diagnostic and Statistical Manual of Mental Disorders* (DSM-IV; American Psychiatric Association, 1994), and the *Diagnostic Classification of Mental Health and Developmental Disorders of Infancy and Early Childhood* (DC: 0–3; Zero to Three/National Center for Clinical Infant Programs, 1994). Although DSM-IV does not focus on the developmental characteristics of infants, toddlers, and preschoolers, the symptoms of traumatized young children can fit the diagnoses of posttraumatic stress disorder, one of the mood disorders, and adjustment disorder with anxiety, depressed mood, and/or conduct problems. By comparison, DC: 0–3 was specifically developed for use with children in infancy and early childhood. The primary diagnosis in this nosology is framed in the context of the child's most salient emotional relationships and developmental level. The diagnostic classification is guided by a decision tree stipulating that the category of traumatic stress response should be used as the first option when the clinical symptoms emerged after the child experienced or witnessed a traumatic event. The manual defines a traumatic stressor as an event or series of events that involve actual or threatened death, serious injury, or danger to the psychological or physical integrity of the child or others.

Traumatic Stress Disorder in Infancy and Early Childhood

The diagnosis of traumatic stress disorder is made when, following a traumatic event, a series of connected traumatic events, or chronic, enduring stress, the child shows clinical symptoms that can be organized in four categories: reexperiencing of the traumatic event, numbing of responsiveness, increased arousal, and new symptoms that were not present before the traumatic event (Zero to Three/National Center for Clinical Infant Programs, 1994). Reexperiencing of the event(s) is manifested through any of the following criteria: posttraumatic play, defined as play that represents a reenactment of some aspect of the trauma, is compulsively driven and fails to relieve anxiety; recurrent recollections of the event outside of play; distress at reminders of the trauma; nightmares; and flashbacks or dissociation. Numbing of responsiveness may involve increased social withdrawal, restricted range of affect, temporary loss of previously acquired developmental skills, and play constriction. Increased arousal is manifested through night terrors, difficulty going to sleep, repeated night wakings, difficulties paying attention or concentrating, hypervigilance, and exaggerated startle responses. New symptoms often involve aggression toward peers, adults, or animals, separation anxiety, fear of the dark or other new fears, inappropriate sexual behavior, pessimism, somatic symptoms, and motor reenactments. All of these symptoms must be understood in the context of the nature of the trauma, the child's constitutional characteristics and temperamental style, the parents' ability to help the child cope with the trauma, and the protective and risk factors in the child's family and broader environment.

Prolonged Bereavement/Grief Reaction

The loss of a parent or primary caregiver through death or permanent separation constitutes a specific traumatic experience for young children because they lack the emotional and cognitive maturity to cope with a major loss without serious disruption to the continuity of their sense of self (Furman, 1974). Following the loss, the child may show a clinical mood disorder characterized by prolonged bereavement and grief (Zero to Three/National Center for Clinical Infant Programs, 1994). This condition is often manifested in the classic sequence of protest, despair, and detachment described by Bowlby (1973). Initial efforts to find the parent through crying, calling, and searching are eventually replaced by lethargy, sadness, emotional withdrawal, and lack of interest in age-appropriate activities. Detachment may eventually be manifested through seeming indifference to reminders of the lost figure. The child may show "selective forgetting," apparently failing to recognize photographs or other reminders of the lost person. Alternatively, the child may become extremely emotionally aroused by exposure to these reminders, or respond with intense distress to themes that have some connection with separation and loss, such as hide-and-seek games or the misplacement of a household object or toy. The content of play may show unrelieved preoccupation with separation, loss, and reunion. These manifestations indicate strong parallels between traumatic stress disorder and prolonged bereavement/grief reaction in the prevalence of symptoms that indicate reexperiencing, affective numbing, increased arousal, and new symptoms. For this reason, bereavement in early childhood can be understood as a specific manifestation of traumatic stress response caused by loss of an emotionally salient person, as eloquently expressed in the phrase "the trauma of loss" used by Bowlby (1980) to describe the emotional toll of losing a loved one in early life.

Comorbidity of Traumatic Stress Disorder and Prolonged Bereavement/Grief Reaction

The severity of the trauma of loss can be conceptualized along a continuum of traumatic experience, depending on the emotional salience of the child's relationship with the person who died, the circumstances of the death, whether or not the child witnessed the death, and the child's developmental stage (Lieberman, Compton, Van Horn, & Ghosh Ippen, 2003). The more extreme manifestations occur when the child witnesses the parent's violent death and the child is at a developmental stage of simultaneous total dependence on the parent and inability to understand the meaning of death. In such a situation, the child is flooded by intense anxiety caused by the sights, sounds, and smells that accompanied the violent death, the frightening events that followed the death, and the inability to comprehend why the parent cannot move or act to alleviate the child's fear and distress. The child's ability to mourn for the parent's death is derailed by intrusive memories of the manner of the death and by traumatic reminders that may maintain the manner of the death continually present in the child's mental representations of the parent (Pynoos et al., 1999). To give proper importance to the different facets of this complex trauma experience, the clinician must use two simultaneous lenses—the lens of trauma and the lens of the trauma of loss—in examining the responses of children who witnessed their parent's violent or sudden death (Lieberman, Compton, et al., 2003).

Applying the Assessment Information: The Feedback Session

The assessment information needs to be conveyed to the parents in a feedback session that clearly describes how the child's functioning has been affected by the traumatic experience. At its best, the feedback session involves a collaborative process, where the parents and the assessor contribute their respective areas of knowledge to the common goal of helping the child recover from trauma. This objective can be more easily attained if the assessor shares information and insights with the parents as these emerge in the course of the assessment, building themes that can be revisited during the feedback session for the purpose of deciding on a course of action.

The decision to recommend treatment is a central component of the feedback session. The clinician is likely to learn from the course of the assessment whether the parents are willing to consider treatment, and the areas of ambivalence or resistance if they are not amenable to intervention. Resistance to treatment is a common response in parents of traumatized children because of the strong wish to believe that the passage of time will alleviate the child's traumatic response. The assessor can be helpful in normalizing the parents' wishes for a spontaneous recovery while providing supportive evidence for the desirability of treatment. Many parents assume that their child needs treatment because they are not "good enough" parents. For this reason, it is important to avoid the appearance of blaming the parents in recommending treatment and to address sympathetically the parents' feelings of guilt or remorse about the traumatic event whenever clinically appropriate.

TREATMENT OF TRAUMATIZED INFANTS, TODDLERS, AND PRESCHOOLERS

The most basic principle in the treatment of early trauma is the establishment of a safe environment for the child and for the caregiving adults. This prerequisite can be challenging, particularly when the trauma involves interpersonal violence within the family, in the neighborhood, or in the larger social context, and when the threat of violence is ongoing. The creation of safe external conditions is often beyond the scope of what the clinician can undertake to achieve. Nevertheless, it is important to remember the therapeutic value of an unwavering focus on safety, both physical and psychological, and on concrete steps that can be taken to increase safety even if it cannot be totally guaranteed. The effort to increase external safety often becomes a useful port of entry to address internal sources of danger, including unmanageable aggressive impulses, fears of abandonment, and the defenses used to cope with these internal states. Feeling protected, both from external threats and internal impulses, is the cornerstone of recovery. Everything that follows is built on this foundation. For this reason, ensuring and preserving external and internal safety is the first principle of trauma treatment.

The second principle in the treatment of traumatized young children is the importance of framing the therapeutic intervention in the context of the child's relationships with parents, attachment figures, and/or primary caregivers. Infants, toddlers, and preschoolers are completely dependent on adults for their physical care and psychological well-being, and rely on their attachment figures both as a safe haven in danger situations and as a secure base from which to explore (Ainsworth, Blehar, Waters, & Walls, 1979). Trauma derails the child's developmental expectation that the parents will be effective protectors and may engender in the parents feelings of guilt and self-deprecation that interfere with their ability to help the child in the aftermath of the traumatic event. The quality of emotional support between the parent and the child and among family members may be gravely affected by these responses. There is empirical evidence that the symptoms of preschoolers exposed to traumatic situations are predicted by their mothers' psychological functioning (Laor, Wolmer, & Cohen, 2001; Linares et al., 2001; Lieberman, Van Horn, & Ozer, 2003). It follows that enhancing mothers' ability to help their children cope with trauma should have a beneficial effect on the child's recovery. Although there is no systematic evidence about the role of fathers in early trauma recovery, clinical experience supports the premise that parents of both genders can be of great help in the treatment process. A major focus of treatment is to create or restore feelings of closeness and intimacy between the child and the parents as a backdrop to the ongoing resolution of the traumatic stress responses.

The third principle of trauma treatment is the focus on concurrent developmental tasks that are derailed by the traumatic experience. In the first years of life, the developmental tasks affected by trauma include the establishment and consolidation of psychobiological rhythms, the development of secure attachments, the balance between attachment and autonomy, the regulation of emotion, the achievement of age-appropriate socialization skills, the acquisition of gender identity, and readiness to explore the environment and learn (Drell, Gaensbauer, Siegel, & Sugar, 1995; Marans & Adelman, 1997). Treatment needs to incorporate intervention strategies that promote a return to normal development and engagement with age-appropriate activities (Marmar, Foy, Kagan, & Pynoos, 1993).

The fourth principle of treatment is attention to the potential effect of trauma on future development. The symptoms of traumatic stress include increased arousal as well numbness of responsiveness, two patterns of affective dysregulation that interfere with the adaptive deployment of attention and the capacity to focus and concentrate. These patterns can have extensive negative effects on subsequent development by interfering with the child's ability to form satisfying relationships with teachers and peers and to distinguish between cues to safety and danger in exploring the environment, as well as his or her readiness to learn. Therapeutic interventions should take into account how the child's present symptoms are likely to affect future development, in order to prioritize specific treatment goals and to implement preventive measures when appropriate.

Treatment Goals

Defining clear treatment goals enables the clinician to maintain a balanced therapeutic perspective as the treatment unfolds. The overarching treatment goal is to help the child and the family return to the level of functioning that was achieved prior to the trauma (Gaensbauer & Siegel, 1995). This goal needs to be expanded when the child lives in family circumstances characterized by chronic turmoil and acute stress. If family dysfunction has contributed to the child's trauma, the therapeutic goal needs to encompass the improvement of the child's parenting environment to alleviate the sequelae of the trauma and to prevent retraumatization in the future.

Different approaches to the treatment of trauma, for children as well as adults, are characterized by commonalities of goals and the mechanisms proposed to achieve these goals (Marmar et al., 1993). These commonalities target the main symptoms of traumatic response and are described below:

1. *Encouraging a return to normal development, adaptive coping, and engagement with present activities and future goals.* As stated above, this is the overarching goal of treatment, both for children and adults. In working

with traumatized infants, toddlers, and preschoolers, the clinician supports the child and the parent in practicing developmentally appropriate activities, striving for normative achievements, and attempting new and adaptive ways of functioning.

2. *Fostering a realistic response to threat.* The experience of trauma impairs the ability to appraise accurately cues to danger and safety, leading to underestimating threat or overreacting to benign stimuli. The clinician focuses on promoting more accurate perceptions of danger and more appropriate responses to it.

3. *Maintaining regular levels of affective arousal.* The typical traumatic stress responses—numbing, avoidance, and hyperarousal—interfere with the ability to rely on others for help and with the spontaneous extinction of learned conditioning, creating a "biopsychosocial trap" because neurophysiological disruptions in affective arousal negatively affect other self-regulatory systems (Shalev, 1996). A major goal of treatment is to help the child gain increasing trust in bodily sensations by establishing and reinforcing daily routines, structured activities, and self-regulation mechanisms that help the child acquire better control of affect dysregulation and the negative emotions that accompany it.

4. *Building reciprocity in intimate relationships.* One of the most damaging by-products of early trauma is the loss of the parents as a safe haven from danger and a secure base from which to explore. Treatment involves identifying and practicing ways of repairing this loss of trust by fostering empathic recognition and response to social and emotional cues between the parent and the child.

5. *Normalization of the traumatic response.* Traumatic responses can be of such intensity as to impair self-recognition and self-esteem, leading to fears of being "crazy," "bad," and "unlovable" in children as well as adults. Validating the traumatic responses as legitimate and universal reactions to an overwhelming event provides a frame of meaning that promotes self-worth and supports momentum toward healthy development.

6. *Encouraging a differentiation between reliving and remembering.* Children reenact the traumatic experience through action or through play and may become increasingly confused about remembering and reexperiencing the trauma. The treatment aims at increasing their capacity to make the connection between what they are feeling in the moment and the traumatic experience of the past, emphasizing the concrete differences between their subjective experience and their present surroundings.

7. *Placing the traumatic experience in perspective.* Treatment focuses on helping children and parents achieve a balance where the memory of the trauma is not eradicated but is integrated with other life experiences instead of remaining a central preoccupation. The person is encouraged to take pleasure in rewarding life events and personal achievements, and to appreciate the enriching aspects of his or her life.

Treatment Modalities

Treatment may take a variety of formats, depending on the presenting problem, family circumstances and preferences, and the clinician's preferred treatment approach and area of expertise. Different theoretical orientations may inform the treatment, including psychodynamic, attachment, cognitive-behavioral, and social-learning approaches. In large measure, however, interventions with infants, toddlers, and preschoolers integrate a variety of theoretical approaches and stress the developmental appropriateness rather than the theoretical origins of specific intervention strategies. Some prevailing modalities are described below.

Developmental Guidance

This modality consists of individual sessions with the parent to provide information about the meaning of the child's symptoms and to recommend strategies for responding to the child's symptoms and organizing the child's daily routine. This approach is indicated when the traumatic event is circumscribed, the child's response to the trauma is of mild-to-moderate intensity, the protective factors in the child's environment outweigh the sources of concern, and the parent is motivated and able to implement the clinician's recommendations.

Example. Michael, age 9 months, suffered second-degree burns in his leg when he lurched forward suddenly from his mother's lap and reached toward the coffee pot as his friend's mother was pouring the hot liquid into a cup. He was rushed to the emergency room while his mother held him in the backseat of the car. He cried intermittently but dozed off when his mother rocked him and sang to him. In the emergency room, Michael cried intensely when he was separated from his mother for medical intervention for approximately 30 minutes and continued to cry at the top of his lungs for the entire duration of the procedure. He calmed down quickly when his mother returned to the room and nursed him. That night Michael was hospitalized for observation and his mother stayed with him. Upon discharge, the mother called an infant specialist who was also a friend and asked for advice about how to help Michael. The infant specialist recommended that the mother take time off from work and told her to anticipate and respond to expectable behavioral regressions such as increased clinginess and night wakings. During the following week, Michael was particularly sensitized to his mother being out of his sight and responded with crying, which quickly subsided when he was held. He woke up crying during the nights and was promptly brought to his parents' bed, where he fell asleep easily until the next morning. He whimpered when his bandages were changed but did not seem to be in pain during the rest of the time. He did become more demanding and forceful in his signals, but he ate well and continued to take pleasure in play. The mother kept in touch with the infant specialist over the phone, but Michael's manageable intensity of response and quick return to normative functioning precluded the need for further intervention.

Individual Child Psychotherapy with Collateral Sessions with the Parents

This modality is recommended in three circumstances: (1) when the parent is unable to tolerate a therapeutic focus on the child because of his or her psychological makeup or personal traumatic stress response; (2) when the child is unable to give expression to the traumatic experiences in front of the parent because of fear of hurting the parent's feelings or fear of the parent; and (3) when the child needs help in attaining greater autonomy and social competence because of excessive reliance on the parent and corresponding parental overprotectiveness. Under these conditions, collateral sessions need to be built into the child's treatment in order to enhance the parent's ability to respond to the child's developmental needs.

Example. Ben, age 3½, witnessed severe episodes of marital violence where his father kicked and punched the mother and then threw her against the wall. After the parents separated, the mother asked for assessment and treatment of the child because of Ben's lack of language and social withdrawal in preschool. The preschool teacher reported that Ben stayed by himself the whole day, did not approach his peers, and turned his back on other children when they tried to engage him. He allowed the teacher, a very gentle and affectionate man, to be near him but did not initiate interaction with him. The mother reported that Ben spoke clearly and was friendly and affectionate when he was alone with her. This report was confirmed during the assessment, when Ben was observed from behind a one-way mirror talking freely and playing with his mother when he was alone with her but was silent and reserved while the male assessor was in the room.

Treatment started with sessions involving Ben, his mother, and the therapist, where he was encouraged to play with a range of toys that included a family of dolls, figures of baby animals and their parents, blocks, and drawing materials. The therapist and the mother jointly explained to Ben that the mother did not want to live with Ben's father because he did scary things that hurt the mother and frightened Ben. The mother added that Ben's father loved the child but had not learned how to be angry without hurting the mother and scaring Ben. Ben listened attentively but did not respond. His behavior was painfully inhibited during these sessions. His movements were slow and deliberate, his facial expression was blank, and he did not speak.

After approximately six weekly sessions, the clinician told Ben that he wanted to spend time alone with him so that Ben could learn that he and his mother would be safe even when they were away from each other. The therapist explained that the mother would be in the next room and would watch Ben and the therapist through the one-way mirror. Ben listened quietly as the therapist spoke, but did not respond. He followed the mother to the door as she prepared to leave, but he did not protest her departure after she said, "I'll be back," and closed the door behind her.

The decision to see Ben individually was based on the observation that he suffered from a massive constriction of affect that affected every area of his development. He recoiled from any reminder of conflict or anger, and relied on his mother's unfailing sensitivity and attunement to his needs to feel safe. When he was away from her, he was bereft of autonomous skills to cope with what he perceived as a dangerous and unpredictable world.

For the ensuing 6 months, the therapist and Ben spent part of each session together while the mother watched through the one-way mirror. After 40 minutes the mother returned, and for the final 20 minutes of the session all three met together, playing and discussing what Ben and the therapist had done. The sessions between Ben and the therapist focused on helping Ben tolerate gradually increasing amounts of excitement and affect through play. The therapist read feeling books with him, asked him playfully to repeat feeling words and to name objects, had puppets speak among themselves and to Ben about being "sad, mad, and glad" as they enacted lively social encounters, and encouraged physical activity (within the constraints of the playroom) by tossing a ball back and forth and responding with heightened expressions of pleasure or frustration to getting the ball or missing it. Very gradually, Ben's affective repertoire increased. Although he remained a basically quiet and reserved little boy by the end of treatment, he made one friend at preschool and began to speak in short sentences to his teacher. His mother was hopeful that she could continue to encourage his development on her own by becoming less solicitous and overresponsive and by encouraging him to try new things on his own instead of doing them for him.

It was noteworthy that Ben never used the play props to enact the scenes of violence that he witnessed between his father and his mother. The therapist made the decision not to take the initiative in encouraging symbolic reenactment for fear of increasing Ben's self-protective emotional withdrawal by making the sessions feel dangerous to him. On follow-up 6 months after the termination of treatment, Ben's mother reported that he continued to progress slowly in becoming more sociable at school.

Child–Parent Model

The presence of the parent during the treatment of traumatized infants, toddlers, and preschoolers is well documented in the literature (Gaensbauer

& Siegel, 1995). It has the purpose of incorporating into the treatment the parent's knowledge of the traumatic event and of the child's reaction to it, using the parent's presence as a source of comfort during the sessions and helping the parent participate in the therapeutic reworking of the traumatic experience. When significant problems in the parent–child relationship preceded the traumatic event or contributed to it, the preferred mode of treatment is infant–parent psychotherapy (Fraiberg, 1980; Lieberman, 1999; Lieberman, Silverman, & Pawl, 2000) or child–parent psychotherapy (Lieberman & Van Horn, 1998) in order to foster the caregiving conditions necessary to enhance and maintain the child's mental health. The therapeutic focus of these relationship-based interventions is on helping the child regain developmental momentum by promoting a psychological partnership between the child and the parent where the child's reality testing, capacity for relatedness, affect regulation, and readiness to learn are supported by the parent's increased ability to provide concrete protection and emotional reciprocity (Lieberman, Compton, et al., 2003).

Example. Antonia, 30 months old, was referred for treatment because she showed physical aggression toward her mother, excessive separation anxiety, and multiple fears following numerous scenes of loud fighting between her parents, accompanied by pushing and shoving, which culminated in her mother's suicide attempt. Although Antonia had not witnessed the suicide attempt, which took place outside the house, she overheard agitated talk between her father and his relatives in which the words "killing herself" and "dead" were repeatedly used. The mother was hospitalized for a week, and Antonia did not see her during that time. The referral was made 6 months after the mother's discharge from the hospital by the child's pediatrician.

The first assessment session consisted of an individual meeting with the mother, where she reported that when Antonia first saw her after her discharge, the child screamed at her, "You are crazy! You died! You killed yourself!" The verbal skills of this young child were clearly very advanced, and she was echoing what she heard her father and her aunt say in her presence. During this first reunion, which took place in the family home, the mother was accompanied by a policeman, who stood by as the mother retrieved Antonia's things and then took Antonia and the mother to their new home. The father was present but did not interfere. By the mother's report, Antonia looked very sad and had big dark circles under her eyes. She had been pining for her mother all through the week, and it seemed as if she had not been given a reassuring explanation of what had happened by her father and aunt, who were too self-absorbed in their pain and anger to be aware of the child's experience.

Antonia saw her father frequently, and the visits went apparently well. However, he was distraught about his wife's leaving him, and 3 months after she left he broke into a family gathering to beg her to return home. He became increasingly more threatening when she refused, the police were called, and he was handcuffed and taken away while screaming out of control. Antonia witnessed this scene and was very upset by it, crying and asking if her father was being hurt. After this scene, the father started psychotherapy and psychotropic medication, and calmed down considerably. Antonia spent weekends with him, and the mother reported that the child enjoyed spending time with her father.

Antonia's symptoms included acute separation anxiety when leaving both her mother and her father. She insisted on sleeping with her mother, having her mother's arms wrapped tightly around her. If the mother interrupted physical contact, Antonia woke up crying until the mother held her tightly again. During the day, she showed intense aggression toward her mother. She hit and bit the mother, and called her "crazy" and "dead." One time she took a kitchen knife and lunged at her mother, saying "I kill you!" She was hypervigilant and remembered vividly the two scenes where policemen came to the home. Whenever there was an unusual noise, she stopped what she was doing and asked anxiously, "Is that the police?" She often said that she hated the police and that she would kill the police.

Treatment consisted of weekly joint sessions with Antonia, the mother, and the therapist; collateral meetings with the mother took place every other week. Treatment lasted 6 months and took place in the home because the mother was in the final months of pregnancy and transportation was difficult. Two sessions will be reported: the first joint session and a session from the middle of treatment.

In the first session, the therapist set up a doll family constellation comprising the mother doll, father doll, a girl doll, and a baby doll. Antonia moved quickly to the dolls, held each doll in turn, and said, "This is my mommy, this is my daddy, this is me, this is my baby brother." She had the mother and father dolls lie together, holding hands, then put the father doll in another part of the room, saying "He has another house." She then switched to scribbling with crayons on a piece of paper, which she gave to the mother, saying: "This is a drawing to tell you that I love you very much." She looked at the therapist, pointed to her mother, and said, "She killed herself." Then she took the mother doll and dropped her from up high several times, saying "She fell." After this she said that she would throw all the toys away and scrambled them together. The therapist commented that things can get very messy but they can get better again, adding that she would help Antonia and her mother. The child listened quietly and then proceeded to put the dolls together one next to the other, singing a lullaby.

In this first session, Antonia spontaneously presented the major emotional themes of her life: her wish to have her parents live together in harmony, her father's departure, her love and anger at her mother, her worry about the mother's suicide attempt and the ensuing falling apart of the family, and her hope for reparation. She also incorporated her unborn baby brother as an integral part of the family. This session illustrates the importance of letting children describe their own internal states without prejudging where the focus of treatment needs to be. Like many traumatized children, Antonia showed a remarkable ability to understand the therapist's job of helping to cope with difficult feelings, and she became an ally in her own treatment.

During the first 8 weeks of treatment, Antonia's conflicted feelings of love, anger, and worry toward her mother were the most salient themes of the sessions. During the session, the therapist helped the mother explain to Antonia that she had hurt herself but that she was not crazy and was not dead. The mother also told Antonia that she was sorry that she could not see Antonia when she was in the hospital, that she missed her, and that she would not leave her again. During the collateral sessions with the mother, the therapist helped her find firm ways of stopping and redirecting Antonia's aggression toward her in the course of everyday life. Antonia's separation anxiety and her aggression toward her mother declined significantly during this period, and she began to use words to say she was angry at her mother.

At the end of the second month of treatment, the father's frightening side appeared in the sessions, along with Antonia's ambivalent love and sense of responsibility for protecting him. In one play scene, the Antonia doll did not want to go to the father's house. She said, "A wolf lives there. If I don't go, the police won't come." But in the next scene, the police did come. Antonia yelled, "The police is here. I don't like the police. I will kill the police." She stamped and trampled on the invisible police, and asked the therapist to help her. She smiled in delight when the therapist joined in trampling the police, but she soon became anxious and asked worriedly, "The police is not really here, right?" The therapist answered, "No, it is a game." Antonia relaxed and gleefully continued the game, at times pretending to be Superman to have total power over the police. At the end of the session, she drew the father's house and asked the therapist to put locks in it. "What are the locks for?" asked the therapist. "So that the police won't come," said Antonia. This session represented Antonia's disguised fear of her father and her simultaneous wish to protect him from the police, including the wish to be as strong as Superman to do away with the danger.

During the next 4 months, the themes of detecting anger and trampling and killing the source of danger continued unabated, largely uninterrupted by the birth of Antonia's baby brother, to which she responded with an appropriate range of affect that was remarkably well modulated. Antonia was clearly preoccupied by her own internal struggles involving her mother and her father and the violent scenes that she witnessed. The external reality of the baby brother did little to divert her from her efforts to master the psychological tasks that were most salient for her, namely, integrating her love for her father with her fear of his aggression. Neverthe-less, Antonia did spend at least part of each session after her brother's birth playing out scenes of putting a baby doll in the trash and then throwing it away. This interweaving of developmentally appropriate themes and con-cerns with reworking of the trauma is a regular feature of children's treat-ment.

The therapist's role consisted of supporting Antonia's freedom to play, reassuring the mother that this was a necessary component of the child's re-covery when the mother became frightened by the intensity of the child's emotions. The therapist sometimes translated the symbolic themes into the real-life scenes that Antonia had witnessed, but Antonia showed little inter-est in these translations. Working on the symbolic realm seemed the appro-priate course of action for her. After 4 months of active work on themes of aggression and punishment, the tone of the sessions began to change. The play acquired a more domestic character, with daily routines of cooking, feeding the baby, and going to market taking center stage. The mother and father dolls were used interchangeably as caregiving figures. Simulta-neously, Antonia's symptoms of hypervigilance decreased noticeably. As the theme of ending treatment was brought up, Antonia's gains were main-tained and games of hide-and-seek took up major portions of the session. During the last session, Antonia said, "I'm sad you are leaving. Will you write to me?" This ability to express feeling and her wonderful faith in the continuity of relationships bode well for Antonia's future emotional health.

Mental Health Child-Care Consultation

The child's traumatic response might be exacerbated by child-care practices that are not geared to the child's individual needs or continue to expose the child to traumatic reminders. Group practices, such as napping time or shared toileting, might elicit in the traumatized child strong responses that may seem disruptive or developmentally inappropriate when the child-care providers are not aware of the child's trauma experience. Informed child-care providers can be powerful allies in helping children recover from trau-ma. When the home setting is unpredictable or harshly punitive, the child-care setting can become a safe haven when the providers are responsive to the child's emotional needs.

Mental health consultation in the child-care setting needs to be guided by confidentiality considerations that are worked out collaboratively with the parents. Within this framework of agreements about what is private and what can be shared, the clinician can inform the child-care provider about developmentally predictable responses to trauma and about the child's individual responses in particular. By finding meaning in the child's outbursts of anger, social avoidance, or other seemingly inappropriate be-haviors, the child-care provider can become more appropriately responsive, both in her management of the child's behavior in the moment and in organizing the child's daily routine in ways that minimize exposure to traumatic reminders.

Observation of the child in the child-care setting helps the clinician gain valuable information about the range of the child's responses to trauma and the extent and manifestations of developmental impairment. When appropriate, therapeutic interventions in the child-care setting help the child in the moment and provide a model for the caregiver about how to intervene in response to aggressive, unmodulated, or disruptive behavior. When the child's behavior is consistently disruptive, interventions such as a "shadow" in the form of a companion that anticipates, prevents, and responds to inappropriate behavior can be implemented.

Example. Mental health consultation to the preschool was an integral component of the treatment of Ben, 3½ years old (see the earlier subsection on individual child psychotherapy). The therapist visited Ben's child-care classroom to observe his behavior and spoke with Ben's teacher about the child's behavior in the classroom and at home. The therapist found out that the teacher made a practice of staying close to Ben during the day but did not attempt to entice Ben into group activities for fear of appearing to single him out and making him self-conscious. The therapist described Ben's fear of taking the initiative for fear that it would trigger an angry reaction in the adult. Using this information as an organizing principle, the preschool teacher decided to become active in encouraging Ben's social engagement, explicitly inviting him to join an activity and staying near him during the activity in order to support and prolong Ben's ability to stay engaged.

Therapeutic Commonalities across Treatment Modalities

A common thread across different early trauma treatment modalities is the dual focus on the child's individual functioning and on the child's relationships. In concrete terms, this dual focus involves addressing the specific caregiving routines that have been disrupted by the trauma, with the goal of increasing a harmonious reciprocity between the child and the caregivers in going through daily life. Different approaches may give preeminence to either the individual or the relationship dimension, and a particular focus might predominate within any one modality when one of the dimensions is particularly salient in the child's experience. Saxe and Grant-Knight (2002) consider this dual focus in terms of two dimensions: (1) a gradient of neurobiological dysregulation and (2) a gradient of social-environmental instability. Within the interplay between these two dimensions, Saxe and Grant-Knight describe five phases of treatment: "surviving," "stabilizing," "enduring," "understanding," and "transcending" the trauma. These treatment phases are guided by goals that are consistent with those described by Marmar et al. (1993) of encouraging a return to normal development, establishing safety, tolerating and regulating emotion, placing the trauma in the perspective of a broader life experience, and deriving meaning from the traumatic experience. Simultaneous attention to the child's individual functioning and to the matrix of the child's interpersonal relationships and broader ecological context are essential in achieving these therapeutic goals.

Another commonality among different approaches to early trauma treatment is the integration of intervention strategies that address body sensations, feelings, and cognitions. The growing evidence for alterations in brain structure and function following trauma provides support for van der Kolk's (1994) position that "the body keeps the score" by continuing to respond with stress reactions long after the trauma is past. For this reason, interventions that focus on bringing a calm alignment of the body and the mind can be very helpful. When used with young children, these interventions teach the child relaxation, self-discipline, and spiritual practices that can become lifelong sources of comfort. Young children can be remarkably adept at learning yoga, guided breathing, meditation, and prayer when these are introduced and practiced in age-appropriate ways. Massage and safe and affectionate forms of touching can give the child new trust in body sensations. Martial arts training can help the child discharge and channel aggressive impulses in consciously modulated ways. When also conducted by the parents, these or other practices can create a shared experience where the parent and the child work together to endure, cope with, and transcend the disorganizing impact of the trauma. The use of psychotropic medication is recommended by some practitioners when the child is in acute distress and unable to profit initially from other interventions, although the side effects and long-term consequences of medicating very young children are not known (Gaensbauer & Siegel, 1995; Harmon & Riggs, 1996).

Identifying traumatic reminders and helping the child respond more adaptively to them is another common thread across therapeutic modalities. This work can take a variety of forms. Removing a specific traumatic reminder from the child's environment is the most parsimonious way of helping a distraught child in an acute phase of trauma reaction. For example, a 3-year-old who slept with her mother developed severe nightmares and sleep terror after her mother died and she continued to sleep in the same bed, now with her grandmother. Moving to a different bedroom had a beneficial effect on this child's sleeping patterns. When removing a traumatic reminder is not feasible, the intervention needs to aim at enhancing the child's ability to cope more adaptively with exposure to it. Strategies may involve gradual exposure for the purpose of desensitization, helping the child make the connection between the traumatic reminder and the original trauma, anticipating her reactions in being exposed to the reminder, and practicing coping strategies such as "telling" the traumatic reminder what is on her mind.

Finally, versatility in the use of therapeutic tools is a characteristic of most early trauma treatment. As mentioned earlier, body–mind interventions such as massage, physical contact, martial arts practice, breathing, meditation, and prayer are natural adjuncts to other therapeutic strategies. Other tools involve play with evocative and therapeutic toys; games that evoke or repair childhood stresses, such as peek-a-boo and hide-and-seek; drawing experiences relevant to the child's life; reading age-appropriate books about feelings and trauma; storytelling with relevant themes that end in ways that offer hope; making feeling charts; and dictating and writing letters describing the child's feelings. The list of possibilities is inexhaustible, limited only by the therapist's and the child's creative imagination.

In conclusion, the treatment of early trauma is, like all therapeutic interventions, a deeply collaborative endeavor between the child, the family, and the intervenor. Common threads have emerged in the course of decades of clinical practice and research that stress the importance of a focus on establishing safety, restoring developmental momentum, and maintaining a dual focus on the child's individual functioning and on the child's matrix of interpersonal relationships. Within these commonalities, each treatment represents a unique effort among the participants to create a joint narrative that will help the child and the family give meaning to the traumatic experience and integrate it within the larger context of their lives.

REFERENCES

Ainsworth, M. D., Blehar, M., Waters, E., & Walls, S. (1979). *Patterns of attachment.* Hillsdale, NJ: Erlbaum.

American Psychiatric Association. (1994). *Diagnostic and statistical manual of mental disorders* (4th ed.). Washington DC: Author.

Beeghly, M., & Cicchetti, D. (1987). An organizational approach to symbolic development in children with Down syndrome. *New Directions for Child Development, 36,* 5–29.

Beeghly, M., & Cicchetti, D. (1994). Child maltreatment, attachment, and the self-system: Emergence of an internal state lexicon in toddlers at high social risk. *Development and Psychopathology, 6,* 5–30.

Bowlby, J. (1973). *Attachment and loss: Vol. 2. Separation.* New York: Basic Books.

Bowlby, J. (1980). *Attachment and loss: Vol. 3. Loss, sadness and depression.* New York: Basic Books.

Cicchetti, D., & Barnett, D. (1991). Toward the development of a scientific nosology of child maltreatment. In W. Grove & D. Cicchetti (Eds.), *Thinking clearly about psychology: Essays in honor of Paul E. Meehl: Vol. 2. Personality and psychopathology* (pp. 346–377). Minneapolis: University of Minnesota Press.

Cicchetti, D., & Cohen, D. J. (Eds.). (1995). *Developmental psychopathology: Vol. 2. Risk, disorder, and adaptation.* New York:Wiley.

Cicchetti, D., & Howes, P. W. (1991). Developmental psychopathology in the context of the family: Illustrations from the study of child maltreatment. *Canadian Journal of Behavioural Science, 23*(3), 257–281.

Cohen, J. A., Perel, J. M., DeBellis, M. D., Friedman, M. J., & Putman, F. W. (2002). Treating traumatized children: Clinical implications of the psychobiology of PTSD. *Trauma, Violence and Abuse, 3,* 91–108.

Drell, M. J., Gaensbauer, T. J., Siegel, C. H., & Sugar, M. (1995). Clinical round table: A case of trauma to a 21–month-old girl. *Infant Mental Health Journal, 16*(4), 318–333.

Emde, R. N., Bingham, R. D., & Harmon, R. J. (1993). Classification and the diagnostic process in infancy. In C. H. Zeanah (Ed.), *Handbook of infant mental health* (pp. 225–235). New York: Guilford Press.

Erickson, M. F., Egeland, B., & Pianta, R. (1989). The effects of maltreatment on the development of young children. In D. Cicchetti & V. Carlson (Eds.), *Child maltreatment: Theory and research on the causes and consequences of child abuse and neglect* (pp. 647–684). New York: Cambridge University Press.

Fivush, R. (1994). *Long-term retention of infant memories.* London: Erlbaum.

Fraiberg, S. (Ed.). (1980). *Clinical studies in infant mental health.* New York: Basic Books.

Furman, E. (1974). *A child's parent dies: Studies in childhood bereavement.* New Haven, CT: Yale University Press.

Gaensbauer, T. J. (1995). Trauma in the preverbal period: Symptoms, memories, and developmental impact. *Psychoanalytic Study of the Child, 50,* 122–149.

Gaensbauer, T. J., & Siegel, C. H. (1995). Therapeutic approaches to posttraumatic stress disorder in infants and toddlers. *Infant Mental Health Journal, 16*(4), 292–305.

Harmon, R. J., & Riggs, P. D.(1996). Clonidine for post-traumatic stress disorder in preschool children. *Journal of the American Academy of Child and Adolescent Psychiatry, 35*(9), 1247–1249.

Kleinman, A. (1980). *Patients and healers in the context of culture.* Berkeley: University of California Press.

Laor, N., Wolmer, L., & Cohen, D. J. (2001). Mother's functioning and children's symptoms 5 years after a SCUD missile attack. *American Journal of Psychiatry, 158*(2), 1020–1026.

Lieberman, A. F. (1999). Negative maternal attributions: Effects on toddlers' sense of self. *Psychoanalytic Inquiry, 19,* 737–756.

Lieberman, A. F., Compton, N., Van Horn, P., & Ghosh Ippen, C. (2003). *Losing a parent to death in the early years: Guidelines for the treatment of traumatic bereavement in infancy and early childhood.* Washington, DC: Zero to Three Press.

Lieberman, A. F., Silverman, R., & Pawl, J. H. (2000). Infant–parent psychotherapy: Core concepts and recent developments. In C. H. Zeanah (Ed.), *Handbook of infant mental health* (2nd ed., pp. 472–484). New York: Guilford Press.

Lieberman, A. F., & Van Horn, P. (1998). Attachment, trauma, and domestic violence: Implications for child custody. *Child and Adolescent Psychiatric Clinics of North America, 7*(2), 423–443.

Lieberman, A. F., Van Horn, P., & Ozer, E. (2003). *Preschooler witnesses of marital violence: Predictors and mediators of child behavior problems.* Manuscript in preparation.

Linares, L. O., Heeren, T., Bronfman, E., Zuckerman, B., Augustyn, M., & Tronick, E. (2001). A mediational model for the impact of exposure to community violence on early child behavior problems. *Child Development, 72,* 639–652.

Main, M., & George, C. (1985). Response of abused and disadvantaged toddlers to distress in agemates: A study in the day care setting. *Developmental Psychology, 21,* 407–412.

Marans, S., & Adelman, A. (1997). Experiencing violence in a developmental context. In J. D. Osofsky (Ed.), *Children in a violent society* (pp. 202–222). New York: Guilford Press.

Marmar, C., Foy, D., Kagan, B., & Pynoos, R. S. (1993). An integrated approach for treating posttraumatic stress. In J. M. Oldham, & A. Talman (Eds.), *American Psychiatric Association review of psychiatry* (Vol. 12, pp. 238–272). Washington, DC: American Psychiatric Press.

National Center on Child Abuse and Neglect. (1995). *Study findings: National study of incidence and severity of child abuse and neglect.* Washington, DC: U.S. Department of Health, Education, and Welfare.

Nelson, C. A. (1994). Neural correlates of recognition memory in the first postnatal year of life. In G. Dawson & K. Fischer (Eds.), *Human behavior and the developing brain* (pp. 269–313). New York: Guilford Press.

Osofsky, J. D. (Ed.). (1997a). *Children in a violent society.* New York: Guilford Press.

Osofsky, J. D. (1997b). Community-based approaches to violence prevention. *Journal of Developmental and Behavioral Pediatrics, 18*(6), 405–407.

Pynoos, R. S. (1990). Posttraumatic stress disorder in children and adolescents. In B. D. Garfinkel, G. A. Carlson, E. B. Weller, & B. F. Weller (Eds.), *Psychiatric disorders in children and adolescents.* Philadelphia: Saunders.

Pynoos, R. S., & Nader, D. (1993). Issues in the treatment of post-traumatic stress in children and adolescents. In J. P. Wilson & B. Raphael (Eds.), *International handbook of traumatic stress syndromes* (pp. 535–549). New York: Plenum.

Pynoos, R. S., Steinberg, A. M., & Piacentini, J. C. (1999). A developmental psychopathology model of childhood traumatic stress and intersection with anxiety disorders. *Biological Psychiatry, 46,* 1542–1554.

Pynoos, R. S., Steinberg, A. M., & Wraith, R. (1995). A developmental model of childhood traumatic stress. In D. Cicchetti & D. Cohen (Eds.), *Manual of developmental psychopathology: Vol. 2. Risk, disorder, and adaptation* (pp. 72–95). New York: Wiley.

Saxe, G. N., & Grant-Knight, W. (2002). *Proceedings of the annual meeting of the International Society of Traumatic Stress Studies,* Baltimore.

Schacter, D. L. (1987). Implicit memory: History and current status. *Journal of Experimental Psychology: Learning, Memory, and Cognition, 13*(3), 501–518.

Shalev, A. Y. (1996). Stress vs. traumatic stress: From acute homeostatic reactions to chronic psychopathology. In B. A. van der Kolk, A. C. MacFarlane, & L. Weisaeth (Eds.), *Traumatic stress* (pp. 77–101). New York: Guilford Press.

Shonkoff, J., & Phillips, D. (2000). *From neurons to neighborhoods: The study of early childhood development.* Washington, DC: National Academy Press.

Stern, D. N. (1985). *The interpersonal world of the infant: A view form psychoanalysis and developmental psychology.* New York: Basic Books.

Sugar, M. (1992). Toddlers' traumatic memories. *Infant Mental Health Journal, 13*(3), 245–251.

Terr, L. C. (1988). The child psychiatrist and the child witness: Traveling companions by necessity, if not by design. *Annual Progress in Child Psychiatry and Child Development, 1987* (pp. 327–348). New York: Brunner/Mazel.

U.S. Department of Health and Human Services. (1994). *Child maltreatment 1992: Reports from the states to the National Center on Child Abuse and Neglect.* Washington, DC: U.S. Government Printing Office.

van der Kolk, B. A. (1994). The body keeps the score: Memory and the evolving psychobiology of posttraumatic stress. *Harvard Review of Psychiatry, 1,* 253–265.

Zero to Three/National Center for Clinical Infant Programs. (1994). *Diagnostic classification of mental health and developmental disorders of infancy and early childhood.* Arlington, VA: Author.

CHAPTER 5

DIAGNOSTIC AND TREATMENT ISSUES IN CASES OF CHILDHOOD TRAUMA

STACY A. KLAPPER
NANCY S. PLUMMER
ROBERT J. HARMON

You walk into the therapeutic preschool and before you can remove your jacket and set down your bag, a 5-year-old boy with whom you have spent less than 3 hours is somehow inextricably attached to your legs, arms extended for you to carry him. He looks up at you and says, "I want a meeting right now!" In the next hour he spends with you, this boy asks you why he doesn't have a mommy and offers you, a relative stranger, the job.

Across the room, expertly ignoring your presence, is the 3-year-old boy you have been trying to entice to interact with you for weeks. He looks warily in your direction and then throws a toy at the wall. When you gently offer to join in his play, he kicks you and runs out of the room.

A girl tugs insistently on your sleeve. She looks at you with an exasperated quality and says in a manner not at all consistent with her 4 years of age, "Did you know that my dad is back in jail AGAIN?!" Then, without taking a breath, she informs you, "When we play today, I want to be the social worker and I'll ask you for your Medicaid card and make all the decisions."

What do these children have in common? While their surface behavior suggests very different temperaments, personalities, and psychological resources, each are reacting to problems that did not originate in them. These are young children who have been exposed to severe abuse and neglect, and who are experiencing symptoms associated with trauma.

In this chapter we discuss assessment and treatment strategies in working with chronically abused and neglected children, a far too common form of trauma perpetrated on unsuspecting and defenseless children. There are, however, other types of "traumatic experiences" that warrant assessment, diagnosis, and treatment. Single-episode traumas include children being bitten by dogs, being involved in car accidents, and falling down stairs or out of windows. All reasonably healthy parents try to keep their children safe. Unfortunately, accidents do happen and children may need treatment for the psychological sequelae. Many of the assessment and treatment plans discussed here are applicable to children who have experienced any type of traumatic experience. Some, as noted, apply primarily to children who have been abused by those entrusted with their care. Other chapters in this volume focus on individual traumatic events and their treatment. In this chapter, we share our experience of having treated abused and neglected children in a therapeutic preschool setting for more than 10 years.

WHAT IS TRAUMA?

Trauma is described in the fourth edition of the *Diagnostic and Statistical Manual of Mental Disorders* (DSM-IV; American Psychiatric Association, 1994) as an event in which a person "experienced, witnessed, or was confronted with an event or events that involved actual or threatened death or serious injury, or a threat to the physical integrity of self or others, and the person's response involved intense fear, helplessness, or horror" (pp. 427–428). In DC: 0–3 (Zero to Three/National Center for Clinical Infant Programs, 1994), the criteria for traumatic stress disorder require children to have "experience[d] a single event, a series of connected traumatic events, or chronic, enduring stress [which] might include an infant or toddler's direct experience, witnessing, or confrontation with an event or events that involve actual or threatened death or serious injury to the child or others, or a threat to the psychological or physical integrity of the child or others" (p. 18).

WHAT TRAUMA IS NOT

In our work collaborating and training others who work with traumatized children, we are often reminded to clarify the abuse definitions of trauma and discuss what we *do not* mean by trauma. "Psychic trauma," "traumatic loss," "traumatic grief," and the impact of the neonatal intensive care unit (NICU) environment on preterm infants are all clinically relevant concepts, but they do not meet criteria for a traumatic event as described above. For better or worse, "trauma" is currently used conversationally to describe many different experiences (i.e., "He was traumatized by what she said to him"; "Team A's overtime loss to team B was traumatic for hometown fans"). We need to keep our clinical focus clear and concise with regard to the specific diagnostic definition (above), not the vernacular. While the definition of trauma adheres to a specific diagnostic description, the experience of trauma in young children has repercussions on many interconnected areas of development.

A child's experience of the world is inextricably tied to his or her experience in relationships (Bowlby, 1982; Kohut, 1966; Stern, 1985). When caregivers are unpredictable, abusive, or unavailable, children understand this adult behavior as a reflection of themselves. It is both too painful and too cognitively sophisticated a task for young children to differentiate the actions of powerful adult figures from the way these actions make them feel. A child does not easily separate the idea that "Mommy is having a bad day" from the feeling that "It's my fault." Young children are more likely to assume that their abusive or neglectful circumstances result from them being too demanding, too needy, or simply not worthy of having their basic needs met, rather than accept and understand that their caretaker lacks the capacity to be appropriately responsive. Through repeated interactions over time, the way a child feels in important relationships becomes a blueprint for the ongoing development of a sense of self (Bowlby, 1982; Kohut, 1966). This "internal working model" of relationships (Bretherton & Waters, 1985; Sroufe, Carlson, Levy, & Egeland, 1999) sets the stage for later relationship patterns.

The impact of trauma on a child's sense of self is expressed in different ways in different children. Not every child who has been exposed to trauma will exhibit symptoms. Research on resiliency suggests that there are important individual differences that moderate the effects of trauma. Werner (2000) found that physical attractiveness, intelligence, and the availability of at least one nurturing relationship all serve a protective function for children. In children who do exhibit symptoms, these symptoms are likely to be expressed in different ways according to the unique biopsychosocial makeup of the child. The child who seeks out any available attachment figure to have his needs met looks quite different from the child who carefully avoids intimacy and connectedness in an effort to protect himself from further pain. These children are using strategies to make sense of the world around them. While the first child may be described as "indiscriminant" and the second child "avoidant," both have developed ideas about what to expect in relationships that shape their interactions (Ainsworth, 1973; Bowlby,

1982). These strategies allow the child to manage anxious feelings by producing expected reactions in relationships. For example, a child who is accustomed to caregivers responding punitively is likely to test limits in a way that provokes harsh discipline from others. A child who has been neglected may seek to gain control over her environment by adopting a self-contained, pseudomature attitude that discourages others from offering age-appropriate nurturance and warmth. These strategies are employed in the service of a biologically driven need for relationships. In describing the impact of parent–child interventions on relational functioning, Lieberman, Silverman, and Pawl (1993) note that "changes in maladaptive internal representations of the self in relation to attachment are hypothesized to occur both in the parent and in the baby through the transformational power of the therapeutic relationship, insight-oriented interpretation, and the acquisition of new interactive and caregiving behavioral patterns" (p. 476). A relational model of intervention bases its foundation on the research on attachment and relies on a careful process of assessment and diagnosis of problematic relational patterns.

DIAGNOSTIC PROCESS AND CONSIDERATIONS

In diagnosing and treating childhood trauma, a detailed early history is a valuable starting point. Gathering specific information not just about the pregnancy, birth, and achievement of developmental milestones but about early relationships opens a door through which the clinician can engage the family in "wondering together" about elements that may have contributed to the child's development moving offtrack. Many caregivers are not aware about the importance of relationships in early brain development or about the range of emotions present from infancy. The process of taking a careful early history allows the clinician to educate caregivers while obtaining solid diagnostic information.

Often, when clinicians are working with children who have been abused and neglected, a detailed early history is difficult to obtain or simply not available. As a result, clinicians rely on the feelings evoked in interactions with these children as one element of obtaining diagnostic information. As a child marshals his particular relational strategy, the clinician pays attention to the feelings that get stirred up in the dynamic. This countertransference yields data about the child's relational expectancies and may shed some light on the way he has made sense of his relationships and environment. It is then the job of the clinician to offer the child a new model of relationships that provides a different experience and lays the foundation for a new interactional strategy. Unfortunately, this reworking of internal models does not happen quickly, and a child may escalate with provocative behaviors to test the security of the new relational model.

A diagnostic evaluation with a young child often centers on strategies of observation. The clinician makes decisions about diagnosis and treatment primarily based on what is observed in the interaction between the child and the caregivers. Additional information obtained through the clinician's interactions with the child and through the child's reactions to play scenarios and free play, as well as from collateral informants (such as teachers, day care providers, or extended family members), offers a rich source of data that can contribute to a working picture of the child's strengths and challenges. Particularly when trauma is part of the evaluation question, it is important to move beyond the report of problematic behaviors to assess how presenting symptoms may have been impacted by disruptive events.

Most young children present to a psychiatric treatment setting due to disruptive behaviors (Frankel, Klapper, & Harmon, 2002). As a result, the primary complaint often centers on aggression or acting out. Particularly for children who lack solid language skills, acting out becomes their most effective tool for securing adult attention. Uncovering the meaning of the disruptive behavior may provide answers to diagnostic questions. For a clinician, it is generally helpful to allow three to five sessions to complete a diagnostic evaluation (Harmon, 1995a, 1995b). The clinician needs to manage the family's anxiety about finding a solution and engage them in the discovery process. Often, families come to treatment because they are feeling hopeless and they want immediate results. It can be useful to communicate to families that the problems took time to develop and they will take time to resolve. Assisting the family in thinking about early events and developmental processes is likely to provide them with a renewed sense of competence and control. Rather than jumping in with a solution (which may or may not fit with family values, culture, or dynamics), it is important to structure several observations and conduct a thorough assessment that encourages collaborative thinking. This collaborative framework allows the assessment period to combine with a treatment process and may help the family accept the diagnostic formulation. In this way, the initial assessment period becomes a part of the therapeutic intervention. Assisting families in understanding the development of psychological problems encourages a reflective process. Setting the groundwork for openness to reflection allows both the family and the clinician to move beyond the surface presentation of behavior to address underlying causes.

Disruptive behavioral symptoms, when described in the absence of multiple observations and a careful developmental history, can lead the diagnostic process awry. For example, an aggressive child who moves impulsively from toy to toy without keeping focus or sustained interest may be revealing difficulties with impulse control, inattention, poor motor planning, or anxiety. Observing the child's behavior in different relationships over several sessions allows the clinician to clarify diagnostic hypotheses and is likely to result in more appropriate treatment planning. Assigning a diagnosis based on disruptive behavior or acting out may hide other prominent symptoms such as depression or anxiety.

The following case vignette provides a short example of a clinical presentation that may lead in very different diagnostic directions. A 4-year-old boy runs excitedly to the play therapy room. He opens the toy cabinet and pulls out containers of toys, seemingly not caring when they land on his head. He clumsily walks over the scattered toys, falling repeatedly, and then begins to climb on top of the furniture. When you intervene to provide structure in the form of discussing rules about safety, this boy begins to cry and bang his head against the floor. You gather him in your lap and attempt to calm him. The boy struggles away from you and hides under the table, where he rocks himself into a tight ball and cries, "I'm bad" in poorly articulated speech.

An examination of this boy's behavior might lead a clinician down several different diagnostic pathways. His clumsiness could suggest difficulties with motor planning or motor development. His head banging and negative self-appraisal might reveal a depressive process. His scattered behavior and impulsivity looks like difficulties with attention and concentration. His avoidance of relational closeness and comfort might be tied to an attachment problem. His poor articulation suggests a speech delay. Lacking background information about the history that helped to create this boy's current presentation, the clinician may feel overwhelmed by the array of symptoms presented.

If clinicians focus only on symptoms, they may not really understand the underlying diagnostic condition that they are treating. Young children only have a certain repertoire of behavior to express distress, regardless of etiology. As language development expands their ability to express feelings and describe events, they can more specifically communicate to their evaluator and facilitate the diagnostic process. Since crying, aggression (i.e., hitting, biting, bullying), sleep problems, anger, and oppositionality are common to most, if not all, psychological disorders in young children, it is helpful to organize clinical thinking to help us focus on the diagnostic process. The *Diagnostic Classification of Mental Health and Developmental Disorders of Infancy and Early Childhood* (DC: 0–3; Zero to Three/National Center for Clinical Infant Programs, 1994) is one such framework through which a clinician can organize the diagnostic process enabling the evaluator to develop an appropriate treatment plan.

One of the strengths of DC: 0–3 is the emphasis that it takes three to five sessions in order to adequately assess a child within the family, social, community, and cultural context in which young children live (Harmon, 1995a, 1995b). The diagnostic system offers us guidelines to follow as we consider the underlying etiologies of difficult disorders, so we do not forget or neglect important diagnostic considerations. It is beyond the scope of this chapter to discuss the diagnostic process and the details of DC: 0–3 (see Harmon, 1995a, 1995b; Zero to Three/National Center for Clinical Infant Programs, 1994), but we hope to attune readers to the complexity of the diagnostic process with young children.

As the above case vignette illustrates, history taking can be very difficult in young children presenting for assessment, particularly when they have been removed from their family or abandoned. In our work, we believe strongly that to diagnose trauma in young children, there must be clear evidence of a traumatic event that is visibly distressing to the child (i.e., recurring and intrusive memories or distressing dreams of the traumatic event, or behavior as though the traumatic event was recurring): The child's behavior needs to meet DSM-IV criteria for posttraumatic stress disorder (PTSD; American Psychiatric Association, 1994) or DC: 0–3 criteria for traumatic stress disorder (see Scheeringa & Gaensbauer, 2000, and Scheeringa, Peebles, Cook, & Zeanah, 2001, and Scheeringa, Zeanah, Myers, & Putnam, 2003, for further discussion of diagnostic criteria for PTSD in young children). Obviously, if a child presents symptoms consistent with traumatic stress disorder and we have no knowledge of the child's history, it can and should be considered as a part of the differential diagnosis.

The diagnostic guidelines or "decision tree" of DC: 0–3 (Zero to Three/National Center for Clinical Infant Programs, 1994) reminds us to consider the following:

1. If there is a clear severe or significant stressor to account for the disordered behavior or emotions, then traumatic stress disorder should be considered initially.
2. If there is a clear constitutionally or maturational-based sensorimotor, processing, organization, or integration difficulty related to the observed maladaptive behavior and/or emotional pattern, then regulatory disorders should be considered initially.
3. If the presenting problems are mild, less than 4 months in duration, and related to a clear environmental event, then adjustment disorder should be considered initially.
4. If there is neither a clear constitutionally or maturationally based vulnerability nor a severe or significant stress/trauma and the problem is not mild, of short duration, and not related to a clear event, then the categories of mood and affect disorders should be considered initially.
5. Disorders of multiple delays, including communication and social relatedness, are distinct and usually involve chronic patterns of maladaptation (e.g., multisystem developmental disorders) and an ongoing pattern of deprivation (e.g., reactive attachment disorder). Even when underlying constitutional or maturational vulnerabilities or clear stressors are present, these disorders should

take precedence over other categories and are exceptions to the above general rules.

6. If the problem is specific to a certain situation or a relationship to a particular person, adjustment disorder and relationship disorder should be considered.
7. If the problem only involves a relationship without other symptoms, use Axis II instead of Axis I.
8. Reactive attachment disorder is appropriate when there is inadequate basic physical, psychological, and emotional care. Concerns about the relationship or attachment are to be considered in the relationship axis or other diagnoses related to the present symptoms.
9. Assess the underlying basis for common symptoms such as feeding and sleep disorders, which may be separate problems, part of various diagnostic categories, an ongoing relationship pattern, or regulatory and multisystem developmental disorders.
10. In complex cases where there are many elements present and it is difficult to make a diagnosis, try to decide what is the most prominent contributing feature or characteristic and follow the above guidelines.

Clearly, these diagnostic guidelines prioritize the consideration of trauma in shaping diagnostic thinking. Historically, it has seemed that adults have had a difficult time acknowledging pain and suffering in young children and actually believing the extent to which children can be maltreated. It is nearly 40 years since the publication of "the Battered-Child Syndrome" by Kempe, Silverman, Steele, Droegemueller, and Silver (1962) and only less than 10 years since a diagnostic system has focused on trauma in young children. Thus, on the one hand, we need to be sure to look for trauma; on the other hand, we should not impose the diagnosis of a traumatic disorder in cases where trauma is not actually present. If we are lacking a detailed early history and information about early relationships, the diagnostic process must expand to include multidisciplinary assessments.

A complete diagnostic assessment should include collaboration between mental health professionals and other developmental specialists. Psychological testing, in particular, meaningfully informs the diagnostic and treatment process by facilitating an understanding of the cognitive capacities of the child and aids in treatment decisions. It can help to determine whether a child's impulsive behavior is the result of low cognitive skills or difficulties with processing, attention, or anxiety. Information about the child's motivation, level of persistence, compliance in new social settings, and frustration tolerance can be obtained from psychological testing as well. Enlisting a psychological examiner who is not the treating clinician also allows for an additional perspective on the child's functioning that may provide important information about the child's ability to form relationships.

A multidisciplinary team approach is effective in developing a more complete picture in the evaluation of traumatized children. An occupational therapist is likely to notice different symptoms than a sensory integrationist. Each different specialization offers an important evaluative piece that can aid in diagnosis and treatment planning. Particularly when we are assessing trauma in children, it is helpful to determine if developmental delays are present. Physical therapy, occupational therapy, and speech language therapy evaluations are often necessary complements to mental health intervention in young children. In the absence of an established multidisciplinary team, it is useful to access community and school-based resources to create such a team, as trauma can impact many interconnected aspects of development.

Other important collaborations include the child's guardian ad litem and the Human Services caseworker in child abuse and family violence cases. Forming relationships with these contacts early in the treatment process can facilitate information sharing and serve to prevent later conflicts. System issues can produce obstacles to therapeutic outcomes for children. Delays in permanency planning, moves to multiple foster homes, and the preference for reunification with biological families combine to bring conflict between clinicians and systems to the forefront. Being aware of feelings that arise in these situations is critical for developing collaborative, rather than conflictual, relationships. It is often the job of the clinician to educate the caseworkers and legal representatives about the potential consequences of moving a child from a stable home or reunifying a child with a family that is unable to meet the child's needs. While external forces may override therapeutic decisions, it is helpful for a clinician to clearly articulate the "pros and cons" as well as the psychological meanings of these decisions regardless of the impact on final outcomes.

TREATMENT APPROACHES AND TECHNIQUES

Working with the traumatized child provides a unique challenge to family intervention and therapy. A therapeutic alliance requires the clinician to enter into the internal world of the patient. Direct involvement with young victims of abuse and neglect provides a window through which evocative feelings arise. Often, these feelings make it difficult for the clinician to expand his or her empathic connection with the patient to include the family who has perpetrated the abuse and/or neglect. The classic article "Ghosts in the Nursery" by Fraiberg, Adelson, and Shapiro (1975) offers a framework and a touchstone for understanding the intergenerational nature of problematic family dynamics. Aligning with an abusive caretaker in the service of treating the child is not always an easy task. However, little progress is likely to be made in the absence of participation from the family. It is important to remember the power of internal working models of relationships in shaping interactions for both the child and the abusive caretaker in order to effectively assist them in adopting more appropriate relationship models and interaction patterns.

In addition to aligning with caretakers, aligning with traumatized children presents a different set of challenges. Traumatized children often behave provocatively, particularly when feeling vulnerable and exposed in new or changing circumstances. Children who have experienced abuse or neglect typically struggle during transition periods. This is evident during transitions to and from therapy sessions. Assisting a child in successful transitioning is a "trial-and-error" proposition; what works for one child may not be effective for another. However, some themes seem to be helpful as a general rule of thumb. Anxious children benefit from knowing what to expect. Giving a child a preview of upcoming events often helps to contain the child's anxious feelings and prevents acting out. For example:

> "OK," you'll say, looking at the clock, "Time to clean up!" This is when the tantrum will start. You'll set limits, and she will begin the negotiations. "Five more minutes," she'll plead. If you give in and agree to extend the session for a few more minutes, she will decide that she is not ready to give back the toy she is playing with and will hide it in her clothing. Now you have a choice: you can engage in a power struggle, which you are bound to lose, or you can try to understand the meaning behind the behavior.

Simply putting feelings into words is a powerful therapeutic intervention. Informing the child that you understand that she does not feel ready to end the session, that it does not seem fair that she is not in control of how long she can meet with you, and that she feels angry because she has to leave can encourage a sense of shared understanding. Providing updates about what is coming can sometimes assist the child in containing anxious feelings. Telling the child that "in five minutes we are going to clean up and return to the classroom" enlists the child in the process of transitioning and can prevent power struggles. Other strategies include finding an agreed upon place to keep a special toy to promote a sense of place and security as well as offering transitional objects, such as a drawing or a borrowed toy, to take home. Creating a "child-friendly" therapy calendar, marking which days the child attends sessions, also allows the child to develop a regular routine and reduces fears about what will happen next. These relatively simple interventions provide experiences of increased control for children who often feel at the mercy of external forces.

Issues of control can also be expressed through therapy avoidance. Some children may feel too anxious to accompany a strange adult into a new setting. In such a case, you, the clinician, might allow the child to proceed on her own timetable. If possible, you might meet the child with her caretakers to enlist them in creating a sense of safety about what it will be like to meet with you. Spending time with the child in her classroom setting would offer a low-stress, nonthreatening way of introducing yourself to the child. Again, clearly established expectations encourage an increased sense of security in anxious children. If therapy refusal continues, you might try trading off being in charge with the child. For example, tell the young child that you will take turns choosing activities: first the child will choose a game, then it is your turn. This both teaches social skills and offers the child some time in the session to be in charge.

Nondirective play therapy is an effective tool in enlisting the avoidant child to participate in therapy. Following the child's lead ensures that therapy will not push the child into painful or retraumatizing material too quickly. It should be noted that nondirective play therapy requires a basic structure when clinicians are working with traumatized children. These children will benefit from knowing that the clinician will not allow behavior to get out of control and that the clinician is capable of assisting them in containing powerful emotional experiences. While aggressive play communicates important aspects of the child's world, aggression toward self or others should not be encouraged. Instead, allow the child to choose a toy to represent the target of aggression. This allows the child to express her feelings without endangering anyone and reduces the temptation to assign a negative value to difficult feelings.

SUMMARY AND CONCLUSIONS

Although child abuse and trauma were brought to the clinical limelight more than 40 years ago, it has not been addressed in a diagnostic system specifically developed for assessing young children until recently. With the increased awareness of child abuse and trauma, the terms "trauma" and "traumatized" have become commonly used words, which has clouded the clinical understanding of what trauma actually is when conducting a diagnostic assessment of a young child. The definitions of trauma in the criteria for PTSD in DSM-IV and for traumatic stress disorder in DC: 0–3 have helped dispel the confusion for clinicians assessing and treating young victims of abuse and other forms of trauma.

Diagnosing and treating trauma in young children can be a multifaceted and challenging situation for the treating clinician. First, these children present themselves and their symptoms in response to trauma in a variety of ways. Second, there may be other factors, such as a physical illness or developmental delay, that interplay with the child's behavior. By utilizing the DC: 0–3 system and decision tree guidelines as well as information gathered related to the child's history and social and cultural contexts, a clinician is able to conduct a complete assessment and determine that the child's behavior is a result of a traumatic event(s).

Most young children do not have the capacity, emotionally or cognitively, to understand the trauma that they have experienced, nor do they have the tools to appropriately handle their resulting feelings and reactions. Due to their developmental level, young children may not be able to separate the actions of their abusing caregiver from their feelings that they are responsible in some way for the trauma that they have endured. Given that their language skills are not well developed and that traumatized children frequently have language delays, young children tend to express themselves through a broad range of maladaptive behavior. This poses a dilemma for the clinician, since it is not possible to obtain information verbally from the child about the traumatic event(s) as a part of the diagnostic assessment. In addition, the clinician must learn not to focus exclusively on the behavioral symptoms and instead try to ascertain the underlying condition causing these symptoms. Since internal working models of relationships provide the foundation for subsequent interaction patterns, it can be difficult to alter the relationship strategies of children who have suffered abuse and neglect. Our therapeutic goal is to help them adopt more adaptive relationship models, particularly if they have not had a nurturing relationship with a caregiver. It is imperative that the clinician individualizes the treatment approach to the child by taking into consideration the child's developmental level, whether there are comorbid conditions affecting the child, and whether the child's relationship and interaction styles are maladaptive and need to be conformed to more suitable models.

As mentioned earlier, developing a collaborative relationship with the caregivers to obtain the child's historical, developmental, and family information is essential. This also gives the clinician the opportunity to educate the caregivers about the importance of early relationships and their impact on cognitive and socioemotional development. The caregivers need to understand that their child's behavior is not going to be resolved immediately and that it will require time to complete a diagnostic evaluation, which would entail gathering information from other caregivers, observing the child interacting with other children and in different settings, and developing a therapeutic relationship so that the child feels safe and comfortable when expressing feelings openly. The clinician can work with the family to consider different techniques for managing the child's behavior at home and in other settings, as well as partnering with families so that they are an integral part of the child's assessment and treatment.

The involvement of other parties outside the family and therapeutic setting may be required. In addition to having experienced trauma, the child may have a physical, developmental, or emotional disorder, which may be contributing to the child's symptomatology and would need to be addressed in the treatment plan. For example, psychological testing may indicate that the child is below the age-appropriate level for cognitive and motor functioning and provide other important diagnostic information. If it appears that the child has a speech/language or motor delay, a subsequent evaluation by a speech or occupational therapist should be completed. If the child's symptoms are not responding to behavior modification techniques and relationship-based therapy and could be better managed through psychopharmacological treatment, the consultation of a child psychiatrist to prescribe and monitor the appropriate medication may be beneficial (Harmon & Riggs, 1996). In addition, legal representatives and caseworkers are often involved in child abuse and neglect cases, addressing legal and family system issues. By contacting and maintaining regular communication with these parties and the multidisciplinary treatment team members, everyone involved in the case is kept apprised of the child's treatment progress and the clinician can be more aware of any developments occurring outside of the therapeutic setting that may impact the child and the treatment plan.

As the diagnostic phase gradually transforms into the treatment phase, it is imperative that the therapist develop and foster therapeutic alliances with the child and the caregivers for the treatment process to be successful. The intervention methods beneficial to a traumatized child include helping the child with transitions and changes in daily routines, encouraging the expression of strong and difficult emotions through play therapy, providing a safe and stable therapeutic environment, and assisting the child to adopt more adaptive relationship models and interaction strategies. A more difficult task for the clinician may be in developing a therapeutic alliance with the child's caretaker, especially if the caretaker perpetrated the abuse and/or neglect. Enlisting the caretaker's and family's involvement in the child's treatment is important in order for progress to be achieved, and it may entail working with the caretaker and other family members to alter their behavior patterns and also adopt more appropriate relationship models.

Clearly, the diagnostic and treatment process of a case involving a young child exposed to trauma does not entail only the treating clinician and the child victim but most likely requires the involvement and collaborative effort of many individuals, including the child's family, the multidisciplinary evaluation team, and possibly representatives from the legal and human services systems. Use of the diagnostic tools, such as the DC: 0–3 system, is also invaluable in order to complete a more comprehensive assessment and diagnostic formulation. The clinician should keep in mind the diagnostic criteria for trauma and should not assign a trauma disorder as the primary diagnosis on the basis of conversational usage of the term "trauma" or when there is no history of a qualifying traumatic event. Once the underlying conditions at the root of the child's symptomatology have been determined, the clinician can utilize the therapeutic techniques described earlier to help the child overcome the disruptive behaviors and feelings resulting from the traumatic event and adopt relationship models and interaction styles that will lead to more adaptive and healthy relationships.

FUTURE CONSIDERATIONS

While early intervention is essential in treating childhood trauma, prevention is the ultimate goal. Keeping children safe is a major focus of many trauma prevention campaigns, including the use of child safety seats, bicycle helmets, protecting children from dangerous animals, etc. The prevention of child abuse and neglect remains a major health and mental health need and priority. Treating intergenerational family trauma is a powerful education in how such tragic circumstances are contributed to by societal inequities, including poverty, lack of resources, absence of appropriate treatment for drug and alcohol addictions and mental illness, and marginalization of racial and ethnic minority groups. Treatment of childhood trauma is unlikely to satisfactorily address children's needs in the absence of a larger social context that supports the physical and emotional safety and healthy development of all children.

Effective intervention for childhood maltreatment exists. There is extensive scientific research supporting the importance of early intervention in shaping future developmental outcomes, on both an individual and a societal level (Shonkoff & Phillips, 2000). It is hard to argue that the problem lies in a lack of knowledge when clear, empirically validated strategies are available to address the needs of maltreated children. Children who receive early intervention are much more likely to become productive members of society, diminishing the need for future public funding, remediation, and correctional care. Legislative decisions that divert funding away from programs serving the populations most in need and with the least ability to advocate for their own best interests directly contribute to the increasing discrepancy between the families who are receiving appropriate support and treatment services and those who are not.

Budget cuts that deplete funding of existing treatment programs and government-funded services drastically reduce our ability to effectively intervene to produce positive developmental outcomes. Capable, caring foster parents are being overloaded with needy children, inhibiting their ability to provide quality care. Human Services workers find their caseloads reaching unmanageable numbers, resulting in a deficit in their capacity to function as child advocates and protectors of children's basic needs. Guardian ad litems are assigned overwhelmingly large numbers of children to their caseloads, translating into the unfortunate reality that the legal advocate for the child rarely has the opportunity to meet the child for whom he or she advocates. Even well-intentioned, well-informed legislators, Human Services workers, lawyers, and judges cannot make decisions that serve the best interests of children if they are not assisted in understanding the impact of their work on the developmental outcomes of children (see Chapters 9 [by J. D. Osofsky & C. Lederman], 10 [by P. Van Horn & D. J. Hitchens], & 12 [by J. D. Osofsky, J. H. Hammer, N. Freeman, & J. M. Rovaris], this volume, for discussions of innovative programs involving the courts). It is imperative for child psychiatrists, psychologists, infant mental health specialists, and other mental health workers and professionals who work with and treat young children to educate the community and its leaders about the prevalence of childhood trauma and the negative effects on children. In addition, they should strongly endorse increased funding to create and support services dedicated to the prevention and treatment of young children exposed to trauma.

REFERENCES

Ainsworth, M. D. S. (1973). The development of infant–mother attachment. In B. Caldwell & H. Riccuitti (Eds.), *Review of child development research, 3.* Chicago: University of Chicago Press.

American Psychiatric Association. (1994). *Diagnostic and statistical manual of mental disorders* (4th ed.). Washington, DC: Author.

Bowlby, J. (1982). *Attachment and loss: Vol. 1. Attachment* (2nd ed). New York: Basic Books.

Bretherton, I., & Waters, E. (Eds.). (1985). Growing points of attachment theory and research. *Monographs of the Society for Research in Child Development, 50*(1–2, Serial No. 209).

Fraiberg, S., Adelson, E., & Shapiro, V. (1975). Ghosts in the nursery: A psychoanalytic approach to the problems of impaired infant–mother relationships. *Journal of the American Academy of Child Psychiatry, 14*(3), 387–421.

Frankel, K. A., Klapper, S. A., & Harmon, R. J. (2002, December). *Diagnostic characteristics of clinically-referred young children.* Poster presentation at the Zero to Three 17th National Training Institute, Washington, DC.

Harmon, R. J. (1995a). Diagnostic thinking about mental health and developmental disorders in infancy and early childhood: A core skill for infant/family professionals. *Zero to Three, 15*(3), 11–15.

Harmon, R. J. (1995b, October). *Diagnosing mental health and developmental disorders in infants and preschoolers.* Paper presented at the 42nd annual meeting of the American Academy of Child and Adolescent Psychiatry, New Orleans, LA.

Harmon, R. J., & Riggs, P. D. (1996). Clonidine for posttraumatic stress disorder in preschool children. *Journal of the American Academy of Child and Adolescent Psychiatry, 35*(9), 1247–1249.

Kempe, C. H., Silverman, F. N., Steele, B. F., Droegemueller, W., & Silver, H. K. (1962). The battered-child syndrome. *Journal of the American Medical Association, 181*(1), 4–11.

Kohut, H. (1966). Forms and transformations of narcissism. *Journal of the American Psychoanalytic Association, 14,* 243–272.

Lieberman, A. F., Silverman, R., & Pawl, J. (1993). Infant–parent psychotherapy. In C. H. Zeanah (Ed.), *Handbook of infant mental health* (pp. 472–484). New York: Guilford Press.

Scheeringa, M. S., & Gaensbauer, T. J. (2000). Posttraumatic stress disorder. In C. H. Zeanah (Ed.), *Handbook of infant mental health* (2nd ed., pp. 369–381). New York: Guilford Press.

Scheeringa, M. S., Peebles, C. D., Cook, C. A., & Zeanah, C. H. (2001). Toward establishing procedural, criterion and discriminant validity for PTSD in early childhood. *Journal of the American Academy of Child and Adolescent Psychiatry, 40*(1), 52–60.

Scheeringa, M. S., Zeanah, C. H., Myers, L., & Putnam, F. W. (2003). New findings on alternative criteria for PTSD in preschool children. *Journal of the American Academy of Child and Adolescent Psychiatry, 42*(5), 561–570.

Shonkoff, J. P., & Phillips, D. A. (Eds). (2000). *From neurons to neighborhoods: The science of early childhood development.* Washington, DC: National Academy Press.

Sroufe, L. A., Carlson, E. A., Levy, A. K., & Egeland, B. (1999). Implications of attachment theory for developmental psychopathology. *Development and Psychopathology, 11*(1), 1–13.

Stern, D. (1985). *The interpersonal world of the infant: A view from psychoanalysis and developmental psychology.* New York: Basic Books.

Werner, E. E. (2000). Protective factors and individual resilience. In J. P. Shonkoff & S. J. Meisels (Eds.), *Handbook of early intervention* (pp. 115–134). New York: Cambridge University Press.

Zero to Three/National Center for Clinical Infant Programs. (1994). *Diagnostic classification of mental health and developmental disorders of infancy and early childhood.* Arlington, VA: Author.

CHAPTER 6

RELATIONSHIP ASSESSMENT FOR YOUNG TRAUMATIZED CHILDREN

JULIE A. LARRIEU
SHANA M. BELLOW

Many people shun the knowledge that a parent could betray a defenseless child through acts of violence and aggression; the thought of a parent harming his or her own offspring is utterly opposed to the essential core of parenting. Nevertheless, in 1999, state and local Child Protection Services agencies received close to 3 million reports of abuse and neglect. These agencies investigated nearly 2 million reports, representing an estimated 2,315,000 children. After follow-up assessments, officials substantiated that 826,162 children had been abused or neglected. Forty-four percent of these child victims received no services. An estimated 1,137 children died as a result of abuse and neglect in 1999; 42.6% of those children died before their first birthday (Children's Bureau, U.S. Department of Health and Human Services, 2001).

As other chapters have made clear, child abuse and neglect often have deleterious effects on the development of young children (Cicchetti & Toth, 1995). The maltreated children, their families, and society suffer directly and indirectly due to such trauma, and the responsibility for prevention and intervention lies with us all. Maltreatment during childhood, particularly by a parent or significant caregiver, increases the risk for academic difficulties, substance use and abuse, early pregnancy, criminal involvement, and a range of clinical symptomatology or frank disorders, including developmental delays, learning disorders, depression, disruptive behavior disorders, and posttraumatic stress disorder (PTSD) (Kelley, Thornberry, &

Smith, 1997). Children traumatized by maltreatment also have difficulties in relationships, both in terms of attachment relationships with primary caregivers and in interactions with siblings and peers (Crittenden, 1992). Problems in affect regulation and difficulties in understanding and feeling good about the self (i.e., self-efficacy and self-esteem) also have been well documented (Cicchetti & Toth, 1995; Kaufman & Henrich, 2000).

These difficulties can compromise a child's capacities to cope effectively and to experience well-being, even in supportive environments. Compounding the difficulties of the abused child is the fact that maltreatment is related to exposure to domestic violence and community violence (Kaufman & Henrich, 2000), so that the probability of a maltreated child experiencing other traumatic events is increased. Furthermore, as compared to nonabusive parents, parents who abuse or neglect their children are more likely to have experienced trauma, perhaps maltreatment themselves, both in childhood and as adults (James & Neil, 1996). It is not surprising that experiencing abuse as a child is linked to maltreatment of one's own children, particularly if the parent has no model for nurturance and adequate caregiving, and inadequate resources for showing love and affection. While having been abused as a child does not necessarily lead one to abuse, often those who perpetrate abuse have a history of maltreatment. Studies suggest that as many as 75% of abusers have experienced maltreatment themselves (Romano & De Luca, 1997).

Individuals who have been maltreated in childhood also may have distorted perceptions of their childhood experiences, as evidenced by minimizing, rationalizing, forgetting, or identifying with parental punitiveness (Zeanah & Zeanah, 1989). These distorted perceptions frequently manifest themselves in problematic parenting behaviors, including harsh discipline practices; failure to respond appropriately to their children's needs, especially signs of distress; inconsistency in limit setting; and inability to express affection or have enjoyable interactions with their children (Zeanah, Aoki, Heller, & Larrieu, 1999). Parents may try to block awareness of their own early painful experiences, and this defense may cause them to minimize or deny their child's pain and suffering as well.

A RELATIONSHIP-BASED ASSESSMENT FOR TRAUMATIZED YOUNG CHILDREN

Given the problematic behaviors, perceptions, and relationship disruptions typically manifested by maltreating parents and their young children, the need for intensive intervention by trained infant mental health professionals is paramount. In this chapter, we describe a comprehensive assessment procedure and common themes uncovered in our work with maltreating parents and their children, ages birth to 47 months. The work done by our team is individualized to meet the needs of each parent–child dyad with whom we work. The team is staffed by faculty and trainees from a medical school division of child psychiatry who have expertise in infant and child development and developmental psychopathology. The team is composed of child psychiatrists, clinical and developmental psychologists, social workers, pediatricians, and paraprofessionals.

The initial task of the team is to conduct a thorough assessment of each child and family in order to make recommendations about permanency planning for Child Protective Services and the juvenile court. The families we treat have experienced multiple challenges and stressors, often of a longstanding nature. Typically, the parents are poor, unemployed or underemployed, uneducated, were victims of abuse as children, have symptoms of depression and PTSD, abuse substances, have little emotional support, are involved in violent relationships, and/or live in violent neighborhoods (Larrieu & Zeanah, 1998). Our assessment procedure is designed to understand the experiences of the parent and the child that brought them to abuse and neglect as an answer to life's stressors.

RELATIONSHIP ASSESSMENT PROCEDURES

Because the infant–caregiver relationship is primary, it is the centerpiece of our assessment and treatment (Zeanah et al., 1997). We arrive at an understanding of the infant–caregiver dyad by assessing observable behaviors and subjective experiences. The two central procedures we use are a structured interactional play assessment, which reveals how the caregiver actually behaves with the infant, and a structured parent perception interview, which reveals how the caregiver perceives his or her relationship with the child.

The Parent–Infant Interaction Procedure

The parent–infant interaction procedure we use is designed to assess strengths and concerns about the infant–parent relationship. The procedure is derived from the work of Judith A. Crowell and her colleagues and involves a series of episodes, including free play, cleanup, blowing bubbles together, four teaching tasks, and a separation–reunion segment (Crowell & Feldman, 1989; Heller, Aoki, & Schoffner, 1998; Zeanah et al., 1997). Each episode, along with the transitions between them, allows us to observe how the infant seeks and uses support (or not) from the caregiver, how the pair balance the demands of task completion with the opportunity to enjoy one another, the level of comfort the dyad has with one another, how they share affection, their level of cooperation, and how they handle disagreements. The evaluation measures the parent's ability to set limits, provide structure, help the child learn effectively, and provide emotional and instrumental support to the child. The child's compliance with parental requests, ability to show affection, response to the learning situation, and self-regulation are assessed. Following the teaching tasks, the parent leaves the room for a brief separation and then returns, allowing for the assessment of reunion behavior. We observe whether the child seeks proximity to, avoids, or controls the caregiver during the reunion episode.

The Parent Perception Interview (Working Model of the Child Interview)

We also administer the Working Model of the Child Interview to assess the caregiver's subjective experience of his or her relationship with the infant (Zeanah & Benoit, 1995). Specific areas queried include descriptions of the child's personality, how the child is like and unlike each parent, examples of the child's difficult behavior, and descriptions of the caregiver's relationship with the child. The interview assesses features of the parents' subjective representation, including richness, flexibility, coherence, intensity of involvement, emotional integration, and affective tone. This knowledge is integrated with observations of the parents' overt behaviors with the infant, allowing us to understand the goals and meanings of the parents' interactions with the child.

DOMAINS OF THE CAREGIVING RELATIONSHIP

In assessing relationships between maltreating caregivers and their abused and neglected children, we have found numerous common themes. The themes can be conceptualized using the work of Emde (1989) and Zeanah (Zeanah et al., 1997), who described the important domains of the infant–caregiver relationship. The domains are listed below with each parent domain followed by the corresponding infant domain: Emotional Availability, Emotion Regulation; Nurturance/Empathic Responsiveness, Security/Trust/Self-Esteem; Protection, Vigilance/Self-Protection/Safety; Comforting, Comfort Seeking; Teaching, Learning/Curiosity/Mastery; Play, Play/Imagination; Discipline/Limit Setting, Self-Control/Cooperation; and Instrumental Care/Structure/Routines, Self-Regulation/Predictability. The domains provide a helpful model for understanding functions served by the parenting role and corresponding qualities or competencies of the child. In the subsequent sections we outline each domain and their related themes, and provide illustrative case vignettes. Some themes are relevant to several of the domains; they are separated below for heuristic purposes.

Parent: Emotional Availability;
Child: Emotion Regulation

In our maltreated sample, both parents and children have displayed a range of emotional responses. As might be expected, responses usually change as the intervention proceeds. We define emotional availability as the capacity of the parent to share a range of emotional experiences with the child and to label the parent's own feelings, as well as the child's inferred emotional state, within the context of the relationship. We find that the degree to which the parent can be emotionally available to the child is the degree to which the child can identify and regulate her emotional life. We define emotion regulation as the ability to manage emotions, particularly strong emotions, in a productive manner, to express emotions constructively, in order to better understand one's relationship with oneself and with others across a range of situations and contexts. Unfortunately, numbness and isolation of affect are common in some of the children and parents with whom we work. Some parents avoid eye contact with the child and appear preoccupied, while some are depressed and irritable. Likewise, we have seen children who lack responsiveness, appear dull and lifeless, or seem sad and withdrawn.

We also see some dyads in which both members of the pair display rageful feelings and use aggression to protect themselves from fear and pain. Children often identify with the aggressive parent, typically to gain power over their helpless feelings. We have seen children who associate aggression and violence with an expression of caring, and they act in nurturant or loving ways and then immediately display violent acts such as hitting or kicking the caregiver. Some children attempt to provoke aggression and even attack behavior from others, perhaps as a misguided means to achieve mastery over the traumatic event or to comply with the caregivers' negative view of the child as damaged and damaging. A display of violence toward the caregiver may be a response learned from watching the parents be violent with one another, from being the recipient of the parent's punitive discipline, or from seeing its use with siblings. We see an increased tolerance for pain in some of our children. Avoidance and distancing the self from the caregiver or showing mixed messages of approach and avoidance to the caregiver are common. Below is a vignette that describes interactions we observed between a parent and child who each had difficulties with emotional and behavioral regulation.

Mrs. Warner and Paul

Paul, age 44 months, came to our clinic subsequent to being placed in foster care due to being left with an underage babysitter for a prolonged number of days. In the parent–infant interaction procedure, Paul and his mother were able to have fun together, solve the toy tasks, and cooperate to complete the series of procedures asked of them. Mrs. Warner gave Paul clear instructions, coached him to complete the tasks, and praised him frequently. She was a good teacher, and Paul learned from her instruction. At times, Ms. Warner was quite harsh, however, and she teased Paul in a cruel way. Furthermore, during the unstructured interaction time, when Paul became less compliant than he had been in the problem-solving tasks, Mrs. Warner became extremely punitive and emotionally abusive toward him. She used fear to try to control his behavior, such as telling him not to open the door because "a lion would get him." When he became angry and stated that he was "not her son," she reacted by telling him that she had "another son named Paul, a 'good' Paul," while he was "the 'bad' Paul" and she agreed that he was "not her son anymore." Rather than trying to comfort him and take responsibility for changing the emotional climate of the interaction, the two became engaged in a very coercive cycle, which finally ended with Ms. Warner demanding that Paul apologize for the negative interaction that she had actually begun, namely, relating in an aggressive way.

In a later session with his therapist, Paul was pretending to "groom" his therapist, "braiding" the back of his therapist's hair. Because his male therapist had a close cut, this task involved imaginative play. When Paul was finished with the braid, he unexpectedly kissed the back of the therapist's neck in an intimate way. The therapist set a limit, discussing the interaction with Paul. Shortly thereafter, Paul was playing with make-believe "food" and kitchen utensils. He placed a baker's mitt on his hand to remove "brownies" from the stove. He approached his therapist from behind and slapped him forcefully on the side of his head.

This vignette illustrates the difficulties that Mrs. Warner and Paul had in regulating their emotions and dealing with negative affect. Furthermore, Paul associated affection with violence; this connection was explored and dissected in future therapeutic sessions, such that he could dismantle the association between the two and behave in adaptive ways in response to disappointing or painful events.

Parent: Nurturance/Empathic Responsiveness; Child: Security/Trust/Self-Esteem

Developing security and trust in the self and others is an important developmental task, one related to how the child feels about the self. We define security as the feeling of being safe and free from danger or threat. We characterize trust as the confidence that another will behave as one expects. We identify self-esteem as the complex evaluative feelings, positive or negative, that one has about the self. Empathic responsiveness, characterized as the caregiver's sensitive response to the child's emotional experience, is based on the parent's own identification with the child's feelings. We define nurturance as the provision of support and encouragement to promote development throughout the child's life.

Major breakdowns in caregiving can result when parents are unable to put themselves in the place of their infant and view the world from the young child's eyes. Parents often do not trust the system, themselves, or their babies, which leads to profound failures in empathy. Often, maltreating parents use harsh and punishing language or actions in response to their child's display of distress, need for care, and expression of love. The parent may criticize the child for being too dependent or needy when the child is communicating developmentally expectable wishes, when he strives for closeness, or when he attempts to get his survival needs met by the parent. On the other hand, some parents do not reinforce expressions of independence in their children. They interpret as "positive" the child's behaviors that include moving toward them and away from others in the playroom. These parents interpret a child's striving for independence or curiosity about the world as a rejection of the parent, so that when the child explores toys in the playroom the parent feels abandoned and often behaves harshly with the child.

These parental misattributions and callous behaviors frequently leave children feeling insecure, as evidenced by avoidance of the caregiver, resistance to attempts of the caregiver to connect to the child, or clingy behavior without an ability to be soothed, even when distressed. We also see decreased persistence in problem solving and task completion. Children may view themselves as blameworthy and see themselves as responsible for the maltreatment and violence, while viewing the caregiver positively and justified in his or her abuse of the child. Parents who are not secure in themselves cannot accept constructive criticism, admit shortcomings, and commit to making changes to enhance their parenting and their relationship with their child. Thus, maltreated children are at risk for feeling insecure, mistrusting, and ineffective.

The following vignette illustrates a failure of the parent to respond empathically and the effects on a young child when his caregiver is unable to provide the nurturance he requires to build a healthy sense of self.

Mrs. Caldwell and Brian

Brian, 40 months, was referred to our infant mental health clinic due to concerns about dangerous behaviors exhibited toward himself and others, namely, attempting to cut himself and his baby brother. We had significant concern about Mrs. Caldwell's ability to provide a safe and structured environment for Brian. During the parent–infant interaction procedure, Mrs. Caldwell provided some positive reinforcement when Brian completed teaching tasks successfully and Brian responded well to her praise. Brian completed the initial teaching tasks independently and did not seek guidance from his mother. However, when the tasks became developmentally challenging for Brian, he attempted to seek support from his mother. Mrs. Caldwell did not respond to Brian's requests for assistance in completing the more difficult tasks. In fact, she exhibited provocative behaviors that seemed to escalate Brian's frustration. During a matching task, Mrs. Caldwell reveled in her ability to successfully match several pairs of cards, clearly upstaging her son with her skills. Further, she shunned Brian away when he sought help in accomplishing the same task. Mrs. Caldwell made teasing statements toward Brian about his inability to find a match, and he became increasingly frustrated. Eventually Brian kicked his mother's leg as he walked away from the game and refused to play any longer. Brian began to pout and made negative statements about his abilities. Mrs. Caldwell then attempted to soothe Brian, but he had become so upset that her statements provided little comfort.

This vignette illustrates the difficulties that Mrs. Caldwell and Brian experienced in navigating the completion of a difficult task. A breakdown occurred in Mrs. Caldwell's ability to respond empathically to Brian's frustrations in problem solving. As a result, Brian was unable to develop a sense of security and trust in his relationship with his mother, which then negatively impacted his self-esteem.

Parent: Protection;
Child: Vigilance/Self-Protection/Safety

Parents who have maltreated their children have inherently failed to protect them from harm. We define protection as the parents' ability to keep their child out of harm's way, either by avoiding a dangerous situation or defending the child from harm. Protection and vigilance are complementary components for the parent–child dyad (Emde, 1989). We define vigilance as an awareness of one's environment or surroundings, particularly potential risks or threats to safety. The parental role includes protecting the safety of the child, while we recognize that the child sometimes must develop vigilance to survive in a dangerous or chaotic environment. We define safety as being free from harm or imminent danger. Self-protection can be thought of as the ability to keep oneself free from danger or harm. Parents who have maltreated their children may view themselves as unable to be protective, and they may expect the child to care for herself. To further complicate matters, they may expect the child also to care for them, both emotionally and at times physically. This role reversal takes a toll on the child's ability to form a unique and well-differentiated identity apart from the parent's strong expectations for nurturance. As children grow older, their caring for and overprotection of their parents may turn into bossiness and coercive behavior directed toward the parent (Lieberman & Zeanah, 1999). With such a burden placed upon them, coupled with their experience of trauma, we often see children being hypervigilant to outside stimuli that typically are innocuous but that they perceive as potentially threatening. Likewise, the parent may interpret benign stimuli as threatening in an attempt to control the child. Conversely, the parent may project his or her own destructive impulses onto the outside world, including the child. The parent may neglect the child and leave the infant defenseless against internal and external threats. Such parents' homes often are unsafe, and many of these parents do not monitor the child's movement about the house and the neighborhood. We often see these parents blame the child for serving as the impetus for abuse, and frequently they do not hold themselves responsible for failing to protect the child. Many of the children with whom we work are comfortable approaching strangers, and they place themselves in potentially dangerous or harmful situations.

The following vignette illustrates the strategies developed by a young boy after his caregiver failed to protect him from abuse.

Ms. Andy and William

William, age 42 months, was referred to our infant mental health clinic after being removed from his mother's care after an untreated leg fracture was discovered during a routine doctor visit. We had grave concerns about his mother's ability to protect him from subsequent harm. During our assessment, William displayed a mixture of demanding and bossy behaviors toward his mother. In addition, he was extremely hypervigilant to his mother's reactions. In our clinic, when we telephoned Ms. Andy to provide instructions during the parent–infant interaction procedure, William demanded that his mother hang up the telephone and resume play with him. When Ms. Andy was unresponsive to William, he began playing with a toy animal that made a loud noise. Ms. Andy chastised William for creating a commotion. William became frozen with fear and backed away from his mother. When Ms. Andy began preparing the next task and directed attention away from him, William's posture visibly relaxed and he then engaged with her. When Ms. Andy prepared to leave the room for the separation phase of the procedure, William informed her that he would stay in the room while she was gone and would be "just fine."

This vignette illustrates that William had developed strategies to help him assess the safety of his environment and to behave accordingly. He was hypervigilant to changes in his mother's tone of voice and responded by preparing for flight until he was assured that his environment was safe. When engaged in innocuous play with his mother, William tried to control the interaction by behaving in a bossy manner. When his mother seemed perturbed, William became overfocused on her every move. He also informed her of confidence and safety in being alone, despite the fact that he was a youngster in a novel place. William had developed coping mechanisms, including pseudomaturity, to compensate for his mother's inability to serve as a consistent protector.

Parent: Comforting; Child: Comfort Seeking

The ability to soothe and comfort an infant, particularly a distressed one, is at times a challenge for all parents. A comforting caregiver brings solace to a child, such that the youngster feels content and soothed, especially following upsetting or painful events or circumstances. Comfort seeking involves the child's signaling to the caregiver of the need for soothing and solace. The child's age, developmental level, and relationship to the caregiver influence the manner in which these bids for comfort are displayed. The parents involved in our intervention program often present with few skills to comfort their children, many times related to their inability to be in touch with their own unresolved losses and disappointments. These deficits frequently can be traced to their own lack of having received comfort as children. This deprivation from their early years impedes parents' capacity to perceive their child's pain. Recognizing the pain is a call for action and requires attending to their own anguish as well as their child's. Many parents are not up to the task of dealing with their longstanding disillusionment and grief. When caregivers cannot provide comfort to a child, the effects can be devastating. We see infants who are unable to seek comfort effectively or to be soothed. These children may escalate their distress and then reject soothing attempts, or they may engage in self-injurious behaviors instead of seeking comfort. They also may approach strangers for help, rather than their parents. We see babies and toddlers who console their parents instead of themselves, so that indirectly the child is comforted by meeting the caregiver's needs. The price the child pays for failing to attend directly to her own distress includes being out of touch with her own needs and emotions and being unable to connect to others in a vulnerable way. These difficulties place the child at risk for having relationship disturbances with caregivers, siblings, and peers.

The following vignette describes a youngster who came to our clinic after he was found wandering on a busy highway in a metropolitan area, with no adult caregiver in sight. The manner in which he attempted to meet his needs for comfort illustrates the effects of parental failure to protect.

Ms. Cogan and Ronald

Ronald, age 46 months, presented to our clinic after being placed in foster care due to a failure on his parents' part to provide adequate supervision and protection. Ronald had been found unattended in the neighborhood several times, and when he ran onto a major thoroughfare he was removed from his home and placed in the custody of the state. During our parent–infant interaction procedure with his mother, in the free-play episode, Ronald built a very high wall from building blocks, so tall that it loomed over his head. He and his mother were dressed in costumes they had chosen, he as a superhero and she as a queen. His mother complimented him on the wall he had constructed, then ducked behind it and called for his help, waving her feather boa, stating that she was a damsel in distress and needed to be saved. He dutifully walked behind the wall and led her out, at which point she thanked him for being strong and capable.

In a later session, Ronald used a dog puppet to play out a theme of danger to elicit protection. His mother asked why the dog needed to be saved, stating that the dog was safe in spite of Ronald's fears otherwise. Ronald then had the dog die a dramatic death, at which point his mother rejected this scene, stating that it was time to play with another toy. We later discovered that she divulged intimate secrets to him, including difficulties she has had with his father and her desire to dissolve the relationship with his dad.

This vignette illustrates that at this point in the intervention Ronald's mother was unable to see herself as an effective protector and placed her son in a position to care for her emotional needs while ignoring his. When he attempted to express his needs for safety and protection, she rejected his bids in an effort to avoid her own uncomfortable feelings of insecurity and looming danger. Instead, she looked to him to be her comforter.

Parent: Teaching;
Child: Learning/Curiosity/Mastery

Learning about the people, places, objects, and events of life is an essential task of being human. We define learning as the act of gaining knowledge. Learning is a lifelong process that starts at birth, and parents are the first and fundamental teachers of their children. One of the parents' primary roles is teaching; children have a natural curiosity or inquisitiveness about their environment. Discovering life's great potential is often exhilarating for young children. Once locomotion begins, the world often seems full of boundless opportunity and can provide much joy and discovery for a toddler. Intrinsic motivation to achieve is rooted in having learning experiences that are supported and encouraged by parents. Parents who are good teachers present their children with situations and tasks that do not overwhelm the child's capacities but provide enough challenge to be of interest and to allow success. Good teachers ensure that the tasks are those that can be managed, and these accomplishments lead to confidence that allows future attempts and mastery or success in solving problems.

Many of the parents with whom we work have difficulties with some or all aspects of the teaching role. They may be unable to focus their child's attention on the task at hand, break tasks into manageable subcomponents, create excitement about the process of task completion, provide constructive guidance, praise accomplishments and effort, anticipate frustration and help the child tolerate disappointment, allow the child to attempt the task by himself, provide assistance when the child asks for it, give hints, pace tasks appropriately, or change strategies if necessary. Their children often lack curiosity, are unable to tolerate ambiguity or frustration, are noncompliant, lack enthusiasm and enjoyment in performing tasks, fail to persist toward task completion, and do not rely on the parent for assistance. The learning environment created by these deficiencies may produce a child who lacks confidence, dreads learning in a variety of contexts, is unexcited or anxious in school or academic settings, and feels ineffective in solving the problems presented in daily living. Such a situation can generalize to problematic functioning in several arenas of life.

The following vignette illustrates a mother who was unable to understand her child's capacities and limits, his need for information, and his response to her attempts to instruct.

Ms. Fillmore and Derrick

Derrick, age 24 months, entered foster care after he was left alone in an unkempt apartment for several hours. Derrick was engaged with his mother in our parent–infant interaction procedure, and during free play she placed a puppet on her hand and reached out to him, saying "Hi, little boy!" Derrick was curious about the puppet and its "voice" but seemed apprehensive as well, having never encountered a puppet before. He tentatively took a small step toward the puppet to explore it, when his mother made the puppet lunge at him such that he screamed in fear and ran backward. She followed, laughing at his panicked response, and called his name, still wearing the puppet. When she came to understand that he was afraid, she removed the puppet, which immediately fell limp and lifeless in her hand. She attempted to have Derrick touch the puppet, explaining that is was "nothing but cloth and plastic" and that it was "Mommy's hand inside," but Derrick clearly showed dread and avoidance of the puppet and his mother. She chided him for being afraid of a "stupid little puppet."

This vignette illustrates that Ms. Fillmore misunderstood Derrick's cognitive capacities and his signals of distress. She was unable to explain the situation in a manner that Derrick could comprehend. She quickly rejected his communications, and he showed fear and avoidance of the puppet and his mother, neither of which is conducive to his future love of learning or mastery of material.

Parent: Play; Child: Play/Imagination

Play is a fundamental activity for all humans, both adults and children. Play is a pleasurable activity that is engaged in for its own sake (Santrock, 1997). Play is a primary way in which children learn about and explore their environment. Through play, the parent can help the child learn about herself and the world, solve problems, practice various social roles, and have fun. Enjoying one another's company together through play can motivate the dyad to withstand the difficult periods that are present in every relationship. We assess several aspects of caregiver–child play, including whether the caregiver is able to follow the child's lead, engage in fantasy play, stay within the metaphor the child creates, and allow the child some control of the process. We assess whether the child tries to control all aspects of the play, whether she invites the caregiver to join her in play, or whether she is overly reliant on the parent for generating play sequences.

In our observations of play between caregivers and children, several themes have emerged, including the child's need for nurturance, as demonstrated in play sequences that consist of cooking and feeding, as well as establishing physical contact with the caregiver or the clinician. We also see themes of cleansing objects and repairing damage, including "washing" dishes or other toys, "bathing" dolls, cleaning the dollhouse or playroom, or mending broken toys. Themes of mastery are evidenced by building structures or objects, or tasks that involve creative repetitions, as opposed to the stereotypical, rigid play demonstrating symptoms of PTSD. We see the latter type of play as well and note the caregivers' responses to and interventions in these painful sequences. Children evidence the need for security through sitting in or going under containers, rocking dolls to sleep, and wishing to be held themselves. The inherent tension between autonomy and separation is evidenced by hiding and finding, playing hide-and-seek, peek-a-boo, and other games that entail comings and goings. Frequently, themes of loss and grief are displayed by having play figures move, leave, be injured, or die. Discovering how parents and children deal with these issues is paramount in our work.

The following vignette involves an adolescent mother whose daughter was removed from her care after the girl was left with an underage babysitter. This mother's inability to play with her child in a loving way reflects her own neglectful past.

Ms. Taylor and Sharlene

Sharlene, age 32 months, was removed from her mother's care due to inadequate supervision. Her foster parents were very responsive, and they facilitated her expression of emotions. When Sharlene and her biological mother were engaged in our parent–infant interaction procedure, Ms. Taylor responded to Sharlene's wish to play with the toy grocery carts by arranging a "shopping trip" in our playroom. They proceeded through the "grocery aisles," and each filled her basket with several items. When the shopping was interrupted because Sharlene turned to play with the toy kitchen, without Sharlene's knowledge Ms. Taylor took her daughter's grocery cart and hid it behind a chair. When Sharlene returned to the "groceries," she looked startled because her cart was missing. She walked to her mother's cart and began to inspect it. Ms. Taylor immediately shouted, "No, it's mine. Where is yours? This one is mine!" Sharlene began to look around the room for her missing cart, as Ms. Taylor teased her by saying "I have one and you don't have one. This one is mine; where is yours?"

This sequence underscored Ms. Taylor's own need for control and her anger at her daughter for "robbing" her of her youthful freedom. She engaged with her daughter in competitive and teasing play, as a youngster might with a peer or sibling. Sharlene's vulnerability and need for her mother's appropriate caregiving overwhelmed Ms. Taylor's capacities and touched her own feelings of lost childhood.

Parent: Discipline/Limit Setting;
Child: Self-Control/Cooperation

Learning the boundaries of self and others, the extent and limits of one's capacities, and the consequences for one's actions, including the effects of taking risks, are major tasks of childhood. Parents hold a great responsibility for teaching their children these limits. Discipline is the primary mechanism by which parents instill such learning. A key goal of disciplinary techniques is to teach character and instill self-control in the child. We define self-control as the child's ability for internal regulation and limit setting. Learning to work with others for a common cause is the cornerstone for the development of self-control. Often, parents who maltreat their children use overly harsh discipline practices, such that the child has sustained injuries, or they have neglected their responsibilities in this arena and left the child with no intervention, so that the child has to create limits himself. Either end of the continuum is unsafe for the child and impedes his ability to learn self-control and self-regulation.

In our assessment process, we examine how the parent monitors and intervenes when the child does not respond to her wishes or when he displays dangerous or negative behaviors. The degree to which the parent sets limits, does so clearly, and spells out consequences for misbehavior are assessed. Whether the child complies with parental requests, ignores them, or tries to control the parent are examined. Some maltreated children are bossy, aggressive, or involved in role-reversed relationships, such as inappropriate comforting of the parent, and these patterns are examined as well.

The following vignette involves a mother who is unable to set appropriate limits for her young son. In turn, the son shows little cooperation with her and takes control of the interaction.

Ms. Baldwin and Irving

Irving, age 32 months, was referred to our clinic when his mother left him without adult supervision for several days. During the parent–infant interaction procedure, Ms. Baldwin was extremely passive. Irving was irritable and noncompliant with her requests throughout the interaction. He had several temper tantrums when Ms. Baldwin did not respond quickly to him. Ms. Baldwin pleaded with Irving to stop tantruming, and at one point she pretended to cry. During one temper tantrum, Ms. Baldwin made idle threats toward Irving: "That man is going to get you"; "The Easter Bunny is not going to bring you anything." When Ms. Baldwin attempted to verbally discipline Irving, he ignored her comments. During the interaction, Irving raced Ms. Baldwin to the telephone each time it rang (as she received instructions on the tasks) and a tug-of-war over the telephone ensued each time. On one occasion, Ms. Baldwin beat Irving to the telephone and he took it from her hand while Ms. Baldwin was still talking. Ms. Baldwin pleaded unsuccessfully with Irving to give her the telephone back.

This vignette illustrates Ms. Baldwin's inability to provide structure and discipline effectively. She abdicated control to Irving and provided him with little opportunity to learn cooperative skills that he will need to successfully navigate future relationships.

Parent: Instrumental Care/Structure/Routines; Child: Self-Regulation/Predictability

Predictable and consistent parenting practices are important for establishing regulation of states and feelings of trust and security in children. Instrumental care from the parent means meeting the survival needs of the child, including being fed, changed, and put to sleep at bedtime or naptime, as well as providing for other basic needs such as shelter and clothing. Inherent in providing instrumental care is providing a structured and organized environment. It is also necessary for parents to help young children establish a predictable schedule. The consistency that is established through structure and routine help facilitate the child's development of independent regulatory functions. Parents who do not provide reliable care or who do not have or are unable to maintain regular routines can create dysregulation and even distrust in their children. Children learn about their abilities and their boundaries from the expectations and the limits of their parents. Parents without limits, expectations, and schedules teach children that the world is untrustworthy and that one cannot count on others to set standards and uphold guidelines and conventions for behavior. Children often feel devalued and even abandoned when parents do not provide instrumental assistance, routines, and structure. Unpredictability creates confusion and often reinforces insecure or rebellious behavior. Children exposed to unreliable parenting may make poor choices and take unsafe risks as they grow older due to the inability to curb impulses and establish structure in their own lives.

The following vignette illustrates a child's need for consistency and regulation on the part of his parent and how her failure to provide adequate routines affected his ability to keep himself safe.

Ms. Billings and Thomas

Thomas, age 42 months, was placed into foster care when his mother exposed him repeatedly to domestic violence. During the parent–infant interaction procedure, Ms. Billings sat in a corner of the room in a chair, removed from the play area. Thomas explored the room, discovered a box of costumes, and chose a superhero outfit. After struggling to tie the cape, he approached his mother and asked for her help. She silently fastened the cape for him and resumed looking down at her hands. He ran about the room, flapping his arms as he pretended to fly. His "flights" became more and more elaborate, while his mother continued to study her hands. Finally, he yelled, "Mom, look at me," as he climbed on a chair and jumped off. She said quietly, "Don't do that," as he left the room. After he was returned to the room by a staff member, Ms. Billings admitted that when Thomas had lived with her she did not play with him, nor had she established regular mealtimes or bedtime routines; he was left to his own devices much of the time.

This vignette illustrates the negative effects of inadequate structure on a young child's development. Due to her own symptoms of depression and PTSD, Ms. Billings was unable to regulate herself, and this inability made it virtually impossible for her to provide care and structure for her son.

CONCEPTUALIZATION AND INTERVENTION

These parenting domains both guide our assessment process of traumatized maltreated youngsters and their parents and assist us in conceptualizing family functioning. Every family has strengths, and in conducting our assessment we use a strengths analysis upon which to base our intervention. Having at least one individual in whom the parent can potentially place his or her trust is crucial for constructive change to occur. Once a therapeutic relationship is established and work has begun, parents often come into contact with feelings of shame and rage, frequently rooted in their own traumatic experiences as children, as well as the trauma they have experienced in the present.

We use relationship-based treatment, which focuses specifically on the caregiver–child relationship. This form of treatment involves an understanding of the organization of the infant's and the parent's behaviors as indices of the relationship between the two. The relationship mediates risks and protective factors on the infant's development. We frequently can appeal to a parent's wish to change, to have more healthy relationships with her child, and the adults in her life. We also assess and discuss the lost dreams and wishes of the parent and attempt to discover ways the parent can meet her own needs without compromising those of her child.

The goal of therapy is to help the parent and child develop the ability to trust that others will keep them safe, so that the parent can eventually protect herself and her child. Parents must be able to show vulnerability and seek comfort from others, and be in control of their own rage, fear, and pain. Resolving their own traumatic experiences and losses is paramount to developing belief in themselves as safe and effective parents. When parents are able to experience trust and safety, they often no longer see their child as "too needy," aggressive, mean spirited, or all consuming. They are able to reinterpret their child's normal developmental strivings for intimacy and autonomy as expectable and healthy rather than suffocating or rejecting.

Our intervention model is multifaceted and dynamic, in that it attempts to be flexible in meeting the needs of each family with whom we work. We hope to facilitate parents' abilities to recognize their children's needs, to place their children's needs ahead of their own, and to behave responsibly in their role as caregivers. Empirical investigation of our model confirms that it can frequently prevent future abuse and neglect. Following a parent's participation in our program, we have demonstrated a 68% reduction in subsequent maltreatment of the same child and a 75% reduction in maltreatment of another child by the same mother (Zeanah et al., 2001). We believe this model provides hope for the future in supporting loving and nurturant parent–child interactions that are not marred by abuse and neglect.

REFERENCES

Children's Bureau, U.S. Department of Health and Human Services. (2001). *Child maltreatment 1999: Reports from the states to the National Child Abuse and Neglect Data System.* Washington, DC: U.S. Government Printing Office.

Cicchetti, D., & Toth, S. L. (1995). A developmental psychopathology perspective on child abuse and neglect. *Journal of the American Academy of Child and Adolescent Psychiatry, 34,* 541–565.

Crittenden, P. (1992). Children's strategies for coping with adverse home environments:

An interpretation using attachment theory. *Child Abuse and Neglect, 16*, 329–343.

Crowell, J. A., & Feldman, S. S. (1989). Assessment of mothers' working models of relationships: Some clinical implications. *Infant Mental Health Journal, 10*, 173–184.

Emde, R. N. (1989). The infant's relationship experience: Developmental and affective aspects. In A. J. Sameroff & R. N. Emde (Eds.), *Relationship disturbances in early childhood: A developmental approach* (pp. 33–51). New York: Basic Books.

Heller, S. S., Aoki, Y. A., & Schoffner, K. (1998). *Crowell procedure coding manual.* Unpublished manuscript.

James, A. C., & Neil, P. (1996). Juvenile sexual offending: One-year period prevalence study within Oxfordshire. *Child Abuse and Neglect, 6*, 447–485.

Kaufman, J., & Henrich, C. (2000). Exposure to violence and early childhood trauma. In C. H. Zeanah (Ed.), *Handbook of infant mental health* (2nd ed., pp. 195–207). New York: Guilford Press.

Kelley, B. T., Thornberry, T. P., & Smith, C. A. (1997). *In the wake of childhood violence.* Washington, DC: National Institute of Justice.

Larrieu, J. A., & Zeanah, C. H. (1998). Intensive intervention for maltreated infants and toddlers in foster care. *Child and Adolescent Psychiatric Clinics of North America, 7*(2), 357–371.

Lieberman, A. F., & Zeanah, C. H. (1999). Contributions of attachment theory to infant–parent psychotherapy and other interventions with infants and young children. In J. Cassidy & P. R. Shaver (Eds.), *Handbook of attachment* (pp. 555–574). New York: Guilford Press.

Romano, E., & De Luca, R. V. (1997). Exploring the relationship between childhood sexual abuse and adult sexual perpetration. *Journal of Family Violence, 12*(1), 85–98.

Santrock, J. W. (1997). *Life-span development* (6th ed.). Madison, WI: Brown & Benchmark.

Zeanah, C. H., Aoki, Y., Heller, S. S., & Larrieu, J. A. (1999). *Relationship specificity in maltreated toddlers and their birth and foster parents.* Paper presented at the annual meeting of the Society for Research in Child Development, Albuquerque, NM.

Zeanah, C. H., & Benoit, D. (1995). Clinical applications of a parent perception interview. In K. Minde (Ed.), *Child Psychiatric Clinics of North America: Infant psychiatry* (pp. 539–554). Philadelphia: Saunders.

Zeanah, C. H., Boris, N. W., Heller, S. S., Hinshaw-Fuselier, S., Larrieu, J. A., Lewis, M., Palomino, R., Rovaris, M., & Valliere, J. (1997). Relationship assessment in infant mental health. *Infant Mental Health Journal, 18*, 182–197.

Zeanah, C. H., Larrieu, J. A., Heller, S. S., Valliere, J., Hinshaw-Fuselier, S., Aoki, Y., & Drilling, M. (2001). Evaluation of a preventive intervention for maltreated infants and toddlers in foster care. *Journal of the American Academy of Child and Adolescent Psychiatry, 40*, 214–221.

Zeanah, C. H., & Zeanah, P. D. (1989). Intergenerational transmission of maltreatment. *Psychiatry, 52*, 177–196.

CHAPTER 7

IDENTIFICATION, ASSESSMENT, AND INTERVENTION FOR YOUNG TRAUMATIZED CHILDREN WITHIN A PEDIATRIC SETTING

BETSY MCALISTER GROVES
MARILYN AUGUSTYN

Within the past 10 years, the medical community as well as the general public has become more aware and concerned about the prevalence and impact of psychological trauma in the lives of young children. This increased attention is due in part to evolving knowledge about the sensitivity of infants and young children to events and influences in their environment. In particular, there is a growing body of research that documents the impact of trauma on early brain development and the maturation of the central nervous system (Perry, 1997). Studies show that infants from the time of birth are affected by traumatic events in their environments. This research adds to the substantial body of knowledge about the impact of direct abuse on young children (Cichetti & Toth, 1995; Helfer, Kempe, & Krugman, 1999). There has also been a proliferation of studies on the particular impact of domestic violence on children (Edleson, 1999; Groves, 2002; Kitzmann, Gaylord, Holt, & Kenny, 2003). In summary, both research and clinical findings indicate that age does not protect a child from the effects of trauma. The assumption that a young child will "forget" or that it may be better if the child doesn't talk about the trauma has been

173

disproven. In fact, there is virtually no age that a child is immune from the effects of trauma, either direct trauma or violence that is witnessed.

Responding to the new knowledge about the critical importance of the early years of a child's development, advocacy organizations have raised public awareness about the risks of trauma for young children (Osofsky & Fenichel, 1994, 1996, 2000). A number of clinical intervention programs now identify and treat very young children who are affected by trauma.[1] Federal funding has supported research and demonstration programs to develop effective components of intervention.[2]

At the same time that the public's awareness of the vulnerability of young children has increased, it has become more socially acceptable for adult victims of violence, especially domestic violence, to publicly identify themselves and seek help, a trend observed both in human service organizations and in the increased numbers of calls to law enforcement. With more victims identified and as public concern about the impact of violence on children grows, more parents are seeking help for their children who have been exposed to violence.[3]

Also linked with the increased public attention to the impact of trauma on young children is the growing public concern about violent and aggressive behavior in children. Widely publicized school and community shootings have involved adolescent offenders. Books such as *Ghosts from the Nursery* by Karr-Morse and Wiley (1998) seek to establish a link between early trauma and later violent behavior. There is a renewed interest in efforts to identify children who may be vulnerable and to provide early intervention. Proponents of early identification and intervention point out that pediatric settings are perhaps the only institutions that see virtually all children during their early years. As a result, these settings provide a critical opportunity for family screening for a number of social and health risks, including exposure to trauma.

Several studies have made the case for the importance of providing screening in pediatric settings for exposure to trauma. The Adverse Childhood Experiences Study, conducted on a sample of 30,000 members of the Kaiser Health Plan in California, selected a history of child abuse and exposure to violence against a mother as two of seven risk factors to be investigated for adult health problems in later life (Felitti et al., 1998). In this study, 12.5% of respondents reported childhood exposure to domestic violence and 10.8% indicated a history of child abuse. This study underscored the prevalence of direct victimization and exposure to domestic violence in a large nonclinical sample, as well as its relationship to adverse adult health outcomes. A second study, sampling families who used outpatient pediatric health services in an urban hospital serving low-income families, focused on prevalence of exposure to violence in children age 6 and under, using reports from parents (Taylor, Harik, Zuckerman, & Groves, 1994). These researchers found that 10% of the children had witnessed a knifing or shooting by the age of 6; an additional 18% had witnessed "pushing, kicking, hitting or shoving"; parents reported that nearly half the violence their children had witnessed occurred in the home.

The specifics of screening in a pediatric setting have been less well studied. A few studies have examined self-reported practices among providers and found that, though providers recognize domestic violence as a problem requiring attention, few feel comfortable intervening and even fewer have had any training (Erickson, Hill, & Siegel, 2001; Ganetsky, Giardino, Grosz, & Christian, 2002). A limited number of studies have overcome these obstacles. Siegel and colleagues in a suburban hospital-based practice found during a 3-month period that among 154 women screened for domestic violence, 31% revealed domestic violence at some time in their lives, with 17% reporting domestic violence in the last 2 years (Siegel, Hill, Henderson, Ernst, & Boat, 1999). Parkinson and colleagues in a private pediatric practice in Massachusetts found that 14.7% of mothers reported domestic violence in a past relationship and 2.5% in a current relationship (Parkinson, Adams, & Emerling, 2001).

Despite the growing awareness of this need, there are many young children who have histories of trauma that may not be adequately identified within the current pediatric health system. This chapter addresses the importance of screening for trauma in pediatric settings, describes the role of the health provider in identification of children, and proposes a strategy for screening young children and their parents. Finally, we outline interventions and suggest implications for policy and program development.

DEFINITIONS

"Trauma" or "psychological trauma" is a broad term that potentially encompasses a wide range of events or occurrences. In general, traumatic events are described as those that are outside the range of normal stressors and are of such magnitude as to be perceived as life threatening to self or others. Traumatic events evoke feelings of intense helplessness, fear, or horror. The variable of perception is significant. A child's subjective experience of an event is as important as the objective characteristics of that event. What a young child perceives as life threatening may be quite different from what an adolescent or adult may perceive as dangerous.

For purposes of this chapter, we focus on five types of traumatic events that children may be exposed to: child abuse, including child sexual abuse; exposure to adult domestic violence; exposure to community violence; immigrant and refugee trauma, including the trauma of sudden separation from family, community, or familiar surroundings; and exposure to war and political terrorism. While this is not a definitive or mutually exclusive list of traumatic experiences, we choose these specific traumas because they are most likely to be seen in pediatric settings. Trauma induced by injury or medical procedures is also important to the pediatric provider; however, these traumas are beyond the scope of this chapter.

In this chapter, the term "pediatric provider" refers to a range of health professionals: physicians, nurses, nursing assistants, and others who provide direct care to patients and parents; "pediatric health settings" include family health practices, adolescent health settings that include services to young mothers and their children, as well as traditional pediatric settings.

PREVALENCE

Data on the prevalence of child abuse and child sexual abuse are compiled by every state's child protection agency and forwarded to the National Child Abuse and Neglect Data System. According to the 2000 report (the latest available), child victimization rates decline as age increases. The rate of victimization for children in the age group of birth to 3 years old was 15.7 victims per 1,000 children of the same age. With regard to child fatalities, the youngest children were the most vulnerable. Children younger than 1 year old accounted for 44% of child fatalities, and 85% of child fatalities were younger than 6 years of age (National Clearinghouse on Child Abuse and Neglect Information, 2002). Forty percent of all child abuse victims were under the age of 6 (Children's Defense Fund, 2000).

Data on children's exposure to violence are less available and less reliable because of the inconsistency of definitions and methods of collecting the data. Several studies have reported on rates of children's exposure to community violence. In general, children who live in urban areas with high crime rates are at greater risk for exposure to violence in the community. However, as the spate of high-profile school shootings have made clear, no community is free from the risk of public violent incidents. A study in Los Angeles found that children witnessed 60–80% of homicides in that city (Pynoos & Eth, 1985). In a high-crime area of New Orleans, 90% of elementary school-age children had witnessed violence in the community or home (Osofsky, Wewers, Hann, & Fick, 1993). In a study of 6-year-old children in Baltimore, 54% of the children witnessed some form of violence either in or outside the home (Schuler & Nair, 2001). A study in a suburban middle school in Pennsylvania reported that 57% of the sixth graders surveyed had witnessed a robbing, beating, stabbing, shooting, or murder (Campbell & Schwarz, 1996).

Exposure to domestic violence is equally difficult to measure. Estimates of children's exposure to violence range from 3 million upward (Fantuzzo & Mohr, 1999). The wide range of estimates is due to differences in the definitions of "exposure" and "domestic violence." Two studies point to the particular risks of young children's exposure to domestic violence. In a five-city study of police data of domestic violence calls, investigators found that young children (age 5 years and under) were disproportionately represented in homes where there was domestic violence (Fantuzzo, Boruch, Beriama, Atkins, & Marcus, 1997). Another study, in Massachusetts, reviewed restraining order data for the presence of children at the time of a threatened or actual assault and found that 65% of children were 8 years old or younger (Massachusetts Department of Probation, 1995). Since both of these studies rely on police or court data, they do not include any incident of domestic violence that has not come to the attention of the legal system.

Another source of data that highlights the risks to infants and young children of exposure to domestic violence is the research on prevalence of incidents of domestic violence on pregnant women. Three studies have looked at prevalence of abuse during pregnancy, establishing a range of rates between 3.9 and 8.3% (Centers for Disease Control and Prevention, 1994; Gazmarian et al., 1996; Martin, Mackie, Kupper, Buescher, & Moracco, 2000). Other studies document the direct and indirect harm to the mother and child (Cokkinides, Coker, Sanderson, Addy, & Bethea, 1999; Newburger et al., 1992).

There are fewer data available as to the prevalence of immigrant and refugee children's experiences with violence. This population's exposure to violence may be the hardest to quantify. Many immigrants are traumatized initially in their native country, by war or extreme deprivation, often prompting their emigration. On entry into the new country, the poverty and challenges that face these families may further traumatize children and adults. Additionally, many families are loathe to seek mental health services or report problems because of fear of retribution or the fact that other pressing problems assume precedence over mental health intervention (Geltman, Augustyn, Barnett, Klass, & Groves, 2000). All too many immigrant children experience disconcertingly high levels of violence in their new neighborhoods and school settings. In one study of immigrant children, 36% indicated that violence was the thing they liked least about living in the United States (Suarez-Orozco & Suarez-Orozco, 2001).

SCREENING FOR TRAUMA IN PEDIATRIC SETTINGS

Since the publication in 1963 of Henry Kempe and colleagues' landmark study of abused children, public recognition, social policy, and medical practice has changed dramatically with regard to identifying and responding to children who are traumatized through abuse or neglect (Kempe, Silverman, Steele, Droegemuller, & Silver, 1963). Pediatric providers are mandated reporters and, in this role, may use a variety of screening tools, both formal and informal, to assess for child abuse. Many hospitals have multidisciplinary child protection teams, providing specialized consultation and education to providers about child sexual and physical abuse.

However, despite the research findings that document the critical vulnerability of young children to traumatic experiences and the public concern about violent behavior among children, there is little information in the pediatric literature about identifying children's psychological trauma (other than child abuse) or about screening for other trauma. In fact, a literature search of recent pediatric articles found only one article that mentioned assessment of trauma in young patients (Rusch, Gould, Dzierzynski, & Larson, 2002). There were no articles that focused on screening for children's exposure to violence. Medical professional organizations have endorsed screening of adult patients for domestic violence; however the pediatric organizations have been slower to respond.[4]

The American Academy of Pediatrics (Committee on Child Abuse and Neglect) in 1998 published a position statement entitled "The Role of the Pediatrician in Recognizing and Intervening on Behalf of Abused Women." The first sentence of that statement was "The abuse of women is a pediatric issue." The statement presented information about the impact of domestic violence on women and children and the obstacles women face in disclosing that they are victims of domestic violence. One of the recommendations was that "pediatricians should attempt to recognize evidence of family or intimate partner violence in the office setting" (p. 1092). The statement made a strong case for recognizing domestic violence but did not offer specific guidelines for screening or provide discussion about the policy and practice dilemmas that arise when providers implement screening protocols for exposure to domestic violence. Furthermore, it did not recognize the broader areas where children may be exposed to violence, including chronic abuse and neglect, community violence, terrorism, and refugees who may have been traumatized in their country of origin.

In summary, the prevalence data suggest that pediatric providers see many children who may have been affected by trauma, but the problem is underrecognized, underinvestigated, and undertreated. There is growing knowledge of the critical vulnerability of young children to trauma, the importance of the first years of a child's life, and the potential long-term consequences to children of early exposure to trauma. Therefore, we believe that pediatric health settings should be recognized as offering a unique opportunity to identify children who are at risk. They can provide support to the child and family in order to ameliorate the adverse effects of trauma.

BARRIERS TO SCREENING FOR PSYCHOLOGICAL TRAUMA IN PEDIATRIC SETTINGS

Studies on efforts to implement screening protocols for domestic violence in adult health settings may give insight into barriers that exist in pediatric settings for screening for exposure to violence and other traumas. In a recent study, pediatricians were asked to fill out questionnaires about their customary screening practices (Erikson et al., 2001). Of the 547 who responded, 64% were unaware of the aforementioned recommendations of the American Academy of Pediatrics about screening for domestic violence. However, 51% of the respondents screened at least high-risk families, and 49% had identified a case of domestic violence in their practice. Only 8.5% of respondents routinely screened for domestic violence, and 74% had received no specific training in this area. The most commonly perceived barriers to screening were lack of education (61%), lack of office protocol (60%), lack of time (59%), and lack of support staff (55%). Providers with specific training were 10.9 times more likely to screen than those without training.

In other studies, providers have typically enumerated five barriers to providing violence screening in their work with families:

1. The barrier mentioned most often is that of time constraints (Sugg & Inui, 1992). As providers face increasing demands to see large numbers of patients and additional expectations about what to cover as part of anticipatory guidance, they may avoid topics that lead to lengthy discussion or extensive demands for follow-up.

2. A second barrier that is frequently mentioned is inadequate training. In a study of general violence prevention counseling, Borowsky and Ireland (1999) found that 76% of pediatric residents and 83% of practitioners rated their training as inadequate in this area. They reported that 68% of residents and 73% of practitioners never or rarely screen for domestic violence. Although we do not have specific data about pediatric training on early childhood trauma, our clinical experience of having trained many residents and pediatric providers indicates inadequate knowledge about trauma in young children and its associated symptoms or treatment.

3. A third barrier is a sense of powerlessness. Violence is not an easy problem to address, nor do many patients want to talk about it. In addition to experiencing trauma, many families may present with other problems: low income, inadequate housing, and other health or mental health problems. Physicians are unlikely to be able to address any of these issues easily. In one study, for example, 42% of physicians expressed frustration that although they could intervene with advice or referral to resources, ultimately what was actually done was in the hands of the parent (Sugg & Inui, 1992). For professionals whose success depends on efficiently diagnosing and

treating problems, violence may represent a failure or a frustration that leaves them feeling powerless and unsuccessful.

4. A fourth barrier is concern that patients and families will be offended if asked personal questions about safety, relationships, or violent events at home. Providers worry that patients will feel singled out for this line of questioning and will resent it. However, a study done by Siegel et al. (1999) showed that, rather than being offended, many women appreciated the question as to domestic violence and revealed partner violence when screened in the pediatric office setting.

5. A fifth barrier is the presence of children in the room during screening and the related question of who is the patient. This is particularly true when a practitioner is inquiring about domestic violence. The parent is not the direct patient. Pediatric providers may feel uncomfortable inquiring about parental behavior. This concern may occur less often when they are asking about exposure to community or political violence, but providers also have mixed opinions about whether or not to ask these sensitive questions with children present. Some recommend interviewing the parent alone, without the partner or children (King & Strauss, 2000); however, this logistical challenge may be a significant barrier for the provider. There is strong agreement that a woman should not be screened for domestic violence if her partner is in the room. However, there has been no systematic study of whether the presence of children in the exam room affects a provider's comfort in screening or the parent's comfort in talking. Zink (2000) examined this issue using interviews and focus groups with experienced family physicians and pediatricians and found that experts disagreed on the appropriateness of general screening for domestic violence in front of children older than 2–3 years. The majority thought that general questions were appropriate but that in-depth questioning should be done in private. This is the only study to date examining this issue.

THE ROLE OF THE HEALTH PROVIDER IN RECOGNIZING SYMPTOMS ASSOCIATED WITH TRAUMA IN YOUNG CHILDREN

The most common way that a pediatric provider may become concerned about a child's exposure to violence is through his or her symptoms. In a retrospective chart review of children age 6 and under who were referred to an outpatient mental health program for children who witness violence, three symptoms were mentioned most frequently by parents: increased aggression, sleep difficulties, and increased separation anxiety (Groves, Acker, & Hennessey, 2002). Children who are exposed to violence, particularly chronic episodes of violence, often show symptoms associated with posttraumatic stress disorder (PTSD). One study found that children's exposure to domestic violence (without being directly victimized) was sufficiently traumatic to precipitate moderate to severe symptoms of posttraumatic stress in 85% of the children in the study (Kilpatrick, Litt, & Williams, 1997).

Diagnostic criteria for PTSD in very young children are less well documented and agreed upon than criteria for older children and adults (Perrin, Smith, & Yule, 2000). Based on their research on children age 48 months and younger, Scheeringa and Zeanah (1995) have proposed a modified set of symptom criteria that are more sensitive to the developmental profiles of very young children. Their criteria include the following:

- The presence of an external stressor or traumatic event
- Symptoms of reexperiencing the event, which for young children may be seen as repetitive play with themes from the traumatic event, or directly reenacting aspects of the traumatic experience; recurrent memories of aspects of the event
- Symptoms of avoidance, including constriction of emotion; withdrawal; loss of previously acquired developmental skills
- Symptoms of arousal, including sleep difficulties, nightmares, night terrors, hypervigilance, exaggerated startle response, decreased concentration
- Developmental regressions
- Onset of new fears; new aggressive behavior

The DC: 0–3 diagnostic classification system includes "posttraumatic stress syndrome" as a proposed diagnostic classification for children age birth to 3 (Zero to Three/National Center for Clinical Infant Programs, 1994; see also S. A. Klapper, N. S. Plummer, & R. J. Harmon, Chapter 5, this volume, for an elaboration of the DC: 0–3 classification system).

In addition to the behavioral and emotional symptoms that young children may experience, their cognitive abilities, beliefs, and learning of social skills are adversely affected by exposure to violence, especially domestic violence (Edleson, 1999). Children who grow up with violence in their homes learn early and powerful lessons about the use of violence in interpersonal relationships. They learn that violent behavior is acceptable, that it is an effective means to get one's way or to discharge stress. These children also learn that violence may be an inherent part of loving relationships. Exposure to violence may provide a justification for children to use violence in their own relationships. Similarly, children who are exposed to violence in the community draw the same conclusion: an effective way to settle a disagreement is through force.

Studies have shown that some children may be affected by exposure to violence more than others. Variables such as age, temperament, gender, proximity to the violence, and frequency and severity of the violence may affect children's responses (Pynoos et al., 1987). In addition, the response of the caregiver, characteristics of the family, and community may affect children's responses.

STRATEGIES FOR SCREENING YOUNG CHILDREN AND THEIR PARENTS

When a provider decides to begin screening for children's exposure to violence, several steps should be undertaken:

1. *Examine your own biases and beliefs about children's exposure to violence.* Have you been affected by violence or trauma in your life? Do you know anyone personally who was a victim of violence? Is it difficult to talk about domestic violence or child abuse with your patients? Do you feel that physical violence is an appropriate response in some settings?

2. *Learn how to talk with families about violence.* There is not yet broad agreement in the literature as to the optimal way of administering a screening. Some suggest that direct oral assessment is superior to written questionnaire assessment for case finding (e.g., Kimberg, 2001). Others suggest that written questionnaires are better than face-to-face questioning (e.g., Thompson et al., 2000). To add another dimension, recent studies have shown that computer-based interviewing has the potential to reduce biases, improve measurement validity, and generally provide improved responses compared with either of the above (Kissinger et al., 1999).

We recommend a direct face-to-face inquiry (Groves, 1995; Groves, Augustyn, Lee, & Sawires, 2002). The pediatric provider's direct discussion about safety at home and in the community tells the patient that this is an important topic and one that belongs in the realm of pediatric care. A written question is also effective, but using this method alone may not communicate the same message to the patient. Oral assessment also allows the provider to consider the patient's emotional response to the question.

3. *Integrate assessment into routine history taking and into health maintenance for children.* Questions can be asked routinely in the course of taking the social history. Sample introductions might include: "I have begun to ask all of the parents in my practice about their family life as it affects their health and safety and that of their children. May I ask you a few questions?"; or "Violence is an issue that affects everyone today, and so I have begun to ask all my families about their exposure to violence. May I ask you a few questions?"

Some questions that could be asked of all parents at well-child visits:

- Has your child ever witnessed a scary or unsafe event in the neighborhood or at home?
- Has your child ever been the victim of a violent incident?
- How do you resolve conflict with other adults in your home?
- Do you feel safe in your home and community?
- Have you been hurt or threatened by anyone since our last visit?

In some practices, these questions will be asked by a nurse assistant or a social worker; in others, they will be asked by the physician or nurse practitioner. There is no evidence that one way is better than the other.

These questions may be asked with the child in the room. Children under the age of 3 are less likely to understand verbal content of questions, although they are sensitive to the reactions, emotions, and mood of their caregiver. For older children, the provider must be sensitive to the mother's cues. If the mother is uncomfortable, inquire about contacting her at another time. Her discomfort does not necessarily mean that she is currently a victim of violence, but it is necessary to pursue these questions in a more confidential and safe setting.

4. *If you know or suspect that a child is being exposed to violence, schedule follow-up care.* One of the most important messages you as a pediatric provider may send to a family is that you recognize their trauma and want to be available to help as needed. Certain situations may raise your concern that a child is at risk, for example, when a child presents frequently to the practice with minor medical concerns or stress-related symptoms such as chronic headaches or stomachaches; similarly a parent who brings a child for frequent visits to the emergency department, particularly at night, may be using such visits to escape from a dangerous situation at home.

5. *Know the resources in your community.* The American Academy of Pediatrics recommends that pediatricians should have a protocol or action plan that has been reviewed with local authorities on domestic violence. In cases where a woman acknowledges that she is a victim of domestic violence, appropriate follow-up should include further assessment, intervention, and documentation (Warshaw & Ganley, 1998). Assessment consists of taking a history about the violence, with attention to the immediate risk of injury to the woman and the safety of the child. This assessment will likely include making a decision about notifying child protection services. In some settings a social worker or other counselor provides this assessment; in others, the pediatric provider must provide it. In cases where a family may reveal exposure to community violence, resources may be less available. Working with a social worker or family housing advocate may be important in these situations. In cases where children may have suffered significant trauma in their country of origin, referral to a mental health

agency that has experience in treating cases of refugee trauma might well be required. In cases of suspected child abuse and neglect, mandated reporting to child protective services may be indicated.

Documentation of disclosures of domestic violence and intervention should be done carefully, because both parents may have access to the child's records and these records may provide future evidence against the batterer.

INTERVENTION IN THE PEDIATRIC SETTING

Pediatric providers play a vital role in providing education and anticipatory guidance to all parents about the vulnerability of infants and young children to traumatic experiences. Providers might ask about how parents handle child discipline, how parents handle arguments or conflict within the home, and the role of television in the home, assuming that these are issues that all families face. Pediatricians can educate parents about the sensitivity of infants and young children to adults' emotional states, and can also provide active support to parents. Some pediatricians advocate incorporating violence awareness/prevention into newborn visits and then revisiting the issue with parents and the child at each developmental juncture throughout the child's life (Stringham, 1998).

As researchers have learned about the impact of trauma on young children, they have also learned a great deal about intervention. The importance of intervention has been well documented in such publications as *From Neurons to Neighborhoods,* a comprehensive review of the literature on child development, including early trauma and intervention conducted by the National Academy of Sciences (Shonkoff & Phillips, 2000). Because young children depend almost exclusively on their parents for emotional support and protection, many experts believe that the best way to help the young child affected by trauma is to help the parent by providing education, advocacy, and support. In some instances, specialized intervention with the child may be indicated; however, the first focus of the pediatric provider should be the parent.

In a pediatric setting, intervention has four components: support, education, safety planning, and referrals. Support may include acknowledging the family's fear, confusion, uncertainty about their child, and expressing concern about safety. Education includes providing information about resources, legal remedies, housing, and support. Safety planning provides a brief assessment of the potential dangerousness of the situation and helps guide the provider and family to think about the next steps. If the pediatric provider identifies that a young child has been affected by trauma, he or she should provide direct assistance to the parent and may decide with the parent about whether a referral for special services is indicated. The primary goal of intervention is to stabilize the environment for the family and support the parent's ability to provide consistent emotional support to the child. Education includes giving parents specific information about how trauma may affect young children, including a review of the common symptoms and assistance in managing specific behaviors. This can be reassuring to parents who may be alarmed by the change in behaviors that are observed in the child. Assuring parents that symptoms associated with trauma are normal reactions to abnormal events is important. If parents need specific referrals for legal advocacy, immigration assistance, or domestic violence services, the provider should make the appropriate referrals.

REFERRALS FOR SPECIALIZED SERVICES

The pediatric provider may consider referring a young child for additional mental health or early intervention services in the following instances:

1. If the symptoms have lasted for longer than 3 months and are interfering substantially in the child's life/functioning
2. If the parent is traumatized or otherwise compromised in her or his ability to respond to the child
3. If the trauma involves the loss of a parent or significant caretaker

If it is possible to refer to an early childhood mental health specialist, this is most appropriate. These specialists understand the developmental issues of young children and many are experienced in working with traumatized children. They are not widely available, however. Early intervention services or mental health consultants for child-care settings may also provide important resources for children.

CASE EXAMPLES OF PEDIATRIC
IDENTIFICATION AND INTERVENTION

Case 1

A young mother brought her 13-month-old daughter to the pediatrician because the child "was not eating enough." Upon examination, the child was of normal weight and had not lost weight since the last visit. As the pediatrician inquired about the immediate history of the mother's concerns about her child's appetite, the mother stated that she had been worried for the past 2 weeks. When asked about any stresses or particular events that may have affected the child, the mother began to cry and confided that she and her husband had just separated. The physician asked,

"Do you have any worries about your safety?" The mother replied that the reason for the separation was that her husband had hit her in front of her daughter. The assault resulted in a cut and bruises on her face. She called the police, who responded and arrested the father. She had since sought a restraining order and filed for separation. She said that she had told no one other than her immediate family because she was ashamed that this had happened to her.

The pediatrician asked several detailed questions about what the child had witnessed and what her responses had been. The child had been playing in the room when the parents began to argue and was exposed to the increasingly heated argument and the assault. The child began to scream during the altercation. The father left the home once the police were summoned and the child did not see the arrest. The mother reported that she had blood on her face, which was quite upsetting to the child. She cleaned it up immediately and declined medical assistance offered by the police.

In addition to the concern about eating, the mother also reported that her daughter was awaking at night screaming and that it was difficult to get her back to sleep. The child also experienced intense distress when separated from her mother, even if the mother was in the next room. Mother reported that all of these symptoms began after the violent incident.

The pediatrician explained to the mother that these symptoms were common responses that young children had to extremely frightening events. Although the mother assumed the symptoms were associated with the assault and the stresses of the separation, she was nonetheless reassured that these were not unusual responses and that her doctor was familiar with them. The physician asked about support for the mother. Was she going to be involved with court proceedings? Did she have an attorney? He asked about her immediate concerns, particularly who was supporting her, and offered to refer her to the local domestic violence service agency. He found out that her sister was staying with her temporarily and that her family who lived nearby was providing assistance. He also reassured the mother that her daughter's appetite and eating habits would likely return to normal with the passage of time, particularly if the child felt that her environment had stabilized. The pediatrician discussed with the mother some specific ideas for supporting her daughter: trying to minimize prolonged separations from her; leaving a nightlight on in the child's bedroom to help with sleep (a suggestion the mother made). He scheduled a follow-up visit for 2 weeks. At the follow-up visit, the child was eating normally again and was more comfortable separating from her mother. She still had sleep difficulties, although they were less frequent.

In this case, the pediatric provider identified early trauma and provided supportive and sensitive intervention to the parent. The inquiry about safety provided the opportunity for the mother to share a difficult and personal experience. The emphasis on taking a careful history of the specifics of exposure to violence yielded important information about what the child had experienced. The provider gave concrete information about the child's symptoms that reassured the mother. He found out about existing supports for the mother and offered additional resources. He provided follow-up for the family. This intervention provided early identification of the problem and a sensitive response that likely assisted this mother in being attuned to her child's emotional needs and helped the mother feel less stressed about her situation.

Case 2

Renée, an 8-year-old girl, was brought to her pediatrician by her grandmother with the complaint of chronic headaches and difficulty sleeping at night. Her grandmother stated that these symptoms began about 2 weeks ago when someone threw a brick through their front window. The grandmother stated that the family who lived in the apartment upstairs was involved in gang and drug-related activities, and she believed that the intruders "missed" in hitting her apartment instead. In spite of her reassuring Renée about this, the girl continued to be frightened, slept poorly, and often wanted to stay home from school because "her head hurt."

The pediatrician had provided medical care for Renée since she was 6 years old. On the initial visit, Renée's grandmother reported that the child's mother had died of a violent injury when Renée was 18 months old. No other details of the mother's death were known. With this new traumatic event, the pediatrician asked the grandmother again about the specifics of the death of Renée's mother. Wondering with the grandmother if perhaps this new trauma may have triggered something in Renée's past, the pediatrician found out that Renée had in fact been in her mother's arms when her biological father shot her mother, then fled the home. He was later incarcerated for the murder. Renée had never been told the details of the murder. Instead, she had been told that her mother and father were both "dead." Other members of the family, including young cousins, did know part of the "true story" and the grandmother admitted that it was possible that Renée may have heard some of the details (correct or incorrect) from other family members or friends. The pediatrician met with the grandmother for several visits to talk about posttraumatic symptoms and repressed memory, helping the grandmother plan a way to tell Renée the truth about her parents and to help her feel safe again in her home. She then referred the family for individual counseling for Renée and family counseling with her grandmother.

In this case, the pediatric provider used knowledge of the child's history and knowledge of the impact of early trauma to sensitively interview the grandmother about the deeper causes of these new somatic symptoms. She helped the child and grandmother learn new coping and communication methods and referred the family for more intensive therapy to help Renée resolve a significant trauma and loss of a parent.

DILEMMAS FOR PROVIDERS WHO SCREEN FOR TRAUMA IN YOUNG CHILDREN

When pediatric practitioners screen families for trauma, they may face dilemmas about reporting suspected abuse of children or reporting injuries of adult victims. Although laws in most states require medical reporting of specified injuries and wounds in adults, these laws are unlikely to apply in the pediatric setting when the health provider is treating the child. In the pediatric visit, where the parent is not the patient and is not seeking treatment, the provider likely would have no legal obligation to report parent injuries or abuse detected during routine screening. Then, again, the question of making a report of suspected child abuse/neglect to child protection services in cases where a child has witnessed domestic violence is somewhat more complicated. Whenever a child is abused either intentionally or unintentionally as a result of domestic violence, the pediatric provider, as a mandated reporter, must notify the appropriate agency. However, state laws are less clear as to whether exposure to domestic violence in the absence of injury or serious risk of injury requires mandated reporting. The provider should be familiar with the state laws as they pertain to reporting in cases of domestic violence. In states that allow more discretion to the reporter, it becomes important for the provider to carefully assess whether the child has been abused, the potential for dangerousness in the home, whether the abuser has made direct threats to the child, and the capacity of the mother to keep the child safe. For a full discussion of the issues of reporting suspected abuse of children or reporting injuries of adult victims, consult the consensus guidelines published by the Family Violence Prevention Fund for responding to domestic violence in child and adolescent health settings (Groves, Augustyn, et al., 2002).

IMPLICATIONS FOR POLICY, TRAINING, AND PROGRAM DEVELOPMENT

In this chapter we have made a case for using pediatric health settings to screen young children for trauma and proposed specific guidelines to assist health providers in doing so. Both the prevalence of trauma in children and the potential adverse outcomes for children lend urgency to the task of identifying children who are at risk. A decision to implement universal screening in a health setting would have significant ramifications for policy and practice. One strong benefit of more comprehensive screening would be increased knowledge of the extent of the problem. As was stated at the beginning of this chapter, estimates about prevalence of exposure to violence or trauma are difficult to obtain because of different definitions and sampling strategies. We don't have enough knowledge about the kinds of traumas young children experience; systematic inquiry would fill an important gap in the data.

At the same time, it must be recognized that systematic inquiry would also create a greater demand for services. Resources for children's mental health, especially for very young children, are woefully lacking in most states. Increased screening would further strain a fragile and inadequate system. In addition, it is likely that a greater burden would be placed on child protection systems, as more children would be discovered to be at risk for abuse or neglect. As we learn more about the nature and extent of trauma in very young children, we must use that knowledge to vigorously advocate for increased services.

Finally, the ultimate success of screening depends on adequate training and education of medical providers. Pediatric providers must acquire basic knowledge about risks to early child development, as well as learn the symptoms and characteristics of trauma in children. They must acquire skills in interviewing and in accessing community resources to support families. Such education requires skilled teaching and a solid commitment from the medical education system.

The rewards for building capacity for early identification of children affected by trauma are potentially significant: early identification can lead to early intervention and, we hope, a reduction in the adverse consequences for children of living with chronic violence. Screening for these exposures in pediatric and family health settings is a component of quality health care that we can no longer afford to neglect.

NOTES

1. For example, the Early Trauma Treatment Network, funded by the U.S. Substance Abuse and Mental Health Services Administration is a collaboration of four treatment centers that provide mental health treatment to young children affected by violence. The four sites include the Child Trauma Research Project at the University of California/San Francisco General Hospital; the Child Violence Exposure Program at Louisiana State University Health Science Center; the Child Witness to Violence Project at Boston Medical Center; and the Jefferson Parish Human Services Authority Infant Team/Tulane University.

2. Recent federal initiatives include the National Center for Children Exposed to Violence/ Safe Start Initiative, funded by the U.S. Department of Justice; the National Child Traumatic Stress Network, funded by the U.S. Substance Abuse and Mental Health Services Administration; and a recent initiative for research on children exposed to violence, funded by the National Institute of Child Health and Human Development.

3. The Child Witness to Violence Project at Boston Medical Center has seen a steady increase in numbers of self-referrals to the program over the last 10 years. Currently 25% of refer-

rals are self-referred, the majority from mothers who are concerned that their children have been affected by exposure to domestic violence.
4. Health professional associations that have published position statements about family violence include the American Academy of Family Physicians, the American Academy of Pediatrics, the American College of Obstetricians and Gynecologists, and the American Medical Association (a partial listing).

REFERENCES

American Academy of Pediatrics (Committee on Child Abuse and Neglect). (1998). The role of the pediatrician in recognizing and intervening on behalf of abused women. *Pediatrics, 101*(6), 1091–1092.

Borowsky, I. W., & Ireland, M. (1999). National survey of pediatricians' violence prevention counseling. *Archives of Pediatric and Adolescent Medicine, 153*, 1170–1176.

Campbell, C., & Schwarz, D. (1996). Prevalence and impact of exposure to interpersonal violence among suburban and urban middle school students. *Pediatrics, 98*, 396–402.

Centers for Disease Control and Prevention. (1994). Physical violence during the 12 months preceding childbirth: Alaska, Maine, Oklahoma and West Virginia, 1990–1991. *MMWR Morbidity and Mortality Weekly Report, 43*, 132–137.

Cichetti, D., & Toth, S. L. (1995). A developmental psychology perspective on child abuse and neglect. *Journal of the American Academy of Child and Adolescent Psychiatry, 34*(5), 541–565.

Children's Defense Fund. (2000). *Child abuse and neglect.* Retrieved May 19, 2003, from *http://www. childrensdefense. org/ss_chabuse_fs. php*

Cokkinides, V. E., Coker, A. L., Sanderson, M., Addy, C., & Bethea, L. (1999). Physical violence during pregnancy: Maternal complications and birth outcomes. *Obstetrics and Gynecology, 93*(5), 661–666.

Edleson, J. (1999). Children's witnessing of adult domestic violence. *Journal of Interpersonal Violence, 14*(8), 839–870.

Erikson, M. J., Hill, T. D., & Siegel, R. M. (2001). Barriers to domestic violence screening in the pediatric setting. *Pediatrics, 108*(1), 98–102.

Fantuzzo, J., Boruch, R., Beriama, A., Atkins, M., & Marcus, S. (1997). Domestic violence and children: Prevalence and risk in five major U.S. cities. *Journal of the American Academy of Child and Adolescent Psychiatry, 36*(1), 116–122.

Fantuzzo, J. W., & Mohr, W. K. (1999). Prevalence and effects of child exposure to domestic violence. In R. Behrman (Ed.), *The future of children: Vol. 9, No. 3. Domestic violence and children* (pp. 21–32). Los Altos, CA: David and Lucile Packard Foundation.

Felitti, V. J., Anda, R. F., Nordenberg, D., Williamson, D. F., Spitz, A. M., Edwards, V., Koss, J., & Marks, L. (1998). Relationship of childhood abuse and household dysfunction to many of the leading causes of death in adults. *American Journal of Preventive Medicine, 14*(4), 245–258.

Ganetsky, M., Giardino, A., Grosz, P., & Christian, C. (2002, May). *General pediatricians' approaches to domestic violence in the office setting.* Presented at the annual meeting of the Pediatric Academic Society, Baltimore, MD.

Gazmarian, J. A., Lazorik, S., Spitz, A. M., Ballard, T. J., Saltzman, L. E., & Marks, J. S. (1996). Prevalence of violence against pregnant women. *Journal of the American Medical Association, 275,* 1915–1920.

Geltman, P. L., Augustyn, M., Barnett, E. D., Klass, P. E., & Groves, B. M. (2000). War trauma experience and behavioral screening of Bosnian refugee children resettled in Massachusetts. *Journal of Developmental and Behavioral Pediatrics, 21,* 257–263.

Groves, B. M. (1995). Witness to violence. In S. Parker & B. Zuckerman (Eds.), *Behavioral and developmental pediatrics: A handbook for primary care.* Boston: Little, Brown.

Groves, B. M. (2002). *Children who see too much: Lessons from the Child Witness to Violence Project.* Boston: Beacon Press.

Groves, B. M., Acker, M., & Hennessey, C. (2002, August). *Profiles of the youngest referrals to the Child Witness to Violence Project.* Paper presented at the International Family Violence Conference, Durham, NH.

Groves, B. M., Augustyn, M., Lee, D., & Sawires, P. (2002). *Identifying and responding to domestic violence: Consensus recommendations for child and adolescent health.* San Francisco: Family Violence Prevention Fund.

Helfer, M. E., Kempe, R. S., & Krugman, R. E. (Eds.). (1999). *The battered child.* Chicago: University of Chicago Press.

Karr-Morse, R. & Wiley, M. S. (1998). *Ghosts from the nursery: Tracing the roots of violence.* New York: Atlantic Monthly Press.

Kempe, C. H., Silverman, F. N., Steele, B. F., Droegemueller, W., & Silver, H. K. (1963). The battered-child syndrome. *Journal of the American Medical Association, 181,* 17–24.

Kilpatrick, K. I., Litt, M., & Williams, L. (1997). Post-traumatic stress disorder in child witnesses to domestic violence. *American Journal of Orthopsychiatry, 67*(4), 639–644.

Kimberg, L. (2001). Addressing intimate partner violence in primary care practice. *Medscape Women's Health eJournal, 6*(1). Retrieved May 19, 2003, from *http:// www. medscape. com/viewarticle/408937*

King, H. S., & Strauss, M. (2000). *Routine screening for domestic violence in pediatric practice.* Newton, MA: Newton Wellesley Hospital.

Kissinger, P., Rice, J., Farley, T., Trim, S. Jewitt, K., Margavio, V., & Martin, D. (1999). Application of computer-assisted interviews to sexual behavior research. *American Journal of Epidemiology, 149,* 950–954.

Kitzmann, K. M., Gaylord, N. K., Holt, A. R., & Kenny, E. D. (2003). Child witnessing to domestic violence: A meta-analytic review. *Journal of Consulting and Clinical Psychology, 71*(2), 339–352.

Martin, S., Mackie, L., Kupper, L. L., Buescher, P., & Moracco, K. (2000). Physical abuse of women before, during, and after pregnancy. *Journal of the American Medical Association, 285,* 1581–1584.

Massachusetts Department of Probation. (1995). *The tragedies of domestic violence: A qualitative analysis of civil restraining orders in Massachusetts.* Boston: Office of the Commissioner of Probation.

National Clearinghouse on Child Abuse and Neglect Information. (2002). *National Child Abuse and Neglect Data System (NCANDS) summary of key findings from calendar year 2000*. Retrieved May 19, 2003, from *http://www. calib. com/nccanch/pubs/factsheets/canstats. cfm*

Newburger, E. H., Barkan, S. E., Lieberman, E. S., McCormick, M. C., Yllo, K., Gary, L. T., & Schecter, S. (1992). Abuse of pregnant women and adverse health outcomes: Current knowledge and implications for practice. *Journal of the American Medical Association, 267*, 2370–2372.

Osofsky, J. D., & Fenichel, E. (Eds.). (1994). *Hurt, healing and hope: Caring for infants and toddlers in violent environments*. Arlington, VA: Zero to Three/National Center for Clinical Infant Programs.

Osofsky, J. D., & Fenichel, E. (Eds.). (1996). *Islands of safety: Assessing and treating young victims of violence*. Washington, DC: National Center for Infants, Toddlers and Families.

Osofsky, J. D., & Fenichel, E. (Eds.). (2000). *Protecting young children in violent environments: Building staff and community strengths*. Washington, DC: Zero to Three.

Osofsky, J. D., Wewers, S., Hann, D. M., & Fick, A. C. (1993). Chronic community violence: What is happening to our children? *Psychiatry, 56*, 7–21.

Parkinson, G. W., Adams, R. C., & Emerling, F. G. (2001). Maternal domestic violence screening in an office-based pediatric practice. *Pediatrics, 108*(3), e43. Retrieved May 19, 2003, from *http://www. pediatrics. org/cgi/content/full/108/3/e43*

Perrin, S., Smith, P., & Yule, W. (2000). Practitioner review: Assessment of posttraumatic disorder in children and adolescents. *Journal of Child Psychology and Psychiatry, 41*(3), 277–289.

Perry, B. D. (1997). Incubated in terror: Neurodevelopmental factors in the "cycle of violence. " In J. D. Osofsky (Ed.), *Children in a violent society* (pp. 124–149). New York: Guilford Press.

Pynoos, R. S., & Eth, S. (1985). Children traumatized by witnessing acts of personal violence: Homicide, rape, or suicide behavior. In S. Eth & R. S. Pynoos (Eds.), *Posttraumatic stress disorders in children* (pp. 19–43). Washington, DC: American Psychiatric Press.

Pynoos, R. S., Frederick, C., Nader, K., Arroyo, W., Steinberg, A., Eth, S., Nunez, F., & Fairbanks, L. (1987). Life threat and posttraumatic stress in school-age children. *Archives of General Psychiatry, 44*, 1057–1063.

Rusch, M. D., Gould, L. J., Dzierzynski, W. W., & Larson, D. L. (2002). Psychological impact of traumatic injuries: What the surgeon can do. *Plastic and Reconstructive Surgery, 109*(1), 18–24.

Scheeringa, M. S., & Zeanah, C. (1995). Symptom expression and trauma variables in children under 48 months of age. *Infant Mental Health Journal, 16*, 259–270.

Schuler, M. E., & Nair, P. (2001). Witnessing violence among inner-city children of substance-abusing and non-substance-abusing women. *Archives of Pediatric and Adolescent Medicine, 155*, 342–346.

Shonkoff, J. P., & Phillips, D. A. (Eds.). (2000). *From neurons to neighborhoods: The science of early childhood development*. Washington, DC: National Academy Press.

Siegel, R. M., Hill, T. D., Henderson, V. A., Ernst, H. M., & Boat, B. W. (1999).

Screening for domestic violence in the community pediatric setting. *Pediatrics*, *104*(4), 874–877.

Stringham, P. (1998). Violence anticipatory guidance. *Pediatric Clinics of North America, 45,* 439–488.

Suarez-Orozco, C., & Suarez-Orozco, M. (2001). *Children of immigration.* Cambridge, MA: Harvard University Press.

Sugg, N. K., & Inui, T. (1992). Primary care physicians' response to domestic violence: Opening Pandora's box. *Journal of the American Medical Association, 267,* 3157–3160.

Taylor, L., Harik, V., Zuckerman, B., & Groves, B. (1994). Exposure to violence among inner city children. *Developmental and Behavioral Pediatrics, 15,* 120–123.

Thompson, R. S., Rivera, F. P., Thompson, D. C., Barlow, W. E. Sugg, N. K., Maiuro, R. D., & Rubanowice, D. (2000). Identification and management of domestic violence: A randomized trial. *American Journal of Preventive Medicine, 19*(4), 253–263.

Warshaw, C., & Ganley, A. (1998). In D. Lee, N. Duburow, & P. Salber (Eds.), *Improving the health care response to violence: A resource manual for health care providers.* San Francisco: Family Violence Prevention Fund.

Zero to Three/National Center for Clinical Infant Programs. (1994). *Diagnostic classification of mental health and developmental disorders of infancy and early childhood.* Arlington, VA: Author.

Zink, T. (2000). Should children be in the room when the mother is screened for partner violence? *Journal of Family Practice, 49*(2), 130–136.

CHAPTER 8

TRAUMATIZED YOUNG CHILDREN

Assessment and Treatment Processes

THEODORE J. GAENSBAUER

This chapter illustrates the ways in which our understanding of early trauma, as outlined in previous chapters, can be translated into actual practice. It begins with a general overview of the processes of evaluation and treatment as I have experienced them in my work with traumatized young children and their families, followed by the description of a clinical case exemplifying my approach to therapy.

Given the diverse nature of traumatic events and their background settings, no single description can capture the range of therapeutic interventions that might be helpful in a given case. It is important therefore to place the approaches described here in their clinical context. Working as I do in a private practice setting, the types of trauma I tend to see are circumscribed in nature, generally involving unintentional injuries such as those caused by medical illnesses and/or treatments or accidents of various types. Where abuse or violence has occurred, the perpetrator is likely to have been someone outside the nuclear family rather than the parents. Family settings are generally stable, and parents are able to provide relatively uncomplicated support around the trauma. This contrasts with situations of parental abuse where work with the parents is complicated by their direct responsibility for the child's trauma and where the child's loss of trust in adults has been doubly damaged by the knowledge that the trauma was intentionally inflicted on him or her by those upon whom he or she most depended.

The therapeutic needs of children who have experienced a single trauma in the context of an otherwise normal developmental course will be very different from those of children who have experienced repeated traumas, particularly if those traumas have been inflicted by caregivers. Further complications arise when traumas occur in the context of other developmental stressors, such as emotional and physical neglect, chaotic and/or precarious living situations, and numerous losses, all of which will create their own pressing therapeutic needs. Because of these differences, the question frequently comes up as to whether treatment principles applicable in an advantaged setting are relevant to clinicians working with less-advantaged children. I would argue that they are. Although removed from the harsh realities that clinicians working in settings with children exposed to family and/or community violence will face, work with the kind of case to be described here allows examination of the symptomatic and developmental impact of trauma in relative isolation from other pathogenic influences. It also facilitates the identification of effective interventions that are trauma specific, in contrast to situations where the trauma issues are embedded within multiple and ongoing stressors. Since trauma work with multiply stressed children and their families can often lead to professional "burnout" and therapeutic pessimism (Osofsky, 1996), knowledge of the degree to which therapeutic interventions can promote recovery in responsive children and their families can also help therapists to retain a sense of optimism and conviction about their ability to be effective in doing trauma work. In the discussion section concluding this chapter, I return to the issue of the applicability of the treatment approaches described here to children who have been more severely traumatized and who lack stable caregiving support.

GENERAL DESCRIPTION
OF THE EVALUATION PROCESS

In cases involving a relatively discrete trauma, the overall goal of treatment is, as much as possible, to return the patient's and family's functioning to its pretrauma level. In order to accomplish this, the therapist must be concerned not just with posttraumatic stress disorder (PTSD) symptoms themselves but with the full range of symptomatic, developmental, and interactional disturbances resulting from the trauma, as well as the overall impact on the family system (Gaensbauer & Siegel, 1995). The therapist will need to work closely with both children and their parents/caregivers.[1]

I generally begin the evaluation process by interviewing the parents without the child being present. In my questioning, I encourage parents to assume that any changes that have occurred subsequent to a trauma are related to the trauma unless proven otherwise. This assumption helps ensure that subtle traumatic effects will not be overlooked. I gather information in the following areas: (1) a sequential and detailed description from the parents of every aspect of the child's traumatic experience, not only the traumatic events themselves but all of the events surrounding the trauma that will influence the internal meanings that the trauma will have for this particular child; (2) the child's symptoms and behavioral changes from the time of the trauma up to the present, including the expectable posttraumatic symptoms and manifestations of developmental regression that are generally observed with any traumatic experience (Scheeringa, Zeanah, Drell, & Larrieu, 1995; Scheeringa and Gaensbauer, 2000; see also S. A. Klapper, N. S. Plummer, & R. J. Harmon, Chapter 5, this volume); (3) the impact of the trauma on broader developmental tasks such as the child's sense of trust and autonomy, modulation of aggression, capacities for exploration, bodily integrity and gender identity, relationships with peers, and capacities for learning (Gaensbauer, 1995; Pynoos, Steinberg, & Wraith, 1995); (4) any relational disturbances or interactional difficulties with other family members that have resulted from the trauma (Gaensbauer & Sands, 1979; Gaensbauer, 1994); (5) the effect of the child's symptoms on the family's functioning and the degree to which the family's responses to the trauma and to the child's symptomatic behaviors are ameliorating, perpetuating, or even exacerbating the child's symptoms (Green & Solnit, 1964; Figley, 1983, 1989; Scheeringa & Zeanah, 2001); and (6) parents' personal reactions to the child's trauma, as well as general indicators of the family's ability to support therapeutic work with the child, including an assessment of the family's overall stability, cohesiveness, and emotional strength (Terr, 1989; Lewis, 1996).

In addition to these trauma-focused issues, I also gather information about the child's developmental history. Areas of emphasis include the overall quality of the child's attachment relationships, the presence of any major developmental issues and/or areas of emotional conflict that would likely be intertwined with the current traumatic feelings, and whether there have been any prior traumatic experiences that the current trauma might be rekindling (Zeanah, 1994; Zeanah & Scheeringa, 1996). Finally, given parents' understandable sense of urgency about the child's needs being addressed, I spend time in these initial parental meetings providing educational information about PTSD in early childhood and lay out in broad terms the kinds of interventions that we know will be helpful. I particularly emphasize the crucial role parents will play in their child's recovery.

Once having developed a sense of the child's and family's needs for therapeutic work, based on my judgment of the severity of symptoms and whether or not they are likely to resolve themselves without intervention, I then meet with the child, almost always with one of the parents present. I initially encourage the child to explore and play spontaneously, in order to observe variables related to the child's overall developmental functioning, such as the child's cognitive and language attainments, capacities for emotional regulation, quality of play, relatedness to adults, and comfort level in the sessions (Benham, 2000). All of these factors will have enormous influence in determining the kinds of therapeutic interventions the child will be able to make use of. Focusing specifically on issues of trauma, it has been my experience that in the course of the initial evaluative sessions the trauma will come up, either spontaneously or through some natural entrée, in a way that opens the door to an inquiry about the child's experience. Because young children's abilities to provide verbal descriptions of their memories and feelings are limited, their communication will be significantly enhanced by active cueing on the part of adults (Fivush, 1993; Gaensbauer, 2000). For this reason, structuring of the play situation has been recognized as an extremely helpful therapeutic technique for working with traumatized young children as far back as the pioneering work of David Levy (1939).

It goes without saying that throughout treatment, but especially in the beginning, one must be particularly careful in regard to the presentation of stimuli likely to elicit traumatic feelings. While symptoms of emotional distress during or following a session can be a useful diagnostic indicator that trauma feelings are unresolved, it is important not to overwhelm the child. If the distress elicited by a traumatic stimulus is more than the child or the caregiving environment is able to handle, the effect will be to retraumatize the child rather than to facilitate therapeutic processing. As a consequence, both the parents and the child will be understandably resistant to further treatment. Sufficient psychological distance from the trauma and the establishment of a sense of safety, both within the therapeutic setting and in the home environment, are essential preconditions for any therapeutic work. This was illustrated by the case of a 19-month-old child who had been recently discharged from the hospital and who had begun to be comfortable in our sessions until, on a routine visit to his pediatrician, it was decided at the last minute that a blood test needed to be done. This surprise medical procedure so undermined the child's confidence about coming to my office that we were unable to continue. The younger the child the greater will be the difficulty in differentiating trauma-focused discussions and/or play from the risk of actual trauma.

Having parents present during the sessions, if they are able to handle the emotional material that will emerge, offers multiple advantages (Gaensbauer & Siegel, 1995). Young children are much more comfortable when their parents are present. Parents can also provide crucial historical information that helps the clinician to understand the child's play, particularly when there are references to the child's traumatic experience that the therapist might not otherwise recognize. In addition, seeing how the child is continuing to be affected by the traumatic experience helps the parents recognize the need for treatment and promotes their participation in addressing the child's symptoms at home. Throughout the therapeutic work, as discussions and reenactment play mobilize "relived" traumatic feelings, the parents are able to provide comfort in ways that they were not able to at the time of the original trauma. This helps to rebuild the loss of trust that resulted from the parents' failure to prevent the trauma in the first place. Finally, since young children do not engage in sustained thematic play, there can be a natural moving back and forth between focus on the child's play and discussions with the parents. In this way one can keep abreast of ongoing developments and address problems occurring at home, while also monitoring the parents' reactions.

At the same time, it is important to note that having the parents present is not without risks. The child's reenactment of a traumatic event can be emotionally overwhelming to parents, particularly for those who had assumed that the details of the trauma would be forgotten. I have had several cases where parents did not follow through with treatment recommendations because of their difficulties in handling the feelings that the child's traumatic play evoked in them.

GENERAL OBSERVATIONS ON THERAPY

Therapeutic work in the case of relatively discrete traumas often follows a similar sequence. Initial phases of therapy will generally be focused on acute or enduring PTSD symptoms such as nightmares, recurrent imagery, distressed reliving, emotional fragility, avoidance and emotional withdrawal, and symptoms of increased arousal. As PTSD symptoms begin to diminish, the therapist will see more clearly the particular psychological meanings that the trauma has had for the child. Over time the trauma's effects on the child's overall developmental trajectory, both at the time of the trauma and subsequently, will become more evident and can be incorporated into the therapeutic work. The interplay between trauma effects and preexisting parent–child issues will come into sharper focus as well. Although this progression could theoretically lead to an expansion of therapeutic focus beyond the immediate trauma issues, it has been my experience that parents generally decide to terminate at the point when the trauma issues are satisfactorily resolved. Flexibility in fitting goals to the family's needs, identifying effective therapeutic techniques, and in determining who should be seen in sessions will be required throughout the process. Thus a variety of treatment modalities will be utilized in any therapeutic work, depending on the therapeutic issues that are most pressing at any given moment and the modalities that will be most effective in addressing them. These will include parent-counseling sessions, family and parent–infant therapy, the development of behavioral management strategies and desensitization protocols, and individual work with the child utilizing a full range of cognitive-behavioral and play therapy techniques (Terr, 1995).[2]

With the therapist taking care to ensure that the emotions that are elicited are manageable, the cornerstone of treatment for trauma at all ages has been psychotherapeutic work that allows patients to communicate and to reprocess their traumatic experience in the context of a supportive environment (Pynoos, 1990). For very young children, communicative vehicles that allow children to demonstrate their memories and emotional reactions but that are not dependent on language will often be necessary, such as actual situational reexposure, structured and/or spontaneous play, behavioral reenactments, and drawings (Terr, 1988; Gaensbauer & Siegel, 1995). The reliving of a traumatic experience can serve a variety of therapeutic purposes including abreaction, desensitization to traumatic feelings, development of a coherent narrative, and ultimately integration and mastery. It can also be retraumatizing. In therapeutic work both in sessions and at home, the child will return again and again to traumatic play themes in order to process various aspects of the experience. Whether repeated play reenactments or other forms of reliving are therapeutic or whether they serve to fixate the trauma in the child's mind may be judged by the extent to which the child is able to identify and process the important affects associated with the trauma and whether the forms of reexperiencing are dynamic and evolve over time, as opposed to being rigid and unchanging.

Helping the child to develop a coherent and accurate narrative about the traumatic events by linking fragmented traumatic memories into an intelligible picture will be particularly important in correcting children's almost inevitable misunderstandings and cognitive distortions about the trauma (Terr, 1988, 1990). A child may assume, for example, that the trauma was a punishment for having been bad. In this process of developing a narrative, parents can play a crucial role at home. Even in the absence of fluent expressive language, children's receptive language is often quite advanced. Thus "storytelling" can be a particularly valuable technique for enabling parents to fill in details, provide explanatory background, identify the child's feelings, and convey their own thoughts and feelings in order to help the child realize that they were distressed as well. The child's participation in the storytelling facilitates a co-constructed narrative that can serve as a basis for ongoing family dialogue (Fivush & Fromhoff, 1988).

Even though many symptoms will be significantly relieved through therapeutic work in the office, probably the most important contribution we can make as therapists to the child's recovery is to help parents to deal with the child's symptoms in the home environment. Having to deal with a child's intense posttraumatic symptoms, often in the context of their own emotional turmoil, can place extraordinary demands on caregivers. Since behavioral disturbances are an inevitable manifestation of trauma in young children, helping parents to respond empathically and to develop effective behavioral management techniques will be essential aspects of therapy. This is particularly true since many symptoms, such as clinginess and emotional fragility, the need for parental support around sleep, aggressive behavior, and needs to control the environment will, because of secondary reinforcement, have a tendency to continue even after the intensity of the original traumatic feelings is reduced. The establishment of firm limits with appropriate consequences will thus be necessary to interrupt traumatically driven behaviors. At the same time, it will be crucial for parents to keep in mind that the child's acting out is a function of traumatic experience rather than simply the product of willful misbehavior, for two important reasons. In the first place, it promotes disciplinary actions that are carried out with empathy and minimal punitive anger, thereby reducing the risk of escalation. Secondly, it opens the door to further resolution of traumatic feelings. When traumatically driven behavioral acting out is interrupted, the underlying feelings that are driving the behavior will emerge. For example, if the child who wishes to sleep with parents is taken back to his or her own bed, the anxieties about the trauma that have been relieved by being close to the parents will come to the surface. Similarly, as the child is prevented from acting out aggression in destructive ways, the traumatically derived anger will remain.

I thus recommend what I describe to parents as a "two-layered" approach to behavioral acting out. In the process of setting limits I encourage parents to articulate and empathize with the underlying traumatic feelings that are coming to the surface. For example, if children are becoming fearful as they are being returned to their own beds, in the midst of reassuring them parents can take the opportunity to link these fears to the traumatic experience and help children talk about the memories that are causing them to be afraid. Similarly, in the midst of providing appropriate restraint and consequences for out-of-control anger, parents can share their understanding of the traumatic source of the child's angry feelings and help the child to express them in more adaptive ways. In this way, sensitive behavioral management can serve to facilitate parent–child communication, internal processing, and mastery.

Parents' awareness of the connection between the child's symptoms and the traumatic experience is thus the cornerstone for the desensitization and processing of traumatic affects in the home setting. Just as in therapy sessions where children need to return again and again to a traumatic theme in order to gain mastery, so too in the home children will require repeated exposures to situations associated with a traumatic event before they will be able to regain the confidence that the traumatic event will not recur. Even if the source of the distress is not specifically identified, each time the child is exposed to traumatic stimulus triggers and is effectively reassured, the intensity of the traumatic affects will likely be desensitized to some degree.[3] Because traumatic reliving will often occur in the context of everyday situations, specific desensitization approaches that reduce the intensity of the disruptive affects and behaviors that are evoked can be very useful. Desensitization can occur naturalistically as parents comfort the distressed child in situations that precipitated traumatic distress, but desensitization can also be significantly facilitated if done in an active and planned way (Wallick, 1979). Among helpful strategies to be considered would be the use of graduated exposure protocols to reduce the child's distress in specific situations, such as those used by Chatoor (1991) for traumatic feeding disorders. These involve stepwise exposure to stimuli associated with the trauma, beginning with relatively nonthreatening stimuli and leading to a full exposure to the anxiety-provoking situation. To counteract fear reactions and promote more positive associations, each step is designed to be as pleasurable as possible and one does not move from one step to the next until the child is ready.

Reduction in the intensity of traumatically driven affects through concrete situation-specific exposures will be particularly important for children who are unable to utilize symbolic play, either because they are developmentally impaired, too young, or because such play is too anxiety provoking. Taking an example from my practice, a 2-year-old who had been physically abused by a female baby-sitter avoided any participation in a play scene that represented the situation at the baby-sitter's because of his anxiety and difficulty separating the scene from his actual experience. Therefore, the bulk of the therapeutic work took place at home in the context of interactions with his mother, whom he would intermittently confuse with the perpetrator (as a result of stimulus triggers that we generally could not identify). At these moments he would reenact the abuse with her in some form, such as through aggressive behavior, fearful responses, and/or withdrawal. His mother dealt with these transference reenactments with great patience, providing containment while utilizing them to connect his behavior with the baby-sitter's abuse, reassuring him that she would never hurt him, and empathizing with his frightening and anger-provoking experience. These repeated "reliving" sequences that would conclude with his mother being able to comfort him in his distress served the purpose both of desensitization and traumatic reprocessing, and were the primary vehicle leading to a resolution of his traumatic symptoms.

In summary, whether occurring naturalistically or in a structured context, every instance in which children manifest symptomatic behavior secondary to the trauma can be seen not only as an opportunity for desensitization but also as an opportunity to help them recognize that their emotional upset and behavioral acting out are being driven by traumatic feelings from the past rather than the current situation. As children get older and such connections can be verbalized more easily, they establish a pattern of communication about the trauma that can be invaluable in the future in the likely case that traumatic feelings will resurface at subsequent points in development.

The case description that follows will serve to illustrate the various points made in this overview discussion.

CASE EXAMPLE

Katy's parents consulted me because of their concerns about her reactions following an auto accident that had occurred a month earlier. I met with the parents for three sessions over a 1-month period prior to meeting with Katy herself. The entire therapy involved 14 sessions extending over approximately 6 months.

Katy had just turned 3 when the car in which she, her mother, and her baby sister were driving was broadsided by another car as they were going through an intersection. In car seats, Katy experienced a mild whiplash and contusions to her chest and her baby sister was unhurt. Their mother, however, was knocked unconscious and bled from her head and arm. Regaining consciousness at the scene, the mother was taken to the hospital by ambulance. Katy and her sister were taken by separate ambulance. In the emergency room, Katy saw her mother briefly prior to the mother's transfer to the intensive care unit (ICU) but did not want to approach her. When the family visited the mother the next day, Amy, Katy's 4-year-old sister, who had not been in the accident, got up on the bed and gave her mother a kiss whereas Katy refused. The mother was hospitalized for a week and then remained at Katy's grandmother's house for an additional 2 weeks to recover from postconcussive symptoms prior to returning home.

At the time of the initial interview with the parents, Katy was showing a number of PTSD symptoms. She was fearful of riding in the car and was very sensitive to loud noises. She had difficulty going to sleep and described nightmares of monsters trying to hurt her to the point where she hid under the bed. Although she frequently complained of "owies" following the accident, rather than seeking comfort she would want to be left alone. Her feelings were easily hurt, and she would refuse to speak and retreat to her room over very slight disappointments. She also became uncharacteristically aggressive, slapping and pushing her siblings. Developmental regressions were reflected in constant, almost obsessive use of her pacifier (prior use had been confined to her room and the car) and several bladder accidents in the weeks following the accident. Of greatest concern to the parents, however, was the marked change in Katy's relationship with her mother. During visits to the hospital and during the daily visits with the mother at her grandmother's house, Katy had continued to pull back from her mother, not wanting a hug or a kiss. Although initially happy when her mother returned home, her anger continued. She clung to her father and refused to let her mother comfort her. She would say, "I don't like you, Mom," and repeatedly scolded her mother for "driving on the grass."

Katy's developmental history had been relatively unremarkable. There had been no problems during pregnancy or delivery and she was described as a very "mellow" baby. Developmental milestones had all been within normal limits. Family life had been stable, and the mother had remained home with Katy and her sisters. There was some rivalry with her elder sister Amy, but overall her sibling relations were good. There had been a brief regression in toilet training following the birth of her younger sister 6 months earlier. The most notable developmental event was a "feeding strike" that occurred when she was 4 months of age: introduced at this time to commercially prepared milk, she vomited to the point of requiring emergency intravenous rehydration. Although she ate solid foods without difficulty, for the next week she refused to take either a bottle or breast. Her parents were able to work with her over the next several weeks to help her to nurse again. The only carryover they noted to other areas of her functioning or to persisting effects was that it was at this point that she began to use a pacifier. (Although it did not have direct applicability to the therapy at the time, one could hypothesize that this experience had relevance for understanding Katy's response to the trauma. Did the feeding refusal, for example, reflect a temperament-based tendency to withdraw that presaged the reaction pattern observed following the accident? Or were the vomiting and the medical treatments traumatic in themselves, priming Katy for a more intense affective and physiological reaction than she might have experienced otherwise?)

During the initial sessions with her parents, it was clear that Katy came from a resourceful and supportive family. Katy's father had been able to take considerable time off from work during his wife's convalescence, and close friends and relatives, including her mother's parents, provided assistance throughout the recovery period. Her mother, although still in the process of recovering from her own head injuries with periods of fatigue and need for quiet, was attuned to her children's feelings. On one occasion, noting Katy's frustration as she threw a toy train on the ground, her mother commented that she thought Katy was mad because of the accident. Katy gave a big sigh, nodded, and said, "Mommy, you drove up on the grass and I was crying and crying, and the police came and said it's okay and then the fire trucks came." In spite of being aware that Katy's reactions were connected to the accident, her parents had not actively talked with her about it except to respond supportively whenever the subject came up. In particular, they had not attempted to explain how the accident had happened.

Beginning with the first session, I spent time educating the parents about how Katy's symptoms were consistent with a traumatic reaction and made several suggestions relating to how they could help Katy at home. In particular, I encouraged them to take the initiative in talking with Katy about the accident. I highlighted various moments in addition to the collision itself that I believed would have been quite frightening to Katy and that I thought would be important to address, such as seeing her mother unconscious and bleeding after the accident or the scene in the emergency room. I also encouraged them to give Katy an accurate picture of what had actually occurred in order to correct her belief that her mother had been responsible for the accident by driving up on the grass. From a behavioral management standpoint, I attempted to relieve pressure on Katy by encouraging her parents to not make an issue of the pacifier or her toileting accidents at this point in time, as they were beginning to do. I tried to reassure them that as we were able to help Katy with her traumatic feelings these regressive behaviors would diminish. Finally, I conveyed my optimism that Katy's symptoms could be significantly helped.

In the course of the three sessions with the parents, even prior to my seeing Katy, as her parents began to talk more directly with her about her feelings, they reported significant progress. For example, as her mother was talking to Katy about how upset she had been when her pacifier had been left in the damaged car, Katy responded, "I hold on to it tight so that I won't ever lose it again." Her mother empathized with how much Katy did not want something like that to ever happen again. At the end of the discussion Katy threw both arms around her mother and gave her a big hug. On another occasion they played out the accident with cars and the mother demonstrated how the other car had gone through a red light and hit their car. As a result, Katy began to describe how "Mommy was pushed onto the grass" rather than "Mommy drove onto the grass." Whereas previously Katy would become sulky when the accident came up, she was now more able to talk about it. She even began to demonstrate it on her own, showing how the car was hit and "flopped around" and describing how her mom's head fell over and that she had "red spots all over the place."

The week after the first session with the parents, Katy's great grandmother died. This loss was not only painful in itself but stimulated associations to the mother's injuries. At bedtime, Katy frequently brought up the issue of dying. Her mother took the opportunity both to explain the concept of death and to help Katy understand that her great grandmother's death was the result of aging and that her mother was not going to die for a long, long time. During a conversation at dinner, the whole family talked together about how the great grandmother's death had reminded them all of their fears for Katy's mother. Helping to validate the children's feelings about the accident, Katy's father expressed how worried he had been until he arrived at the hospital and saw that Katy's mother was okay. This stimulated Katy's elder sibling Amy to describe how worried she had been as well. Katy did not participate in this discussion.

Given the fact that the family situation had stabilized with her mother's return home and her great grandmother's funeral, and the fact that significant symptoms were still present although much improved, I felt that it was time to meet directly with Katy. Sucking on a large pacifier as she arrived for our first session with her mother, Katy presented as a very engaging little girl. Although quiet, she seemed comfortable as she entered my office playroom. As a result of her parents' previous discussions at home, we were able to move relatively quickly to a focus on the accident.

While Katy explored the playroom, her mother began by describing the children's upset about the caretaker who came during the day to help out with the children. She then described how she had told Katy that she was coming to see me to talk about the accident. Katy initially did not respond to my questions about how she felt about these events, but she seemed to be listening carefully. She tacitly acknowledged my observation that these were difficult things to talk about.

Her mother went on to describe how she and Katy had been able to talk about certain parts of the accident at home but that it was very hard for Katy to talk about the period when her mother was at the hospital. At this point, we again turned to Katy and asked if she had been worried when her mom was at the hospital. She nodded affirmatively. I asked Katy's mother to review the kinds of things they had talked about. As her mother mentioned several details, such as how the seats in the car had been broken and how Katy had described seeing her mommy flopping on the ground, Katy moved over by her mother's chair and leaned against her mother's knee. Sensing the anxious reaction to her mother's description of what she had seen, I asked her if she had seen her mother when her mother was asleep and she again nodded. When I asked if that was really scary she again nodded "yes." She then moved away from her mother to the toy cupboard, but soon thereafter came back to climb into her mother's lap, laying her head on her mother's shoulder for comfort as her mother and I empathized with how frightening it had been. This interchange seemed an important example of a point made earlier, namely, that having parents in the sessions allows them to "be there" with the child's traumatic feelings in ways they were not able to be at the time of the original trauma, thus helping to restore the child's trust. Katy's initial moving close and then away clearly reflected her conflict about her mother's availability as a source of comfort. It seemed to me a very positive step that she was able to return quickly, nestle in her mother's arms, and experience her mother's reassurance in the face of her frightening memories.

I asked if Katy and her mother could describe for me exactly what had happened. As they did so, in order to help decrease her reactivity to the physical sensations associated with the trauma, together we acted out the noise of the collision and the body movements of being shaken about. Katy herself described how scary it had been when the crash occurred and nodded as we empathized with how her pacifier helped her feel better. Toward the end of the session, Katy drew a stick-figure-like design on a blackboard and then handed the chalk to me. Knowing that seeing her mother at the hospital had been a particularly difficult moment, I drew a stick figure in a bed, then added a little girl figure standing by the bed with a sad face. Katy immediately evidenced her distress about this moment by erasing the picture. Although I tried to provide reassurance by drawing a new stick figure representing her mother standing up with a smile to remind her that her mother had recovered, it was clear that Katy was not ready to discuss the scene at the hospital.

Continued reworking of the trauma both at home and in the office continued over the next month. The morning after our first session Katy told her mother that she didn't want her to go away. Her mother asked, "You mean like when I went away in the fire truck?" Katy replied, "Yes." Together they drew a picture of her mother in the ambulance being taken to the hospital. Katy immediately went to get her pacifier and blanket and then, letting her mother hold her as they remembered the scene, related how she cried as her mother was taken away. During the sessions, as Katy and her mother described their discussions, I would ask them to elaborate on the details and would try to elicit Katy's feelings. She became an increasingly active participant. For example, as her mother told me how Katy had described the accident to her sister Amy and then told her sister that she had wanted to ride in the ambulance with her mother, Katy interrupted her mother's recounting to explain specifically to me, "That made me sad."

As is frequently the case in the course of trauma treatment, as Katy's feelings about the accident were being brought to the surface, there were moments when she seemed even more emotionally vulnerable than before. Some new signs of regression appeared both at home and during the sessions, including baby talk, silliness, and hyperactivity. Although not to a point where it became a serious obstacle to progress, it was difficult for Katy's mother to let go of her concerns about these behaviors, and I could see a potential for escalating angry interactions around use of the pacifier and toileting accidents. For example, following several toileting accidents in 1 week, her mother became quite frustrated. When Katy refused to go to the potty at her mother's request, her mother angrily threatened to put diapers back on her, which was quite upsetting to Katy. Since these episodes were infrequent and generally resolved in a reasonable way, I felt comfortable conveying my belief that these symptom breakthroughs were expectable aspects of the therapy and that they would diminish over time. Not without difficulty, her mother was able to accept this reassurance. It was only at the end of treatment, when Katy's symptoms had indeed resolved, that her mother realized that her sense of urgency had been largely driven by feelings of guilt and anxiety that these regressive behaviors meant that Katy had been permanently damaged by the accident.

A significant turning point in the form of a play reenactment occurred several sessions into our work together, as we talked about how Katy and her family had visited her mother at the hospital after the accident. Katy commented spontaneously that "Amy got up on the bed and I didn't." When we asked why she hadn't gotten up on the bed she replied, "I was scared." Her mother asked sensitively, "Were you scared because Mommy looked different?" Katy said, "Yes." We then encouraged her to describe how her mother looked. She described the bump on her mother's head. As her mother gestured toward where she had been bleeding, Katy touched her mother's head gently on that spot. She then touched her mother's hand, leg, and knee, referencing all the areas where mother had had "red spots."

Thinking it would be helpful to dramatize the discussion with play materials, with Katy's assistance I brought out various toy cars, ambulances, fire trucks, and small dolls in order to set the scene. As Katy and her mother played out the accident, Katy put the mother doll on the ground to show where her mother had lain following the collision. With a marker I drew red spots on the mother doll to help desensitize Katy to the frightening experience of the blood (in a previous session when I had asked about putting "red spots" on a drawing of her mother, Katy had indicated that I should put them on a separate sheet of paper). After we put the mother doll in the ambulance, Katy very purposefully placed the doll representing herself in the same ambulance with her mother. I then set up a hospital scene with play hospital equipment and placed the doll representing Katy alongside the mother doll's bed. Katy immediately took the "Katy" doll and laid it next to the mother doll on the bed. These actions on Katy's part allowed us to interpret how much she had wanted to be with her mother in the ambulance and how much she had in fact wanted to climb up on the bed to be close to her mother but had been too frightened. Katy then took out several tiny medicine bottles and put them to the mother doll's mouth. I picked up the theme of helping mother by suggesting we bandage her mother's "owies." Katy participated enthusiastically in taping small pieces of tissue to her mother's hand and head and then proceeded with additional caretaking, setting up a toy TV set for the mother and putting the father doll and other figures by the mother doll's bed. Her mother was struck by how actively engaged Katy was in the session as compared to at home and commented that this was the first time Katy had talked about her feelings related to seeing her mother at the hospital.

Her mother described a "big breakthrough" following this session, with a major improvement in Katy's symptoms and her relationship with her mother. This opportunity to deal with the frightening image of her mother as she looked with her facial injuries and in the medical surrounding seemed enormously helpful. In particular, the opportunity in play to carry out "reparative fantasies" of placing herself alongside her mother in the ambulance and in the bed and of aiding her mother in the hospital was significantly helpful in relieving the feelings of alienation and guilt that had resulted from her inability to approach her mother in the hospital because of her fear.

As a result of Katy's significant improvement, the therapeutic focus began to shift to address some of the larger trauma-related issues that were confronting the entire family. These included the family's reactions to the fact that the mother needed continued help in the home as well as increased behavioral upset on the part of Katy's elder sister Amy. The mother reported: "Whenever the nanny comes, everyone falls apart." Katy would cry and hold onto her mother's leg, while Amy would have huge temper tantrums. Even apart from the nanny's arrival, Amy was showing considerable distress of her own in the form of defiance and angry outbursts.

The entire family came to the next session to discuss these issues together. I took the opportunity to share with Katy's father and sister the kinds of discussions that Katy, her mother, and I had been having about the accident. My goal was to promote the family's ability to talk about the trauma together and, more specifically, to open the door for Katy's sister Amy to talk about her own feelings about the accident. In the course of the meeting I got out the play materials. With Katy taking the lead, we played out the whole sequence again for Amy's benefit. Amy was very articulate in describing how sad and worried she had been, including reporting a bad dream she had had the evening of the accident that her mother had died. Like Katy, Amy too described how scared she had been to see her mother looking so different at the hospital, but also how relieved she had been that her mother was alive. She poignantly described how, when thinking of that time "sometimes my body gets so scared I get the shivers."

As has frequently been my experience with traumatized young children (Gaensbauer, 1994, 2000), although Katy and Amy were able to talk about being frightened and sad, they both had difficulty acknowledging feelings of anger. For example, when I asked Amy what kinds of feelings she had when she was kicking and screaming on the floor in an obvious temper tantrum, she said that she was feeling scared. I attempted to validate feelings of anger by describing to Amy how common it was for kids who had experienced "bad things" to be angry. Amy continued nonetheless to insist that she was not mad. She did, however, acknowledge that she got "frustrated" sometimes. I encouraged the family to talk together about these frustrated feelings.

Following this family session, Katy's mother described that there had been a marked decrease in temper outbursts as they had been able to talk about these issues as a family. Most dramatically, the mother also reported that both children had started "to be able to play and fantasize again." After observing the children engage in imaginative play the evening after the family session, she had realized that she had not seen that kind of play since the accident. I commented on how often a trauma can interfere with children's ability to fantasize because of the danger that traumatic images and feelings might intrude (Terr, 1984; Pynoos, 1990). In support of this hypothesis, the mother observed that as the children had begun to play again they played out the accident with many different scenarios, including scenarios where their mother died. In other words, they were able to confront this worst-case scenario in their imagination without being overwhelmed.

The next few sessions with Katy and her mother served to consolidate Katy's gains. As she continued to play out elements of the accident, especially the "spread part" (i.e., the separation), consistently placing herself in the ambulance and on the hospital bed with her mother, her play over time became more expansive, less accident focused, and more symbolically rich in nature. She began to line the toy cars up in parking places and to drive them around without indicators of anxiety or needs to replay car crashes. Her spontaneous play resumed very age-appropriate themes as she used dolls to enact positive mother–child interactions in caregiving situations. That the turbulence of being shaken by the collision was beginning to be sublimated into more symbolic forms was suggested by Katy's drawing of several oblong shapes which she happily described as "upside-down mountains."

At home, Katy was "doing beautifully" for the most part. There were occasional moments of sadness or withdrawal, but her parents were generally able to bring her out without too much difficulty. Her mother proudly announced that they were at this point "a pacifier-free household" and that Katy had been using a new "lovey" stuffed animal as a comfort object instead. Another indication of Katy's developmental progression was her excited announcement that she was going to be going to a preschool for 3-year-olds where you had to be potty trained to be admitted. Katy's sister, Amy, however, was continuing to show distress, including being very sensitive about "getting less than Katy." She felt that Katy was receiving special attention as a result of being in the accident, including coming to see me. To help with these feelings, I scheduled a follow-up meeting with just Amy and her mother. In this session we discussed her needs to control her mother as her way of dealing with her feelings of sadness and helplessness about the accident and its aftermath, including her anger at feeling abandoned. Her mother also brought up an additional factor contributing to her defiance. Amy, as the eldest, had begun to assume a "mother" role with her younger sisters in the mother's absence. Even prior to the accident she had been showing developmentally expectable competitiveness with her mother. When her mother returned home and began to resume her authority, these competitive feelings were intensified. Amy listened carefully to these interpretations. Although she continued to deny having any angry feelings, she was able to acknowledge that in these interactions with her mother that she had "big feelings" that were more than the immediate situations called for.

In the midst of these sessions with Katy and Amy, a number of changes were moving the family toward resumption of a more normal preaccident pattern of functioning. When the mother's recovery reached the point where the home visitor was no longer needed, both Katy and her sister were able to tolerate being sent to day care without feeling abandoned by their mother. This indicated to me the fundamental solidity of their underlying attachment, as well as their confidence that things were truly getting back to normal. The mother's resumption of driving triggered considerable anxiety and traumatic reexperiencing. On one occasion Katy started crying as her mother pulled into traffic, saying "Don't go this way, Mommy! There are too many cars!" With discussion and reassurance, this anxiety diminished over time. Typical of the ongoing metabolizing of a trauma, everyday events in addition to driving continued to produce unforeseen strong emotions associated with traumatic reminders. Fortunately, these occasions were rare and, given the parents' attunement, able to be identified and processed. For example, when Katy's parents spent a weekend away and Katy stayed with one of her best friends, she was physically aggressive with her friend and sulky both during and immediately after the stay. In thinking about this unusual response, her mother made the connection that the last time Katy had stayed overnight at her friend's house had been the night of the accident. When her mother asked if being there had reminded her of the accident, Katy's face showed an immediate sign of relief and she gave her mother a hug.

The last phase of therapy came about when, after a period of several weeks of things going well, sibling rivalry intensified and Katy reverted to not talking and being upset with her mother about little things. The entire family again came to a session and talked about the changes in the family that seemed to be causing this exacerbation of symptoms. With their mother's recovery, the children's father had begun working more and was less available at home. In addition, Amy had begun piano lessons and Katy was expressing jealousy as her mother would sit with Amy to practice. Although in the family meeting the children played happily together, evidencing their fundamentally close relationship, their rivalry was also quite evident. At one point, as I asked Katy about her new school, Amy interrupted in a competitive fashion. At another point, Katy went to sit on her father's lap whereupon Amy immediately went over to sit on her mother's lap. Seeing Amy on her mother's lap, Katy became quiet and began to pout.

In discussions with the family it became apparent that multiple factors were contributing to this exacerbation of symptoms. As inevitably occurs, the traumatic experience was becoming intertwined with preexisting developmental and interactional patterns, making it difficult, particularly over time, to tease out the degree to which the upsurge in symptoms was attributable to the trauma versus the degree to which other factors were at work. The accident and its immediate aftermath were certainly playing a role. In addition to factors already described, we could identify one additional accident-related circumstance contributing to heightened pressure on Katy. Owing to her head injury, her mother had a reduced tolerance for noise and activity and at times needed to distance herself from highly stimulating situations. Katy, the most active of the children, was the one most frequently asked to play quietly, leading to feelings of criticism and rejection.

Over and above the accident, a number of other factors were playing significant roles. The most important, as I learned at this time, was the existence of a longstanding set of pairings within the family: Amy pairing with her mother, and Katy with her father. On family outings Amy would hold her mother's hand and Katy would hold her father's; during story times, the mother would consistently read to Amy and the father to Katy. Thus, a longstanding pattern of Katy feeling left out of the mother–Amy duo had been exacerbated by the father's return to work and the mother's help with Amy's piano lessons. Katy's position as the middle child, caught between Amy, on the one hand, and her younger sister (who was just beginning to walk), on the other, was also a contributing factor. Additionally, even beyond the mother's concerns about regression, the parents' expectations for behavior were quite high, creating an ongoing potential for conflict. It was my opinion that had the accident not occurred, these various family patterns would not have been overly problematic. However, with the increased vulnerability on everybody's part, they intensified Katy's tendency to express her unhappiness through provocative, negative attention-seeking behaviors to a degree that needed to be actively addressed.

The interventions discussed with the parents were designed to address all of these different factors. From a behavioral standpoint this involved helping them to be consistent in their behavioral expectations while not getting pulled into Katy's pouting and withdrawal. It was also important for them to "pick their spots" as far as discipline was concerned so there would be fewer occasions where Katy might gain attention through negative behavior. I also recommended a switch in the pairing patterns so that the mother would spend more time with Katy and the father more time with Amy. Not surprisingly, this shift was initially resisted by both children, but especially Amy, who wanted to continue to be able to control her mother in ways that left Katy out. We also attempted to help Katy realize that her mother's increased irritability or needs to disengage were related to her process of recovery and not Katy's fault. Finally, I attempted to normalize the entire situation by conveying my sense that the family would be dealing with these issues even if there had not been an accident. It was important to remember that Katy and Amy were both at an age where finding their respective places in the triangle between their mother and father and in their relationship with each other was a normal developmental task, independent of any accident effects. Given the solid relationships on all sides and the parent's responsiveness to the children's feelings and developmental needs, I expressed my confidence that they would be able to work them out over time as a family. This normalization of the issues was particularly helpful to the mother. It was at this point, as she was able to see the children's conflicts in this larger developmental framework, that she realized that her anxiety that the children had been permanently damaged by the accident had caused her to be less tolerant of Katy's misbehavior. She was sure that Katy had picked up on this.

In the remaining sessions, the family continued to focus on these issues to the point where the parents felt that things were very close to being back to normal and that the specific effects of the accident were largely resolved. The family appeared to have an excellent grasp of both the trauma-related and the ongoing developmental issues and was generally able in their discussions to tease out the various contributions of each. The parents were continuing to work on helping the children accept the mother's discipline and switching the parent–child preference patterns. Although neither of these issues was completely settled, the parents felt they were approaching resolution and that they could be dealt with without further therapy. Termination occurred at this point.

Follow-Up

In a follow-up interview almost 5 years later, Katy's mother reported that Katy was doing well and that the relationship between them was close. The accident continued to be a topic of periodic conversation in the family, coming up naturally in the course of everyday events without any indicators of stress. Interestingly, in these discussions Katy had added new details that had not been discussed during the therapy, such as how her baby sister had "cried and cried" in the ambulance on the way to the hospital. Occasional distress associated with traumatic triggers such as sudden loud noises, driving in the car, and seeing ambulances and fire trucks had been observed as long as a year after the accident, although her mother reported that as a result of the therapy they understood what Katy was experiencing and were able to reassure her. There had been no differences in her subsequent development as compared to that of her sisters' that her mother could attribute to the accident. Her mother did feel, however, that Katy had a greater appreciation than most children of the difficult things that can affect people's lives. She was very sensitive to when someone might be hurt, was very empathic to others' feelings, and would express a strong desire to help. She continued to be rather quiet and introverted, with a tendency to withdraw under stress. She also showed an occasional stubborn streak. While it is difficult to say how much the trauma contributed to these enduring personality traits, it had certainly been an influence in their expression at the time that it occurred.

DISCUSSION

The preceding discussion and case report highlight the challenges and rewards of working with traumatized young children and illustrate useful approaches to treatment. As noted in the introduction, the treatment described took place under relatively optimal conditions, involving a circumscribed trauma without permanent disabling effects and a high-functioning child and family. The importance of creating a safe environment, facilitating a child's communication of the experience, identifying and desensitizing traumatic affects, developing an accurate narrative, promoting adaptive processing and integration, monitoring symptom resurgence, and working closely with parents and other family members to address the ripple effects of the trauma in the home environment were all well demonstrated by virtue of the family's ability to make use of them. Katy and her family's experience also illustrates how, even in relatively optimal circumstances, an early trauma can have very significant and enduring effects. If a trauma like Katy's requires 6 months of therapeutic work with extensive family involvement, one can imagine what might be required to resolve more severe and/or repeated traumas.

As alluded to in the introduction, it is important to consider the extent to which the approaches described are relevant to the many children who experience more severe traumas and who do not have the benefit of the kind of family support that Katy enjoyed. Based on my experience, I would assert that the therapeutic principles outlined here are applicable to more severely traumatized children, even those who are dealing with multiple other stressors, but that they need to be applied in more circumscribed contexts. Although repeated traumas in combination with other pathogenic conditions will have their cumulative effects, each significant trauma will nevertheless have its own imprint. In the midst of all the other issues that they are dealing with, children will bring these specific traumas with their specific imprints into therapy in various forms—through behavioral enactments, through play, through their identification with the aggressor, through affective storms, through disorganized behavior, or other means. When this occurs and the clinician can make the connection to a specific trauma by applying in condensed form the types of therapeutic approaches that were helpful to Katy, it should be possible to facilitate some degree of therapeutic processing. Clearly, the amount of time that can be devoted to a single trauma may be extremely limited, given the children's multiple therapeutic needs and the fact that one is rarely able to work with such children in a sustained way over a long period of time. Thus, the goal in working with these more disadvantaged children would not be full resolution of the child's traumas. Instead, it would be to give as much help as possible in the time that the therapist has with the child. The trauma-specific therapeutic techniques described here would likely not come into play in the context of an overall treatment plan for fully resolving a traumatic experience, but rather in more focused moments when some aspect of a specific trauma has presented itself in the material. Given the vulnerability of these children, special care must be taken not to let the child become disorganized or overwhelmed, and techniques of ego building and positive modeling will be called for to a greater extent than in the case of Katy. Within these parameters, however, utilization of the kinds of traditional therapeutic techniques described here provides an opportunity at those moments when traumatic material is presented for some quantity of abreaction, desensitization of traumatic affect, organization of experience, facilitation of adaptive coping mechanisms, and modeling of an empathic relationship, even if it is to a small degree and in short spaces of time before the child moves on to other issues. As was true with Katy's family, as much therapeutic work as possible should also be done to encourage sensitivity in the caregiving environment to the child's traumatic needs (Osofsky, Cohen, & Drell, 1995; Osofsky, 2000).

An analogy drawn by a colleague who had witnessed a very traumatic situation in the course of a disaster response seems very appropriate here. In relating his experience to a group of us at a social occasion and being aware that his description of the scene was painful to imagine, he expressed his appreciation for our willingness to listen. He went on to impart his perspective that the traumatic event for him was akin to a huge mountain. Each time he talked about his experience, whatever the context, a quantity of dirt was removed from the mountain. Although perhaps the mountain would never be leveled, each opportunity to share some aspect of his experience diminished the load he had to carry. Our work with severely and multiply traumatized young children can be conceptualized similarly. We cannot take away the mountain. However, by being sensitive to the manifestation of specific traumatic symptoms when they do occur and allowing the child to share his or her experience in ways that are respectful of the child's ego capacities and social support, we can contribute to a lightening of the child's burden, even if it is in small increments.

NOTES

1. For convenience the term "parents" is used throughout the chapter to refer to the child's caregivers. It is to be understood that in many therapeutic situations, caregivers will be other than the parents.
2. Although at this point in time therapeutic modalities for traumatized young children are almost entirely psychosocial in nature, increasing knowledge about the neurodevelopmental impact of trauma will lead inevitably to potentially beneficial somatic treatments. Although there is to date no systematic research upon which to base pharmacological decisions, in situations where severely disruptive symptoms have persisted despite intensive psychosocial intervention medications that have been useful for older children may be considered.
3. This is one of the reasons that working with children who have experienced repeated traumas is so difficult. Because of the time and effort required before a child can begin to feel confident that the trauma will not recur, if subsequent traumas do occur the child's trust will be much more permanently shattered.

REFERENCES

Benham, A. L. (2000). The observation and assessment of young children including use of the infant–toddler mental status exam. In C. H. Zeanah (Ed.), *Handbook of infant mental health* (2nd ed., pp. 249–265). New York: Guilford Press.

Chatoor, I. (1991). Eating and nutritional disorders of infancy and early childhood. In J. Wiener (Ed.), *Textbook of child and adolescent psychiatry* (pp. 352–361). Washington, DC: Academy of Child and Adolescent Psychiatry Press.

Figley, C. (1983). Catastrophes: An overview of family reactions. In C. R. Figley & H. I. McCubbin (Eds.), *Stress and the family: Vol. 2. Coping with catastrophe.* New York: Brunner/Mazel.

Figley, C. R. (1989). *Helping traumatized families.* San Francisco: Jossey-Bass.

Fivush, R. (1993). Developmental perspectives on autobiographical recall. In G. S. Goodman & B. I. Bottoms (Eds.), *Child victims, child witnesses: Understanding and improving testimony* (pp. 1–24). New York: Guilford Press.

Fivush, R., & Fromhoff, F. (1988). Style and structure in mother–child conversations about the past. *Discourse Processes, 11,* 337–355.

Gaensbauer, T. J. (1994). Therapeutic work with a traumatized toddler. *Psychoanalytic Study of the Child, 49,* 412–433.

Gaensbauer, T. J. (1995). Trauma in the preverbal period: Symptoms, memories, and developmental impact. *Psychoanalytic Study of the Child, 50,* 122–149.

Gaensbauer, T. J. (2000). Psychotherapeutic treatment of traumatized infants and toddlers: A case report. *Clinical Child Psychology and Psychiatry, 5,* 373–385.

Gaensbauer, T. J., & Sands, K. (1979). Distorted affective communications in abused/neglected infants and their potential impact on caretakers. *Journal of the American Academy of Child Psychiatry, 18,* 236–250.

Gaensbauer, T. J., & Siegel, C. H. (1995). Therapeutic approaches to posttraumatic stress disorder in infants and toddlers. *Infant Mental Health Journal, 16,* 292–305.

Green, M., & Solnit, A. J. (1964). Reaction to the threatened loss of a child: A vulnerable child syndrome. *Pediatrics, 34,* 58–66.

Levy, D. (1939). Release therapy. *American Journal of Orthopsychiatry, 9,* 713–736.

Lewis, M. L. (1996). Trauma reverberates: Psychosocial evaluation of the caregiving environment of young children exposed to violence and traumatic loss. In J. D. Osofsky & E. Fenichel (Eds.), *Islands of safety: Assessing and treating young victims of violence* (pp. 21–28). Arlington, VA: Zero to Three/National Center for Clinical Infant Programs.

Osofsky, J. D. (1996). When the helper is hurting: Burnout and countertransference issues in treatment of children exposed to violence. In J. D. Osofsky & E. Fenichel (Eds.), *Islands of Safety: Assessing and Treating Young Victims of Violence* (pp. 35–38). Arlington, VA: Zero to Three/National Center for Clinical Infant Programs.

Osofsky, J. (2000). Infants and violence: Prevention, intervention, and treatment. In J. D. Osofsky & H. E. Fitzgerald (Eds.), *WAIMH handbook of infant mental health: Vol. 4. Infant mental health in groups at high risk* (pp. 161–196). New York: Wiley.

Osofsky, J. D., Cohen, G., & Drell, M. (1995). The effects of trauma on young children: A case of 2-year-old twins. *International Journal of Psychoanalysis, 76,* 595–607.

Pynoos, R. S. (1990). Posttraumatic stress disorder in children and adolescents. In B. Garfinkel, G. Carlson, & E. Weller (Eds.), *Psychiatric disorders in children and adolescents* (pp. 48–63). Philadelphia: Saunders.

Pynoos, R. S., Steinberg, A. M., & Wraith, R. (1995). A developmental model of childhood traumatic stress. In D. Cicchetti & D. Cohen (Eds.), *Developmental psychopathology, Vol. 2. Risk, disorder, and adaptation* (pp. 72–95). New York: Wiley.

Scheeringa, M. S., & Gaensbauer, T. J. (2000). Posttraumatic stress disorder. In C. H. Zeanah (Ed.), *Handbook of infant mental health* (2nd ed., pp. 369–381). New York: Guilford Press.

Scheeringa, M. S., & Zeanah, C. H. (2001). A relational perspective on PTSD in early childhood. *Journal of Traumatic Stress, 14,* 799–815.

Scheeringa, M. S., Zeanah, C. H., Drell, M. J., & Larrieu, J. A. (1995). Two approaches to the diagnosis of posttraumatic stress disorder in infancy and early childhood. *Journal of the American Academy of Child and Adolescent Psychiatry, 34,* 191–200.

Terr, L. (1984). Children at acute risk: Psychic trauma. In L. Grinspoon (Ed.), *Psychiatry update: The American Psychiatric Association annual review* (Vol. 3, pp. 104–120). Washington, DC: American Psychiatric Press.

Terr, L. (1988). What happens to early memories of trauma?: A study of twenty children under five at the time of documented traumatic events. *Journal of the American Academy of Child and Adolescent Psychiatry, 27,* 96–104.

Terr, L. (1989). Family anxiety after traumatic events. *Journal of Clinical Psychiatry, 50,* 15–19.

Terr, L. (1990). *Too scared to cry.* New York: Basic Books.

Terr, L. (1995). Childhood posttraumatic stress disorder. In G. O. Gabbard (Ed.), *Treatments of psychiatric disorders* (2nd ed., Vol. 1, pp. 287–299). Washington, DC: American Psychiatric Press.

Wallick, M. M. (1979). Desensitization therapy with a fearful two-year-old. *American Journal of Psychiatry, 136,* 1325–1326.

Zeanah, C. H. (1994). The assessment and treatment of infants and toddlers exposed to violence. In J. D. Osofsky & E. Fenichel (Eds.), *Caring for infants and toddlers in violent environments: Hurt, healing and hope* (pp. 29–37). Arlington, VA: Zero to Three: National Center for Clinical Infant Programs.

Zeanah, C. H., & Scheeringa, M. (1996). Evaluation of posttraumatic symptomatology in infants and young children exposed to violence. In J. D. Osofsky & E. Fenichel (Eds.), *Islands of safety: Assessing and treating young victims of violence* (pp. 9–14). Arlington, VA: Zero to Three/National Center for Clinical Infant Programs.

PART III

HOW TO REACH
SERIOUSLY TRAUMATIZED
CHILDREN EARLIER

COLLABORATIONS FOR YOUNG TRAUMATIZED CHILDREN WITH JUVENILE COURTS, LAW ENFORCEMENT, AND CHILD WELFARE

Collaborations with "unexpected" professionals (first responders and nontraditional first responders) who come in contact with young traumatized children offer a creative way to support and help the children by reaching them earlier and in nontraditional settings for mental health professions. Juvenile court cases consist of both dependent children (who have been abused and neglected by the very people who are supposed to nurture and love them) and older delinquent youth. Many people think only about the older children who are arrested and charged with a crime. What is unique to the chapters in this section is their focus on the younger children who because of abuse and neglect and family dysfunction are at higher risk for later problems in development and adaptation. These chapters speak in different ways to creative interventions in courts, with law enforcement, and in child welfare.

Chapter 9 by Joy D. Osofsky and Judge Cindy Lederman describes an innovative program that has been put in place in the 11th Circuit Juvenile Court in Miami, Florida, to identify and intervene with and provide services for abused and neglected children and their parents with the goal of improving the relationship, preventing further abuse and neglect, and increasing permanency.

In Chapter 10, Patricia Van Horn and Judge Donna J. Hitchens describe ways to build partnerships for young children in court and different ways to link juvenile court judges with mental health professionals to develop prevention and intervention programs through the court setting. This chapter describes with a case vignette a treatment approach for working with dependent children and their parents.

In Chapter 11, Anna T. Smyke, Valerie Wajda-Johnston, and Charles H. Zeanah, Jr., describe a program working with traumatized children within the child welfare system. They consider the types of trauma seen in infants and toddlers who have come into foster care and discuss the important components of the child welfare system and the ways in which they impact the very young child. Specific types of treatment useful in the management of traumatized infants and toddlers are presented, with case vignettes to illustrate the authors' approach to this important work.

The organizing principle of the work of this group as well as of all the aforementioned approaches in Juvenile Court is to determine the best interests of these very young traumatized children so that their needs are addressed first and foremost. Chapter 12 by Joy D. Osofsky, Jill Hayes Hammer, Nancy Freeman, and J. Michael Rovaris describes ways to build a partnership with law enforcement personnel as first responders to identify and help young traumatized children as early as possible. The authors describe a successful 10-year collaborative program with the New Orleans Police Department that has evolved by building trusting relationships, providing ongoing education, and developing consistent consultation and referral resources for police officers to help traumatized children and families. All of these programs that involve strategies "thinking out of the box" for traumatized children have been able to develop approaches to address their needs more effectively.

CHAPTER 9

HEALING THE CHILD
IN JUVENILE COURT

Joy D. Osofsky
Cindy Lederman

Juvenile court, perhaps unexpectedly nationwide, has become an important place to "heal the child." There were 903,000 substantiated cases of child maltreatment in 2001, most of which involved neglect (U.S. Department of Health and Human Services, 2003). Every day, the courts are making decisions, often irrevocable ones, about children's lives. This situation places a heavy burden on juvenile court judges; at the same time, the decisions have to be made and will be made. Building partnerships between these judges and mental health professionals can be helpful because they provide an important opportunity to help the judges make better—or at least better-informed—decisions about young children's lives. In addition, juvenile court judges can be supported in their difficult work by gaining more knowledge and information about developmental issues for young children as well as referrals and services.

The objectives of this chapter are the following: (1) to describe the plight of young children in the child welfare system as it relates to the work of juvenile court; (2) to review the literature on exposure to domestic violence and child maltreatment that is relevant to young children in dependency court; (3) to elaborate on how collaborations between mental health professionals and judges on behalf of young children can be helpful in juvenile court; and (4) to illustrate the conceptualization and principles of "healing the child" by describing the course of a young child and mother who appeared in juvenile court.

THE JUVENILE COURT AND CHILDREN

Initially, the juvenile court was created in Chicago at the end of the 19th century (Illinois Juvenile Court Act, 1899) and was charged with the responsibility of protecting children from family members who had abused, abandoned, and neglected them as they were unable to fulfill their roles as loving, nurturing parents. Under these circumstances, the juvenile court must intervene to protect and rehabilitate children when all else has failed. The judges have the weighty responsibility of making crucial decisions about the health, safety, and well-being of vast numbers of children every day. The juvenile court is a place of last resort where the state must act to protect the lives of children when there is a compelling reason to intervene in the sanctity and privacy of the relationship between a parent and a child. By the time children appear in juvenile court, tremendous harm has already been done. That is why the juvenile court can become a place to heal in trying to address the negative effects that can only be decreased by giving the child and family opportunity to change their harmful behaviors.

An additional burden for juvenile court today is that the children within the child welfare system increasingly are becoming younger. Of the almost 600,000 children currently in foster care in 2002 in the United States, one in five of them have entered care for the first time during their first year of life (Wulczyn & Hislop, 2002). Furthermore, there has been an unprecedented increase in younger babies entering care, with 1 in 20 in urban areas being birth to 3 months of age. Because babies who enter foster care younger stay in placement longer, it is crucial that those coming in contact with the babies, including judges, lawyers, CASA (court-appointed special advocates), court personnel, and others in the child welfare system, be informed about ways to better protect and promote the healthy development of these innocent children, who can be seen as "silent victims" with no voice. These children are rarely seen in the courtroom; often their parents are unable to recognize their needs. The judges, attorneys, and guardians in court are often overburdened, frequently have little knowledge about child development and the needs of these children, and have limited opportunity to interact with the child.

CO-OCCURRENCE OF YOUNG CHILDREN'S EXPOSURE TO DOMESTIC VIOLENCE AND CHILD MALTREATMENT

Because so many children who appear in dependency court are exposed to both domestic violence and other forms of child maltreatment, a reality that is frequently ignored, a review of relevant literature will be presented to frame our understanding of the potential environment of a dependent child. Since the mid-1970s, researchers have explored the co-occurrence of child maltreatment and domestic violence. In 1975, a national survey was conducted of 1,146 families indicating that 77% of children living in high-violence families were abused during their lifetime (Straus, Gelles, & Steinmetz, 1980). Senate Report No. 101-939 (1990) revealed that in homes where domestic violence occurs children are physically abused and neglected at a rate 15 times higher than the national average. Several studies have found that in 60–75% of families where a woman is battered, children are also battered (Straus et al., 1980; Bowker, 1988; McKibben, DeVos, & Newberger, 1989). According to a recent report, "In Harm's Way: Domestic Violence and Child Maltreatment," researchers have typically used one of two methods to study the overlap (National Clearinghouse on Child Abuse and Neglect Information, 2002). They either identify evidence of woman battering in families where known cases of child abuse exist, using child protection services records, or they search for evidence of child abuse in families where abuse of the mothers has been documented using shelter samples.

Several federally funded studies done in the late 1970s included questions for families about major presenting problems in additional to child maltreatment. Those families reporting domestic violence as a significant co-occurring problem ranged from 11% in a 1977 study to 42% in a 1982 study (Daro & Cohn, 1988). A 1990 review of 200 substantiated cases of child abuse in the Massachusetts Department of Social Services indicated that adult domestic violence was cited in 30% of the cases, with more recent studies indicating the rate may be as high as 48% (Dykstra & Alsop, 1996). A similar review done by English (1998) in Washington State indicated that 55 percent of the physical and emotional abuse referrals involved domestic violence.

In a study of Minnesota child welfare cases, 71% of the families in crisis reported issues related to domestic violence (Shepard & Raschick, 1999). Edleson's 1999 review of 35 published studies of co-occurrence concluded that the majority of the research supports the notion of a high level of overlap ranging from 30 to 60% in most studies. In Margolin's (1998) review of the effects of domestic violence, she noted that 45–70% of children exposed to domestic violence are also victims of physical abuse and that as many as 40% of child victims of physical abuse are also exposed to domestic violence. McCloskey, Figueredo, and Koss (1995) reported that children living with a battered mother are also at serious risk for sexual abuse either by the mother's partner or outside of the home. Beeman, Hegemeister, and Edleson (2001), in their review of police records cross-referenced with child protection referrals, identified that more than 64% of the cases were identified as dual-violence families (see also Edleson, 1999).

As might be expected, negative outcomes are more likely for children who experience both domestic violence and child maltreatment when compared to outcomes for those who experience one form of violence. Further, not infrequently in families where there is domestic violence and child maltreatment, there are also other risk factors including parental mental health problems, substance abuse, divorce, criminality, poverty, and general family dysfunction. Thus, there are many factors that may be contributing to the negative outcomes for children. With the literature indicating that the risk for exposure to domestic violence is higher for younger children who are also more vulnerable to child abuse and neglect, the field could benefit enormously from longitudinal follow-up studies.

Across all of these studies, irrespective of the methodology used, the following conclusions can be drawn

1. Child abuse impacts negatively on children affecting them cognitively, socially, and emotionally.
2. Witnessing violence impacts negatively on children of all ages, regardless of severity or frequency.
3. Being victimized by both child abuse and exposure to domestic violence impacts more negatively on children.

With this information in mind, it is crucial to take into account additional family factors that may mediate to influence outcomes more positively or aggravate the situation leading to more negative child outcomes. These factors include stress, poverty, parental mental illness, substance use, age of the parents, and age of the child. All of these risk factors impact heavily on dependent children and their parents or caregivers.

BUILDING COLLABORATIVE RELATIONSHIPS TO HELP CHILDREN IN JUVENILE COURT

Mental health professionals, particularly those with expertise about child development, can provide assistance to judges and attorneys in several different ways (see Appendix 9.1 for a helpful checklist for judges). First, they can help by providing information and training for people who work in conjunction with the juvenile court about the science of child development and early intervention. Often education can result from expert testimony. Second, they can provide more knowledge about the needs of young children, especially those at considerable risk within the child welfare system. Third, they can provide resources in the form of information, screenings, assessments, evaluations, and therapeutic or other services. Finally, they can also offer assistance in the form of consultation, education, and/or ongoing collaborations.

Many years ago, Lenore Terr (1986) wrote about the baby in court. She emphasized that infant mental health specialists must assist the legal system in understanding the infant's perspective. Direct "evidence" is needed from the baby, which for a young child who cannot talk must come either through careful observations of behaviors and emotions or adult reports. In this way, the baby will be protected and the court will be better informed. Although Terr's article was written in the late 1980s, we have not come a long way since then toward recognizing and intervening for young children who, through no fault of their own, are represented in juvenile court. Very often the representation relates to their well-being, that is, whether they will remain with their parent who often is not providing adequate care or whether parental rights will be terminated and they will be placed with a foster and/or adoptive family. Often the adults in these cases will be very poor reporters, as they may be the perpetrators of abuse and neglect. Developmental and clinical expertise may be needed to protect the baby and better inform the court. It behooves the court to be as well informed as possible about the needs of young children through the science of early childhood development so as to be able to use the law to support "the best interests of the child" (Goldstein, Solnit, Goldstein, & Freud, 1998).

Addressing the needs of the young child in court not only is vitally important so that the infant has a "voice," it is also crucial to prevent more damage from happening by placing the child in a living situation that will fail to nurture his or her development (Lederman & Osofsky, 2004). Brain growth and development are very active during the first few years of life. During the first 3–4 years of life, brain structures that influence cognitive development, social and emotional development, learning, ability to deal with stress, and personality are established and strengthened. The abuse and neglect that causes children to enter foster care, coupled with frequent substance abuse, poor nutrition, lack of stimulation, and exposure to violence, all contribute to impairments in the healthy development of the brain (Shonkoff & Phillips, 2002). The children in the child welfare system are victims of cumulative disadvantages and often live in families where emotional impoverishment is common. Further, early relationship experiences and attachments that optimize emotional development also build self-esteem and form the basis for all later relationships.

Partnering with a developmental mental health specialist can serve several roles for the judge. The specialist can provide information to help the judge make a more informed decision. She can also help the judge learn more about resources for dependent children and their families that may contribute to breaking an intergenerational cycle of abuse, neglect, and violence exposure. Infant mental health specialists can also develop specially tailored evaluations and intervention strategies for court-referred children that will be workable within this system in an effort to heal the child and support the emerging healthier relationships between young children and their caregivers. These collaborations generally work most successfully by first building trust between the judge and the mental health professional.

Then, with mutual respect for the expertise of people from multiple disciplines, a flexible program can be developed that will work in diverse settings. The case presented below illustrates some of these points.

CASE EXAMPLE

Brianna's baby was born in 1999 when she was 12 years old. She had only finished the eighth grade in school. As a child mother, she did not even know she was pregnant until half way through her pregnancy. She did not receive prenatal care. Because Brianna was a minor, the baby was released from the hospital into the custody of her mother. The baby's father was 19 years old and, not unexpectedly, abandoned Brianna and her baby. He had wanted Brianna to have an abortion. After the baby was born, he was arrested for statutory rape.

We know little about Brianna's life before she had the baby; however after the baby was born, her life was extremely chaotic. She lived with her mother, who would not allow her to go to school. They moved from motel room to motel room as her mother tried to find work. Because Brianna's mother was an alcoholic who also used cocaine, contributing to instability, inconsistency, and likely violence, it was difficult for her to find work. One of the ways that Brianna's mother supported her drug habit was by shoplifting—and with little concern for the baby, she took her grandson along and used him as a decoy. Following in her mother's footsteps, Brianna was arrested for petty theft in 2000 and 2001 after first stealing clothing for herself and then jewelry.

In 2001, Brianna's mother was arrested for child neglect and possession of cocaine when Brianna's 2-year-old son was found wandering around a motel parking lot unclothed at 4:00 in the morning. When searched during the arrest, cocaine was found in Brianna's mother's pocket and worms were found in the baby's bottle. Brianna's mother was placed on probation. Apparently, however, the situation worsened and finally the local child protection service (the Department of Children and Families) intervened. At that time, the family had moved to a trailer located in an open field. There was no electricity or water, and the trailer was filthy and overall in deplorable condition. It was insect infested, lacked windows, and had one bed.

At the time Brianna appeared in juvenile court in the spring of 2002, she had not seen or heard from her father in 3 years. She was a 15-year-old mother of a 3-year-old son. When she first appeared in court for the proceedings, she was distraught and confused. At that time, Brianna and her son were adjudicated dependent. Brianna told the court what she truly believed—that she was a good mother who loved her son and that she had not done anything to harm him. She asked over and over again at every hearing, "When can I have my son back?" Because Brianna had never had adequate mothering herself, she did not know what it meant to be a good mother. She had never had a positive parenting role model. What was blatantly evident in court when Brianna appeared was that she did not understand what she had done to result in the removal of her child; however, she was highly motivated to work to get him back.

The judge recognized the strong motivation in this mother and had learned from her collaboration with child development/clinical specialists that change was possible, even when circumstances might seem almost impossible. Therefore, Brianna and her son were asked by the court to participate in an Early Childhood Relationship Assessment to learn more about their current relationship and evaluate the potential for change. The court was particularly concerned about Brianna's son after it was reported to the judge that he had violently killed a cat. The judge believed that the evaluation would help her decide what the prospects might be for success in changing the negative parenting behaviors of this young mother that likely resulted in the consequent very aggressive behaviors of this young child.

During the evaluation, it became obvious very quickly that Brianna had no idea about how to parent her son. How would she have learned to parent a child since her alcohol- and drug-abusing mother rarely if ever showed any positive parenting toward her when she was growing up? Throughout the play period of the evaluation, Brianna tried to engage her son; however, she repeatedly neglected his leads, was very directive, and didn't know how to play with him. This behavior is common in mothers who have received little attention and had negative parenting themselves. Further, Brianna was passive in response to his negative behavior, could not set limits or provide boundaries or guide him, and did not attempt to intervene or comment to him. When he did not want to clean up the toys and refused to surrender the toys he was playing with, Brianna took no action. She had no idea how to set limits, encourage him to comply, or distract or discipline him; she had no idea how to parent her son.

As always, during the evaluation, we look for strengths in the parent and the dyad in addition to the obvious weaknesses. At the end of the evaluation, the psychologist concluded that Brianna was able to keep her composure when dealing with her angry and difficult child, but she failed to set limits for him. There was no spontaneous affection between mother and son.

Brianna had some unusually positive characteristics not often observed in juvenile court. Despite the fact that she could only read at a fourth-grade level, she was engaging and bright. She also was psychologically minded enough to realize that she needed to make changes in her life in order to grow as an individual and as a parent. What was also evident was that she was motivated to change and genuinely wanted to improve her situation for her son. At that time, Brianna was exceptionally fortunate to be in a nurturing foster home where she had a loving relationship with her foster mother.

The Part C screening for her son indicated that he was not only delayed in language development but also in social and emotional development and cognitive skills. At 3 years of age, he could not draw a circle, he did not know his colors, and he did not know his gender. His medical needs had been neglected as well in that he had not received the necessary immunizations.

After the evaluation, Brianna and her son were referred for dyadic child–parent psychotherapy. Both the judge and the therapist observed that there was much strength in the relationship. Brianna clearly loved her son but had little understanding of his developmental needs. Brianna failed to understand how important structure, boundaries, limit setting, and discipline were in the life of a child; yet she was motivated to be a good parent. In dyadic therapy, Brianna was forthcoming with the therapist about her son's behavioral challenges and her weaknesses as a parent. After 15 weeks of dyadic therapy the improvements were significant. Brianna was initiating developmentally appropriate play with her son. Her increasing knowledge of developmental milestones helped her to respond to her child's needs. She was learning to respond to his nonverbal cues. She was able to connect and communicate with her child, showed an ability to follow his lead in play, set limits for the first time, and praised him for appropriate behaviors.

As she made progress in dyadic therapy, the court began to allow an increasing amount of unsupervised visitations between Brianna and her child. The progress was incremental. First Brianna, quite proficient in the use of public transportation, was allowed to transport her child to therapy unsupervised. Later, she was given more and more unsupervised visitation.

Despite her progress, there were some instances of erratic adolescent behavior on Brianna's part that caused concern when she failed to adequately maintain her son's hygiene and when she violated her curfew and stayed out too late. The level of concern heightened significantly when the court was informed that Brianna was dating a 31-year-old man. During more than one of her dates with him, there was police involvement. During therapy, Brianna was praised for her success in therapy but strongly admonished about the dangers in her choice of men. This theme was repeated over and over at every court appearance, in her dyadic therapy, and in her conversations with her foster mother.

Brianna, who did not wish to be reunified with her mother, was at the same time repeating what she had learned from her by exhibiting these erratic behaviors. Brianna's mother still would not accept responsibility for her neglect, substance abuse, and abuse of her daughter and grandchild. She denied any wrongdoing and failed to gain any insight. She wanted her daughter and grandson back.

Brianna had learned enough to know that she did not want to live with her mother or live the life of her mother; however, it was difficult for her to learn that there is another way. Brianna is no longer seeing the 31-year-old man. She seemed to be reached by explaining the effect of an inappropriate partner on her child. Brianna knew from her past how dangerous an imprudent choice of relationship could be on a child. Now, Brianna can be reasoned with by being asked to reflect upon the ramifications of her behavior on her son. The fortunate conjunction of the court intervention, the dyadic therapy, and the nurturing foster mother, together with Brianna's strong interpersonal skills and motivation to provide a better life for her son, all bode well for his future. She has acknowledged after 6 months of dyadic therapy and increasing time with her son that parenting can be difficult! All of this progress and growth has occurred despite the fact that Brianna is still an adolescent.

CONCLUSION

The intergenerational transmission of child maltreatment is a heartbreaking cycle. The abused child who becomes the abusive mother to her baby as a consequence of maltreatment is particularly worrisome to all involved in the child welfare system. Yet, how can we expect a child mother who has never felt safe and never been nurtured to know instinctively how to parent? Our challenge and our hope must be to intervene with young mothers and their infants early in their development. In the late 1980s, Selma Fraiberg and her colleagues (Fraiberg, Adelson, Shapiro, 1987) wrote the groundbreaking paper, "Ghosts in the Nursery," which vividly explicated how unresolved conflicts from the past so often reappear in the present in maladaptive and harmful parenting behaviors. The only way to change these negative patterns is to acknowledge them, come to understand how they have developed, and work them through so that they will not continue to haunt present relationships.

Brianna thought being a parent was simple. From her mother who was neglectful and selfish, Brianna learned that parenting did not take a lot of time and effort. Protecting one's child from inevitable danger was not a parenting skill she had observed. Brianna was trying to be a better parent than her mother but did not know how to accomplish this goal. The court was always aware of Brianna's love for her son and desire to be a good parent, an important foundation not always observed in the dependency court parent population. Only through intensive self-understanding and dyadic child–parent psychotherapy was she able to learn healthy ways to interact with her son and try to meet his needs. One day, Brianna, having progressed to the halfway point in her therapy sessions, came to court for a review hearing. When asked by the judge what she was learning in her dyadic therapy she said, "I am learning that being a good parent is really hard." That is the day it became clear to the court that Brianna could overcome her past and, with continued assistance and services, become a good mother to her child. There is hope that Brianna and her son will overcome their expected destiny and thrive together.

Collaboration between judges and child development/clinical specialists have provided a unique opportunity to "heal the child" in juvenile court. Dependency court can be understood and worked with in several different ways. Some people treat the court as the place of last resort for abused and neglected children who will suffer whether their parents are able to work with the court to achieve permanency or if the children languish for years in the child welfare system while a determination is made about whether there is any way their parents can be deemed adequate. As was mentioned above, very young children remain within the child welfare system longer than older children, often for 2–3 years before achieving some type of stability in their lives. And yet babies "cannot wait" because damage can result very quickly from instability in their lives and relationships in the first few years of their lives. The collaboration described in this chapter, illustrated by the case of Brianna, has led to the development of a successful intervention program in the 11th Circuit Juvenile Court in Miami. By referring young children early for evaluations and introducing dyadic therapy for them and their mothers who are motivated to become better parents, we have seen remarkable changes. We fully understand that it is an "uphill battle" in that these child mothers so often can still be "haunted" by the ghosts from their past and the difficult pressures and circumstances of their current lives. At the same time, we have seen mothers who based on their past life experiences knew nothing about parenting, playing with their children, holding their children, or talking to their children. Although these skills might seem obvious and basic to some, if a woman has never learned them from her own early experiences, it is difficult for her to parent. Further, what such women have most often learned is abuse and neglect and very negative early relationship experiences. Juvenile court is a place for the relearning to start with the support of other systems in the community, including mental health, education, early intervention, and family support services. We have found that this model can be implemented successfully if both the judges and the mental health professionals can join together and make the commitment to change the way the court has treated these cases that come before them every day. Brianna and her child are an excellent example of what can result from these efforts.

As Judge William E. Gladstone has said so wisely, "if we truly value our children and want to prevent the development of violent behaviors and consequent delinquency, it is vital that we put in place supports and prevention programs that address children's needs" (personal communication, July 16, 2001). Judges are generally not exposed to social science literature or child psychology in law school or through judicial training where the law is emphasized almost exclusively. Education in other disciplines is not readily available to judges, many of whom fear that knowing "too much" about a subject may compromise their objectivity. Hence, every chance to help judges learn through testimony, education, and even casual conversation in multidisciplinary professional or social settings is important.

ACKNOWLEDGMENTS

The work reported in this chapter was supported by Miami Safe Start, funded by the Office of Juvenile Justice and Delinquency Prevention (OJJDP), New Orleans Safe Start funded by OJJDP, and the Harris Center for Infant Mental Health, Louisiana State University Medical Center, New Orleans.

REFERENCES

Beeman, S. K., Hagemeister, A. K., & Edleson, J. L. (2001). Case assessment and service receipt in families experiencing both child maltreatment and woman battering. *Journal of Interpersonal Violence, 16*(5), 437–458.

Bowker, L. H. (1988). On the relationship between wife beating and child abuse. In K. M. Bograd (Ed.), *Feminist perspectives on wife abuse.* Newbury Park, CA: Sage.

Daro, D., & Cohn, A. H. (1988). Child maltreatment evaluation efforts: What have we learned? In G. T. Hotaling, D. Finkelhor, J. T. Kirkpatrick, & M. A. Straus (Eds.), *Coping with family violence: Research on policy perspectives* (pp. 275–287). Newbury Park, CA: Sage.

Dykstra, C. H., & Alsop, R. J. (1996). *Domestic violence and child abuse* [Monograph]. Englewood, CO: American Humane Association.

Edleson, J. L. (1999). The overlap between child maltreatment and woman battering. *Violence against Women, 5*(2), 134–154.

English, D. (1998). The extent and consequences of child maltreatment. *The Future of Children, 8*(1), 39–53.

Fraiberg, S., Adelson, E., & Shapiro, V. (1987). Ghosts in the nursery: A psychoanalytic approach to the problems of impaired infant–mother relationships. In S. Fraiberg & L. Fraiberg (Eds.), *Selected writings of Selma Fraiberg* (pp. 164–196). Columbus: Ohio State University Press.

Goldstein, J., Solnit, A., Goldstein, S., & [the late] Freud, A. (1998). *The best interests of the child: The least detrimental alternative.* New York: Free Press.

Illinois Juvenile Court Act. (1899). Ill. Laws (Vol. 132).

Lederman, C., & Osofsky, J. D. (2004). Infant mental health interventions in juvenile court: Ameliorating the effects of maltreatment and deprivation. *Psychology, Public Policy, and the Law, 10*(1), 162–177.

Margolin, G. (1998). Effects of witnessing violence on children. In P. K. Trickett & C.

J. Schellenbach (Eds.), *Violence against children in the family and the community*. Washington, DC: American Psychological Association.

McCloskey, L. A., Figueredo, A. J., & Koss, M. P. (1995). The effects of systemic family violence on children's mental health. *Child Development, 66*, 1239–1261.

McKibben, L., DeVos, E., & Newberger, E. (1989). Victimization of mothers of abused children: A controlled study. *Pediatrics, 84*, 531–535.

National Clearinghouse on Child Abuse and Neglect Information. (2002, February 24). *In harm's way: Domestic violence and child maltreatment*. Rockville, MD: U.S. Department of Health and Human Services, Administration for Children and Families. Available from *http://www.calib.com/nccanch/pubs/otherpubs/harmsway.cfm*

Senate Report No. 101–939. (1990). Hearing, Senate Committee on the Judiciary, 101st Cong.

Shepard, M., & Raschick, M. (1999). How child welfare workers assess and intervene around issues of domestic violence. *Child Maltreatment: Journal of the American Professional Society on the Abuse of Children, 4*(2), 148–156.

Shonkoff, J., & Phillips, D. (2000). *From neurons to neighborhoods: The science of early childhood development*. Washington, DC: National Academy Press.

Straus, M., Gelles, R., & Steinmetz, S. (1980). *Behind closed doors: Violence in the American family*. Garden City, NY: Anchor Books.

Terr, L. (1986). The child psychiatrist and the child witness: Traveling companions by necessity, if not by design. *Journal of the American Academy of Child and Adolescent Psychiatry, 25*(4), 462–472.

U.S. Department of Health and Human Services. (2001). *National statistics on child abuse and neglect*. Rockville, MD: Author.

Wulczyn, F., & Hislop, K. B. (2002). Babies in foster care: The numbers call for attention. *Zero to Three, 22*(5), 14–15.

QUESTIONS EVERY JUDGE AND LAWYER SHOULD ASK ABOUT INFANTS AND TODDLERS IN THE CHILD WELFARE SYSTEM

Joy D. Osofsky
Candice Maze
Cindy Lederman
Martha Grace
Sheryl Dicker

We need to change the culture in our courts. Instead of ignoring babies and toddlers and assuming they are fine despite abuse and neglect, we need to recognize that these children are at risk for developing some sequelae of their maltreatment. Such sequelae can range from short-term emotional problems to lifelong serious behavioral and cognitive impairments impacting learning and adult functioning.

The science of early development is unequivocal: Early intervention can be effective. Substantial evidence indicates that early intervention is most effective during the first 3 years of life when the brain is establishing the foundations for all developmental, social, and cognitive domains. We need to learn about the science of early childhood development and use that knowledge to promote the healthy development of the babies and toddlers who come to court. The juvenile court is the last resort for these children. Let's turn that tragedy into an opportunity and be the place where the healing begins.

We developed the following questions to be a guide for lawyers, judges, and child advocates in the child welfare system and to be a first step at advocacy and intervention for young children. Armed with the questions that need to be asked, and the scientific reasons and research on which they are based, we must use this guide and ask these questions over and over until the needs of maltreated infants and babies are addressed. It is our legal obligation under the Adoption and Safe Families Act of 1997, and it is our moral responsibility to these young children.

INTRODUCTION[1]

Increasing numbers of infants and young children with complicated and serious physical, mental health, and developmental problems are being placed in foster care.[2] The following checklists have been developed for use by judges, attorneys, child advocates, and other child welfare professionals in meeting the wide range of health care needs of this growing population.

PHYSICAL HEALTH

- Has the child received a comprehensive health assessment since entering foster care?

Because children are likely to enter foster care as a result of abuse, neglect, homelessness, poverty, parental substance abuse, or mental illness, all foster children should receive a comprehensive physical examination shortly after placement that addresses all aspects of the child's health. Under the early and periodic screening, diagnosis, and treatment provisions of federal Medicaid law,[3] foster children should receive a comprehensive assessment that can establish a baseline for a child's health status, evaluate whether the child has received necessary immunizations, and identify the need for further screening, treatment, and referral to specialists.[4] A pediatrician or family practice physician knowledgeable about the health care problems of foster children should perform the examination.[5]

Ensuring the healthy development of foster children requires that they receive quality medical care. Such care should be comprehensive, coordinated, continuous, and family supported. One person should be identified who will oversee the child's care across the various agencies and systems, including early childhood services, early intervention services, education, and medical and mental health. Family-supportive care requires sharing the child's health information with the child's caregivers and providing caregivers with education and training programs in order to meet the needs of their foster child.

- Are the child's immunizations complete and up-to-date for his or her age?

Complete, up-to-date immunizations provide the best defense against many childhood diseases that can cause devastating effects. Immunization status is an important measure of vulnerability to childhood illness and can reveal whether the child has had access to basic health care. Incomplete or delayed immunization suggests that the child is not receiving adequate medical care and is not regularly followed by a provider familiar with the child's health needs. A child should have a "well-baby" examination by 2–4 weeks of age. Immunizations are recommended at 2, 4, 6, and 12 months of age. A child should have at least three visits to a pediatrician or family practice physician during the second year of life, with basic immunizations completed by 2 years of age.[6]

- **Has the child received a hearing and vision screen?**

Undetected hearing loss during infancy and early childhood interferes with the development of speech and language skills and can have deleterious effects on overall development, especially learning. Hearing loss during early childhood can result from childhood diseases, significant head trauma, environmental factors such as excessive noise exposure, and insufficient attention paid to health problems that may affect hearing. Studies reveal that 70% of children with hearing impairments are initially referred for assessment by their parents.[7] Because foster care children often lack a consistent caregiver who can observe their development and note areas of concern, they should receive ongoing evaluations of hearing, speech, and language development.

Vision screening is an essential part of preventative health care for children. Problems with vision are the fourth most common disability among children in the United States and the leading cause of impaired conditions in childhood.[8] Early detection and treatment increase the likelihood that a child's vision will develop normally and, if necessary, that the child will receive corrective devices.

- **Has the child been screened for lead exposure?**

Children who are young, low-income, and have poor access to health care are vulnerable to the harmful effects of lead.[9] Ingested or inhaled lead can damage a child's brain, kidneys, and blood-forming organs. Children who are lead poisoned may have behavioral and developmental problems. According to the Centers for Disease Control and Prevention (CDC), however, lead poisoning is one of the most preventable pediatric health problems today. Screening is important to ensure that poisoned children are identified and treated and their environments remediated.

The CDC recommends screening for lead poisoning beginning at 9 months of age for children living in communities with high-risk lead levels. The CDC also recommends targeted screening based on risk assessment during pediatric visits for all other children.

- **Has the child received regular dental services?**

Preventative dentistry means more than a beautiful smile for a child. Children with healthy mouths derive more nutrition from the food they eat, learn to speak more easily, and have a better chance of achieving good health. Every year, thousands of children between 1 to 4 years old suffer from extensive tooth decay caused by sugary liquids—especially in bottles given during the night. Children living below the poverty level have twice the rate of tooth decay as children from higher income levels.[10] Furthermore, poorer children's disease is less likely to be treated.

Early dental care also prevents decay in primary ("baby") teeth, which is currently at epidemic proportions in some U.S. populations and is prevalent among foster children.[11] The American Academy of Pediatric Dentistry recommends that before the age of 1 year a child's basic dental care be addressed during routine well-baby visits with a primary care provider, with referral to a dentist if necessary. For children older than 1 year, the academy recommends a check up at least twice a year with a dental professional.

- Has the child been screened for communicable diseases?

The circumstances associated with the necessity for placement in foster care, such as prenatal drug exposure, poverty, parental substance abuse, poor housing conditions, and inadequate access to health care, can increase a child's risk of exposure to communicable diseases such as HIV/AIDS, congenital syphilis, hepatitis, and tuberculosis.

A General Accounting Office study found that 78% of foster children were at high risk for HIV but only 9% had been tested for the virus.[12] Early identification of HIV is critical to support the lives of infected children and to ensure that they receive modified immunizations. Modified immunizations are necessary to prevent adverse reactions to the vaccines while still providing protection against infectious diseases such as measles and chicken pox. The American Academy of Pediatrics recommends that all prenatally HIV-exposed infants be tested for HIV at birth, at 1–2 months of age, and again at 4 months. If the tests are negative, the child should be retested at 12 months of age or older to document the disappearance of the HIV antibody.

- Does the child have a "medical home" where he or she can receive coordinated, comprehensive, and continuous health care?

All children in foster care should have a "medical home," a single-point-of-contact practitioner knowledgeable about children in foster care who oversees their primary care and periodic reassessments of physical, developmental, and emotional health, and who can make this information available as needed.

DEVELOPMENTAL HEALTH

- Has the child received a developmental evaluation by a provider with experience in child development?

Young foster children often exhibit substantial delays in cognition, language, and behavior. In fact, one half of the children in foster care show developmental delay that is approximately four to five times the rate of delay found in children in the general population.[13] Early evaluation can identify developmental problems and can help caregivers better understand and address the child's needs.

Developmental evaluations provide young children who have identified delays with access to two federal entitlement programs:

1. The Early Intervention Program for children under the age of 3 years, also known as Part C of the Individuals with Disabilities Education Act (IDEA; 20 U.S.C. Section 1431 2000])
2. The Preschool Special Education Grants Program for children with disabilities between the ages of 3–5 years (20 U.S.C. Section 1419[a] [2000])[14]

- Are the child and his or her family receiving the necessary early intervention services (e.g., speech therapy, occupational therapy, educational interventions, or family support)?

Finding help for young children may prevent further developmental delays and may also improve the quality of family life. Substantial evidence indicates that early intervention is most effective during the first 3 years of life when the brain is establishing the foundations for all developmental, social, and cognitive domains: "The course of development can be altered in early childhood by effective interventions that change the balance between risk and protection, thereby shifting the odds in favor of more adaptive outcomes."[15] Children with developmental delays frequently perform more poorly in school, have difficulty understanding and expressing language, misunderstand social cues, and show poor judgment.

Early intervention provides an array of services including hearing and vision screening, occupational, speech and physical therapy, and special instruction for the child, as well as family support services to enable parents to enhance their child's development. Such services can help children benefit from a more successful and satisfying educational experience, including improved peer relationships.[16] Foster children can be referred for early intervention and special education services by parents, health care workers, or social service workers. Early intervention services are an entitlement for all children from birth to 3 years and their families as part of Part C, IDEA. Both biological and foster families can receive early intervention family support services to enhance a child's development.

MENTAL HEALTH

- Has the child received a mental health screening, assessment, or evaluation?

Children enter foster care with adverse life experiences: family violence, neglect, exposure to parental substance abuse or serious mental illness, homelessness, or chronic poverty. Once children are placed in foster care, they must cope with the separation and loss of their family members and the uncertainty of out-of-home care. The cumulative effects of these experiences can create emotional issues that warrant an initial screening and sometimes an assessment or evaluation by a mental health professional. Compared with children from the same socioeconomic background, children in the child welfare system have much higher rates of serious emotional and behavioral problems.[17] It is important to both evaluate them and offer counseling and treatment services when needed so that early difficulties are addressed and later problems are prevented.

Children exhibiting certain behaviors may also signal a need for a mental health assessment and neurological and educational evaluations. Many of the symptoms associated with juvenile emotional and behavioral health problems can be alleviated if addressed early. The American Academy of Child and Adolescent Psychiatry[18] recommends assessments for infants who exhibit fussiness, feeding and sleeping problems, and failure to thrive. For toddlers, the academy recommends assessments for children exhibiting aggressive, defiant, impulsive, and hyperactive behaviors, withdrawal, extreme sadness, and sleep and eating disorders.[19]

- Is the child receiving necessary infant mental health services?

The incidence of emotional, behavioral, and developmental problems among children in foster care is three to six times greater than that among children in the general population.[20] Children with emotional and behavioral problems have a reduced likelihood of reunification or adoption.[21] Children with externalizing disorders (e.g., aggression and acting out) have the lowest probability of exiting foster care.[22] During infancy and early childhood, the foundations are laid for the development of trusting relationships, self-esteem, conscience, empathy, problem solving, focused learning, and impulse control.[23]

To promote and facilitate permanency, children identified with mental health problems should receive care from a mental health professional who can develop a treatment plan to strengthen the child's emotional and behavioral well-being with caregivers. Services may include clinical intervention, home visiting, early care and education, early intervention services, and caregiver support for young children.

EDUCATIONAL/CHILD-CARE SETTING

- Is the child enrolled in a high quality early childhood program?

Children cannot learn unless they are healthy and safe. Children learn best in high-quality settings when they have stable relationships with highly skilled teachers.[24] Such programs nurture children, protect their health and safety, and help ensure that they are ready for school. Early childhood programs also provide much needed support for caregivers. Considerable research has indicated that early education has a positive impact on school and life achievement. Children who participate in early childhood programs have higher rates of high school competition, lower rates of juvenile arrest, fewer violent arrests, and lower rates of dropping out of school.[25] Many foster children are eligible for early childhood programs such as Head Start, Early Head Start, and publicly funded prekindergarten programs for 4-year-olds.

- Is the early childhood program knowledgeable about the needs of children in the child welfare system?

Most children are placed in foster care because of abuse or neglect occurring within the context of parental substance abuse, extreme poverty, mental illness, homelessness, or physical disease (e.g., AIDS). As a result, a disproportionate number of children placed in foster care come from the segment of the population with the fewest psychosocial and financial resources and from families that have few personal and extended sources of support.[26] For all of these reasons, it is very important that these children's child care staff and teachers be well trained and qualified.

PLACEMENT

- Is the child placed with caregivers knowledgeable about the social and emotional needs of infants and toddlers in out-of-home placements, especially young children who have been abused, exposed to violence, or neglected?
- Do the caregivers have access to information and support related to the child's unique needs?
- Are the foster parents able to identify problem behaviors in the child and seek appropriate services?

Childhood abuse increases the odds of future delinquency and adult criminality by 40%.[27] Maltreated infants and toddlers are at risk for insecure attachment, poor self-development, and psychopathology.[28] Children in out-of-home placements often exhibit a variety of problems that may be beyond the skills of persons without special knowledge or training. Therefore, foster parents require and should receive information about the child's history and needs as well as appropriate training.[29] Early interventions are key to minimizing the long-term and permanent effects of traumatic events on the developing brain and on behavioral and emotional development. It is imperative that caregivers seek treatment for their foster children and themselves as soon as possible.[30]

- Are all efforts being made to keep the child in one consistent placement?

An adverse prenatal environment, parental depression or stress, drug exposure, malnutrition, neglect, abuse, or physical or emotional trauma can negatively impact a child's subsequent development. Therefore, it is essential that all children, especially young children, are able to live in a nurturing, supportive, and stimulating environment.[31] It is crucial to try to keep children in one consistent and support-ive placement so that they can develop positive, secure attachment relationships.

> To develop into a psychologically healthy human being, a child must have a relation-ship with an adult who is nurturing, protective, and fosters trust and security. . . . Attachment to a primary caregiver is essential to the development of emotional secu-rity and social conscience.[32]
>
> What happens during the first months and years of life matters a lot, not be-cause this period of development provides an indelible blueprint for adult well-being, but because it sets either a sturdy or fragile stage for what follows.[33]

The material in this appendix was first developed by the National Council of Juve-nile and Family Court Judges' Permanency Planning for Children Department as a Technical Assistance Brief and has been available to the field since January 2003. Since that time, it has been incorporated in over 25 trainings, and more than 4,600 copies have been disseminated nationally to members of the juvenile and family court systems, as well as numerous child welfare professionals. The feedback about this publication has been overwhelmingly positive.

NOTES

1. Several of the questions follow the formats and contain excerpts from the "Checklists for Healthy Development of Foster Children," *Ensuring the healthy development of foster children: A guide for judges, advocates, and child welfare professionals.* New York State Permanent Judicial Commission on Justice for Children, 1999. Excerpted with permis-sion.
2. American Academy of Pediatrics. (2000). Developmental issues for young children in fos-ter care. *Pediatrics, 106*(5), 1145–1150. American Academy of Pediatrics. (2002). Health care of young children in foster care. *Pediatrics, 109*(3), 536–541.
3. 42 U.S.C. Section 1396(a)(10) and (43)(2000); 42 U.S.C. Section 1396d(a) (4) (B) (2000) and 1396 (r).
4. 42 U.S.C. Section 1396(a) (10) (2000); 42 U.S.C. Section 1396d(a) (4) (B) (2000).
5. *Supra* note 1.
6. American Academy of Pediatrics. (2002, June 27). Immunizations and your child. Ameri-can Academy of Pediatrics website.
7. NIH Consensus Statement, Early identification of hearing impairment in infants and young children. Online Mar 1–3, 1993 [cited October 8, 2002]; *11*(1), 1–24.
8. American Academy of Pediatrics. (2001). Developmental surveillance and screening of in-fants and young children. *Pediatrics, 108*(1), 192–196.
9. American Academy of Pediatrics. (1998). Screening for elevated blood lead levels (RE9815). *Pediatrics, 101*(6), 1072–1078.
10. Testimony of Ed Martinez, Chief Executive Officer, San Ysidro Health Center, San Diego, CA, to the Senate Subcommittee on Public Health in support of Senate Bill 1626, June 25, 2002.
11. American Academy of Pediatrics, Early childhood caries reaches epidemic proportions (press release, February 1997).

12. General Accounting Office (1995, May). *Foster care: Health needs of young children are unknown and unmet* (pp. 95–114). Washington, DC: GAO/Health, Education and Human Services Division.

13. Dicker, S., & Gordon, E. (2000). Connecting healthy development and permanency: A pivotal role for child welfare professionals. *Permanency Planning Today, 1*(1), 12–15.

14. Website: *http://www.nectac.org/default.asp*

15. Shonkoff, J. P., & Phillips, D. A. (2000). *From neurons to neighborhoods: Committee on integrating the science of early childhood development.* Washington, DC: National Academy Press.

16. American Speech–Language–Hearing Association. (2002, July). Frequently asked questions: Helping children with communication disorders in the schools—speaking, listening, reading, and writing. American Speech–Language–Hearing Association website.

17. Halfon, N., Berkowitz, G., & Klee, L. (1993). Development of an integrated case management program for vulnerable children. *Child Welfare, 72*(4), 379–396.

18. American Academy of Child and Adolescent Psychiatry. (1997). Practice parameters for the psychiatric assessment of infants and toddlers. *Journal of the American Academy of Child and Adolescent Psychiatry, 36*(10, Suppl.).

19. Ibid.

20. Marsenich, L. (2002, March). *Evidence-based practices in mental health services for foster youth.* Sacramento: California Institute for Mental Health.

21. Ibid.

22. Ibid.

23. Greenough, W., Gunnar, M., Emde, N., Massinga, R., & Shonkoff, J. (2001). The impact of the caregiving environment on young children's development: Different ways of knowing. *Zero to Three, 21,* 16–23.

24. National Association for the Education of Young Children. (1999). Week of the young child: April 18–24. *Early Years Are Learning Years, 99*(6).

25. Reynolds, A., Temple, J., Robertson, D., & Mann, E. (2002). Long-term effects of an early childhood intervention on educational achievement and juvenile arrest: A 15-year follow-up of low-income children in public schools. *Journal of the American Medical Association, 285*(18), 2339–2346.

26. National Commission on Family Foster Care. (1991). *A blueprint for fostering infants, children, and youths in the 1990s.* Washington, DC: Child Welfare League of America.

27. Widom, C. S. (1991). The role of placement experiences in mediating the criminal consequences of early childhood victimization. *American Journal of Orthopsychiatry, 61*(2), 195–209.

28. Widom, C. S. (2000). Motivations and mechanisms in the "cycle of violence." In D. Hansen (Ed.), *Nebraska Symposium on Motivation: Vol. 46. Motivation and child maltreatment* (pp. 1–37). Lincoln: University of Nebraska Press.

29. National Foster Parent Association. (1999). *Board manual: Goals, objectives, position statements, and by-laws.* Gig Harbor, WA: Author.

30. Carnegie Task Force on Meeting the Needs of Young Children. (1994). *Starting points: Meeting the needs of our youngest children.* New York: Carnegie Corporation.

31. *Supra* note 2.

32. Ibid.

33. *Supra* note 15.

CHAPTER 10

PARTNERSHIPS FOR YOUNG CHILDREN IN COURT

How Judges Shape Collaborations Serving Traumatized Children

Patricia Van Horn
Donna J. Hitchens

There is little question that in the United States, instead of
focusing on the needs of children for quality education,
economic opportunities, safe and good homes, and loving
families, all of which go a long way toward preventing
violence, we more quickly opt for punishment after the fact.
There is overwhelming evidence that many of the adolescents
and young adults who first become delinquent and later
develop into criminals were exposed earlier in their lives to
much violence, disorganized families, poor education, and
limited opportunities. What is needed is a shift in thinking
and behaving in our society . . . to helping children develop
the values and respect that comes from within families and
community.

—Osofsky (1997, p. 5)

Scholars and clinicians have long recognized that early childhood experience,
particularly traumatic experience such as interpersonal violence in the
home and community, has a potential negative impact on children's development. Research has shown us that, depending on the impact of the traumatic event on the child's developmental and maturational level and on her
ability to marshal internal or external supports to help with coping, trau-

242

matic experiences may alter the shape and functioning of the child's central nervous system and stress hormone system (De Bellis et al., 1999a, 1999b), may interact with developmentally relevant wishes, impulses, and fears to shape her developing personality (Marans & Adelman, 1997), and may continue to shape her development in the form of traumatic reminders and secondary adversities that flow from the original trauma (Pynoos, Steinberg, & Piacentini, 1999). As traumatic life experiences interact with the child's unfolding developmental processes, risks for psychopathology and other maladaptive outcomes increase (Cicchetti & Cohen, 1995; Osofsky & Scheeringa, 1997). Interventions that help children understand and process the terrifying events that they have witnessed or experienced and that help their parents and teachers restore a sense of order and safety to their worlds diminish these risks (Groves & Zuckerman, 1997).

In spite of all that we know, however, the words that begin this chapter remain relevant. Children in our society continue to be victims of violence. In 2001, more than 400,000 youths between the ages of 10 and 19 were injured in acts of violence and 1 in 28 of these injuries were sufficiently severe to require hospitalization (Centers for Disease Control and Prevention [CDC], 2001). Homicide is the leading cause of death for children in that age group overall, and is the number one cause of death among African American youths (CDC, 2001). Consistent with research findings that traumatic life experiences place the developing child at risk for psychopathology, T. N. Thornton and colleagues identified exposure to violence in the home and community as a major risk factor for youth violence (Thornton, Craft, Dahlberg, Lynch, & Baer, 2000). Abused and neglected children have been reported to have higher rates of arrest for both juvenile and adult criminal behavior than nonabused children (Windom & Maxfield, 1996). And violence among our youth continues to be a disturbing trend. Although the actual number of arrests of youth for serious violent crimes has fallen since their peak in 1993, arrest rates for both serious violent crimes and for homicide are still higher than they were in 1983 (U.S. Department of Health and Human Services, 2001).

As a culture, we continue to respond to the path from victim of violence to violent offender in punitive rather than ameliorative ways. The states spend, on average, three times more per prisoner each year than they do per public school pupil. In California, the ratio of prisoner to pupil spending is 3.7/1 (Children's Defense Fund, 2002). Because of our focus on punishment, our response to violent youth is centered in the courts, where increasingly even children as young as 10 may be tried as adults. Vermont and Kansas have laws allowing 10-year-olds to be tried as adults, Colorado and Missouri set the minimum age at 12, and six other states set the minimum age at 13 (Office of Juvenile Justice and Delinquency Prevention, 2000). If our attention to punishment and our inattention to education, violence prevention, and support for families continue, we can expect that frightened young children will continue to grow into frightening youth and adults.

This chapter tells the story of one court's efforts, in collaboration with public and private partners, to shift the focus of its intervention with children and their families from punishment to amelioration and prevention. We describe in depth the processes that the San Francisco Unified Family Court followed as it developed a model where judicial decision making, the traditional province of courts, was blended with outreach to children's closest support systems: their families. Although many of the interventions that we describe are directed at adolescents and adults, the guiding rationale behind the interventions is that by supporting youth and families, the court could strengthen the nurturing environment for the youngest children. The ultimate aim throughout has been prevention: to prevent the acts of violence that would transform our present generation of infants and toddlers into our next generation of juvenile offenders and adult criminals.

In this chapter we outline the process that San Francisco's Unified Family Court followed as it developed its philosophy of family-focused service and violence prevention intervention. Although it will give an incomplete picture, we focus our description on three specific programs undertaken at the court that are of special relevance to very young children: the Youth Family Violence Court; San Francisco Safe Start's court-based access to family advocacy; and a mental health partnership that makes available court-based assessments of infants, toddlers, and preschoolers. Underlying all of these programs, however, was the original unification of the Superior Court departments that served youth and families, and that is where the story begins.

COURT UNIFICATION: SAN FRANCISCO'S FIRST STEP TOWARD PREVENTIVE INTERVENTION

In 1997, Judge Donna J. Hitchens (the second author) began a process designed to move San Francisco toward the model of "one family—one judge." Until that time, the departments of the court that served youth and families were physically and departmentally divided and communicated with each other poorly, if at all. Dependency judges and commissioners presided over cases in which the child protection system had petitioned the court to assume jurisdiction over children because they were victims of abuse or neglect. Delinquency judges oversaw cases involving youth who were adjudged delinquent because of criminal behavior. Family law judges and commissioners presided over civil petitions for separation and dissolution of marriage, for domestic violence protective orders, and for orders regarding child custody and visitation. Still additional commissioners presided over petitions for child support brought by the county in cases where the custodial parent had received public assistance or where foster care reimbursement funds were sought. The adjunct systems that served families within the court were also divided. There were, for example, two groups of mediators: one that mediated disputes for families whose children were dependents of the court because of abuse or neglect, and another that carried out the mediations required by law in cases where issues of child custody or visitation were disputed by parents. In fact, they were in separate buildings and did not even know each other.

There were times when a single family might have business before several different departments. For example, parents whose children were dependent or delinquent might be seeking a domestic violence restraining order in the family law department. The dependency department, which focused on issues of parents' dangerousness to children, might not even be aware that there was co-occurring violence between the parents. The judge in the family law department would not necessarily know, unless the parents advised him or her, that the children were dependents and would focus exclusively on the behavior of one parent toward the other. Matters became even more complex when the domestic violence matter that formed the basis for the request for a civil restraining order had also been charged as a crime. Then yet another court, the criminal court, became involved with the family. The involvement of multiple departments meant that families were often burdened with multiple court appearances to resolve related issues. It also increased the risk that different departments would make conflicting orders. For example, the criminal domestic violence department might issue a stay-away order that barred the violent parent from any contact with the children. Ignorant of this order (and sometimes ignorant that the matter had been charged as a crime if a self-represented litigant did not advise the family law judge), the family law judge might make an order permitting unsupervised visits with the child. Likewise, a delinquency judge might release a youth from custody to a parent who was the subject of a restraining order prohibiting contact with the child.

The unification of the all of the noncriminal Superior Court departments that served families was designed to remedy these potential conflicts and to make appearing before the court less burdensome and less confusing for families. Unification presented a major challenge for judges and commissioners. Before unification, each judge and commissioner had presided over a department that dealt with a limited range of legal issues. The judge or commissioner could become expert in those issues and in the law that he or she needed to understand in order to resolve the issues that most commonly arose. Movement toward a model of "one family—one judge" meant that each bench officer would need to understand the whole range of issues that might affect the family. The bench officer would be expert not in a particular area of the law but in the particular family and its needs.

Unification has been a long process and it is not complete. Currently in

San Francisco, dependency, delinquency, family law, and child support departments work together in a Unified Family Court. The criminal Domestic Violence Court is not part of this court but has adopted protocols to refer all domestic violence defendants with children to the Unified Family Court so that the services of that court can be made available to all members of the family in a safe setting and so that the criminal and family law departments will not issue conflicting orders regarding contact with children. Moving in the direction of placing the necessity of understanding of the needs of individual families on the same level of importance as the necessity of ruling on legal issues involving members of the family has opened the door for the possibility of creating a court that will act as a collaborative partner to support the individuals before it, even as it exercises the necessary restraints on their behavior.

WHY INVOLVE COURTS IN COLLABORATIONS TO SERVE CHILDREN?

Although courts are sometimes viewed as coercive systems set apart from more traditional service organizations, family courts can also be natural collaborative partners with other agencies and with community-based organizations. First, courts are among the institutions in society where troubled children and families are most likely to be found. Children who are abused or neglected, who are delinquent, or who witness domestic violence are more likely than children who do not face similar stresses to need advocacy and mental health services. Their parents also need services to improve their parenting skills, to deal with their own mental health or substance abuse issues, and to help them escape from dangerous environments or to minimize the danger in their current environments.

Many of these children and families come to court, and if their strengths are not affirmed and their problems not understood and addressed, they will come to court again and again. Abusive parents will not reunify successfully with their children; delinquent youth will repeat their behaviors; parents in violent relationships will continue to be hurt and to expose their children to frightening conflict and violence. When troubled families come to court, a court that has formed good collaborative relationships with service providers will be able to recommend interventions that can break destructive patterns before they become entrenched. This is particularly the case in families with infants, toddlers, and preschoolers. The needs of such young children may be overlooked in these highly stressed families. Parents may not have the skills required to read their young children's signals of distress; they may be so overwhelmed with their own problems that they assume that their young children will be "resilient" and that they will not remember the hardships that they suffer at an early age.

Together, courts and their collaborative service providers can give a voice to young children who might otherwise be overlooked.

In addition, courts are uniquely situated to move beyond merely recommending services. Under some circumstances, courts can use their power to compel participation in recommended programs. Most traditionally, criminal courts and dependency courts have used this power to compel adults or children to take part in services. For example, criminal domestic violence courts now routinely require adult batterers to participate in intervention programs as conditions of their probation. Dependency courts routinely require parents who have abused or neglected their children to take part in substance abuse or mental health treatment as a condition of reunification. They may also compel assessments or treatment for dependent children (see J. D. Osofsky & C. Lederman, Chapter 9, this volume for an example of court-ordered intervention to benefit young children). San Francisco's Unified Family Court is now struggling with a new policy question: How does a court justify using its power to compel parents and children who have not committed criminal acts or acts of abuse or neglect to participate in treatment, advocacy, or assessment services?

EARLY STEPS TOWARD COLLABORATION: WORK WITH SINGLE AGENCIES

Even before the formation of the Unified Family Court, the family law department of the San Francisco Superior Court was pioneering collaborative new ways to serve families. In 1989, a family law judge, in cooperation with a few mental health professionals and a few attorneys, founded Kids' Turn, an agency that offers psychoeducational groups to children between the ages of 4 and 14 whose parents are divorcing, together with groups for parents that help them learn conflict resolution skills and focus on their children's needs following the breakup of the family. Kids' Turn has since expanded its curriculum to add a series of "Early Years" groups for divorcing parents whose children are 3 years of age or younger. The family law department was also instrumental in the foundation of the Rally Project: a center that offers supervised visitation and exchange services in cases where there is high conflict or violence between separating or divorcing parents.

In 1997, the Unified Family Court further solidified its focus on serving very young children when it entered into a collaborative relationship with a university-based research and service program, the Child Trauma Research Project (CTRP). This relationship was fundamentally different from the relationships the court had with Kids' Turn and with the Rally Project, chiefly in that it was broader in scope. CTRP serves children younger than 6 who are witnesses to domestic violence or who have experienced other interpersonal traumas, including child abuse and neglect. CTRP sought out the collaborative relationship with the court as a source of refer-rals for a National Institute of Mental Health (NIMH)-funded study that it was conducting to test the efficacy of a child–parent model of psychothera-py with these young children. The court was pleased to have a place to refer families that needed service and to have a relationship with a group of pro-fessionals that it could call upon to provide training for bench officers and mediators on the impact of violence exposure on young children. As the re-lationship between CTRP and the Unified Family Court developed, a num-ber of problems emerged that appear likely to be present in any collabora-tion to serve young children between a court and an outside mental health agency:

1. How will bench officers and other personnel such as mediators be trained to make referrals to the collaborating partner? How will they know which cases are appropriate for referral? A special problem arises when the referrals are intended to serve infants, toddlers, and preschoolers. Often neither parents nor bench officers are aware of the ways in which these very young children communicate their distress behaviorally; some initial training from collaborative partners with knowledge about child develop-ment and infant mental health may be needed to raise awareness of young children's needs.

2. What kind of feedback from the collaborating agency will the court expect? How do we maintain trust so family members will utilize the ser-vices? Does the bench officer referring the case want substantive informa-tion about the family, or does he or she simply want to know whether or not the family took advantage of the referral? In this regard, how do the bench officer and the collaborating service provider avoid misunderstand-ings about the provider's role in a particular case? Will the provider evalu-ate and report to the court or provide a confidential service? If the provider exchanges confidential information with a mediator, how will that confi-dential information be used?

3. In a research setting, where participation must be voluntary, what role should both the court and the provider play in communicating to the family the fact that the family is not required to participate in a study sim-ply because the court has made a referral for services? How can the service provider help the court understand the distinction between accepting ser-vice and participating in research? If the family declines to participate in the research but seeks out service from a different agency, how can it feel cer-tain that it will not be penalized for this decision in court?

Resolving these issues has been an ongoing process between the Unified Family Court and CTRP that has gone far beyond discussions be-tween the director and clinical coordinator of CTRP and the bench officers and mediators of the Unified Family Court. CTRP has invited court personnel to attend its case conferences so that they can understand the way that CTRP works with families. CTRP personnel have attended court sessions and mediations to become aware of the challenges that court professionals face. Referral protocols and forms were developed to facilitate the communication of referral questions and the nature of feedback that was requested. Once it had a clear idea of exactly what the court wanted in referring a family, CTRP could make those expectations clear to the family so that the family could decide whether or not to use the service. We believe that engaging in the hard work required to surmount these challenges has helped us construct the essential framework of a collaboration: mutual understanding and a respect for one another's needs, strengths, and limitations. This work has also made it clear to both CTRP and the court that together we are stronger and more effective than either of us would be alone, and it has established a template for the child-focused projects described here.

Case Example

Susan and her 3-year-old daughter, Gina, were referred to CTRP by a mediator at the Unified Family Court. The mediator sought therapeutic service for Gina, her mother, and Gina's new baby brother. Susan gave permission for the family's CTRP therapist to talk to the mediator. The therapist began providing weekly home visits to Susan and her children. In the fourth week of the therapy, the door to the home flew open during a session and a man burst in. Gina immediately ducked behind her mother. The man did not introduce himself to the therapist but began shouting demands at Susan, who anxiously reassured him that everything he was asking about would be taken care of before the end of the week. The man threw a stuffed animal onto the bed, nearly hitting the baby, and said, "Here's the toy Gina left at my place." Without another word, he left, slamming the door behind him. As Gina sat behind her mother crying silently, Susan turned to the therapist and said, "See how charming he can be?" The therapist could see that this was neither a rhetorical nor a sarcastic inquiry. Susan really believed that her husband, Carl, had been charming. The therapist said that she had found Carl frightening and that she thought Gina had, too. Susan appeared confused but said, "Maybe it's just that I've seen how bad he can be. This was a lot nicer." Indeed, Carl had been nearly murderous in his past assaults against Susan, though neither Susan nor the physicians from whom she had sought treatment on three different occasions had reported him to the police.

As in any therapy, the therapist talked to Susan and Gina about the danger that she perceived in the situation and explored their reactions. With Susan's permission, she also reported back to the mediator at the family court. She told the mediator that she had had an encounter with Carl and found him to be a very menacing and frightening man. She said that Gina also appeared to be frightened of her father, but that Susan seemed to have difficulty recognizing the danger he presented unless he was being actively violent. The mediator said that she found this information helpful. She had also been frightened by Carl during the mediation, and had been discouraged because Susan seemed to take so much responsibility for the violence on herself and because she agreed to everything Carl demanded, including unsupervised visits with Gina. With the information from the CTRP therapist, the mediator felt better able to work with the family. At the next mediation session, she recommended that a full custody evaluation be conducted. The evaluator determined that Carl was dangerously impulsive, had a long history of violent behavior in and outside his family, and was actively abusing substances. He recommended that Carl be allowed no unsupervised contact with either of his children until he had completed a batterer's intervention program and a substance abuse treatment program.

In this case, the CTRP therapist and the court-based mediator were able to share their concerns about this family and fashion an intervention that was more protective of the children than either would have been able to do alone, greatly enhancing the safety of two young children and their mother.

NEXT STEPS: COMMUNITY COLLABORATION

The Unified Family Court established its willingness to collaborate with a broad range of partners by holding two Family Court Jamborees. The court invited attorneys, mental health professionals, child welfare workers, mediators, bench officers, child custody evaluators, and parents to spend the day together, working in small groups to solve problems related to making the Unified Family Court more accessible and effective. Topics ranged from the way the court handles domestic violence cases, to parent orientation, to improving the court process for self-represented litigants. Many of the work groups continued their work together beyond the day of the Jamboree and made suggestions for improvement that have been incorporated into court practice.

The Jamborees were successful beyond their goal of devising recommendations to improve the Unified Family Court's service to the community. They firmly established the reputation of the Unified Family Court as a group of jurists willing to listen to and incorporate ideas from the litigants, attorneys, and others with a stake in the court's operation. The court's willingness to change in order to become more responsive to the needs of families and others who appear before the court, rather than insisting that all involved accommodate themselves to the court's way of being, made it clear to the community that this court would be a genuine collaborative partner.

COLLABORATIONS FOR CHILDREN:
SPECIFIC PROJECTS

In the past 3 years, the Unified Family Court has deepened its collaborative effort, with a particular focus on youths and young children. One collaborative project, the Youth Family Violence Court, is a collaboration that brings a number of public and private agencies together in the courtroom to effect change in the way in which the court manages certain delinquency cases. The other two projects focus on making community services easily accessible to young children and their families who are litigants in the Unified Family Court. These two projects have less direct impact on court procedures. Instead, in these projects, the court is actively guiding the way in which noncourt agencies work with families.

Youth Family Violence Court was initiated in October 2000, when Supervising Judge Hitchens of the Unified Family Court began the planning process for a special court that would serve adolescents who were adjudicated delinquent because they had assaulted dating partners or members of their families. The vision was to bring together a group that could provide comprehensive services to the youths, their victims, and in cases in which the youths had children of their own, to those children. This is a much broader vision than one generally sees in treatment courts such as this one because it encompasses wraparound services for not only the youths, but also for those family members and dating partners whose lives have been touched by the youths' behavior. The supervising judge was particularly aware that a substantial number of the youths who would appear before the court were already parents of babies and young children or soon would be. She wanted to prevent violence from cycling through another generation by providing interventions that would help such youths understand the impact of their violent behavior on their young children. To accomplish this goal, she included agencies that served young children, Kids' Turn and the CTRP, on the planning team for the Youth Family Violence Court.

The planning process that began in October 2000 involved legal advocates, probation officers, and community service providers.

The collaborative team met together, sometimes monthly and sometimes biweekly, for a full year before the Youth Family Violence Court opened its doors. There were practical and legal issues to be resolved during that period, and as the team grappled with these issues it also received training so that team members would have a common understanding of some of the issues that they would confront. These processes allowed the team to build a cohesive unit, building trust and a common philosophy of managing cases. The attorneys, for example, abandoned their traditional adversarial stance and worked from a position of trying to formulate plea bargains that would both protect the juvenile's basic rights and make the wraparound intervention of the court available to him or her during the probation period. Judge Hitchens, presiding over the court, made it clear to service providers that she did not need or want to be told specifics about what youths were working on in treatment but that she did need to understand whether they were working productively and making changes. Service providers, although they remained clear about their obligation to protect client confidentiality, also began to see themselves as working as a member of a team and as possessing information that could be shared within the team for the good of the client.

The services provided by the court are intensive. For the first months of their probation, youths are required to appear in court—and their probation officer is required to report on their progress—every 2 weeks. Before the court calls the calendar, the team meets to discuss all of the cases that are on that day's calendar. This meeting is attended by the probation officer, the judge, the district attorney, the youth's attorney, and a victim services representative. Treatment providers working with the youths also attend. The discussion for each case focuses on the any problems that the youth is having and on the youth's strengths. The team decides as a group whether any disciplinary actions are warranted (e.g., return to custody or community service hours) and whether there are particular strengths that should be the focus of attention.

When the calendar is called, the youth is present and discusses his or her progress directly with the judge. Service providers report progress in treatment. The court has been able to get gift certificates from a local foundation, and youths with exceptionally good progress reports are given gift certificates in open court to encourage and reinforce their progress. All aspects of progress are considered: how well the youth is doing at home, how well she is doing in school, whether she is working, and whether she is participating well in treatment. As problems arise, new services can be added to help her meet them. Victims and family members are offered services as well. The victims' services representative who attends the court works actively to help victims apply for funding to pay for the treatment they need and to get them engaged with services. Victims are invited to court to give their perspective on how things are going.

In keeping with the focus on preparing youths to be nonviolent parents to their babies and young children, all youths with children were referred to the CTRP for child–parent psychotherapy. The supervising judge also asked Kids' Turn to develop a curriculum that could be presented to all of the youths, whether or not they were parents, to help them understand and reflect on the impact of witnessing violence on young children. As adolescents, the youths were at a critical developmental stage—considering their futures and considering whether they would have families and what kind of adults and parents they wanted to be. The court's vision was to give these youths a group forum in which to discuss these issues and to give them information about the impact of violence on children in order to help them break their own violent patterns. Kids' Turn obtained independent funding and developed a 14-week psychoeducational curriculum that included sessions on child development, the emotional stresses of being a parent, and strategies to help manage anger and other negative emotions. Van Horn (the first author) helped with the development of the curriculum.

The Youth Family Violence Court will be evaluated to assess the degree to which it is more successful than more traditional models in preventing repeat juvenile or adult offenses. We will also be looking at more qualitative measures of outcome by interviewing the youth and members of their families. By observation, however, positive changes are occurring in the lives of the youth and their young children.

Case Example

Jamal, age 16 at the time of his arrest, is an African American youth living with Latifa, his 15-year-old girlfriend; Jamal, Jr., their 10-month-old baby; and Latifa's parents. He was arrested for attempting to strangle Latifa following a fight over her request that Jamal give her more help with the baby. Both of them said that it was the first incident of violence between them. Jamal, however, had a history of gang involvement and was estranged from his own family because he had, at age 12, hit his mother when she tried to enforce his curfew.

Jamal was held in custody for a week following his arrest. When he was released, the court issued a stay-away order excluding him from Latifa's home and from contact with Jamal, Jr. In order that Jamal might receive child–parent psychotherapy to enhance his relationship with his son, the court carved out an exception to the stay-away order to allow for treatment. The therapist met first with Jamal and then with Latifa to explain the treatment. Latifa expressed an interest in being involved in the treatment, initially because she feared that the baby would be frightened if she wasn't there. Later, however, she and Jamal worked actively on issues of coparenting during the course of the treatment. When Latifa and Jamal became upset or angry during sessions, the baby grew agitated and distressed. The therapist pointed out that the baby's agitation always increased when his parents were angry. This enabled Latifa and Jamal to see how distressing their conflict was for their baby. They talked together for the first time about how the baby had screamed with fear when Jamal strangled Latifa. They became able to notice the baby's distress even without intervention from the therapist, and their concern for him motivated them to learn different ways to manage their anger at one another.

Jamal and Latifa received a variety of services through the Youth Family Violence Court. They attended several weeks of couple therapy in which they discussed the future of their relationship and decided that they wanted to try to stay together and make a commitment to resolve their future conflicts without violence. Latifa was able to obtain individual psychotherapy funded by Victim Services to help her deal with the nightmares and intrusive thoughts that she experienced after the assault. At Latifa's request and with her parents' permission, the stay-away order was lifted and Jamal moved back into their home. The child–parent therapist offered home visits, and sometimes included Latifa's mother, who cared for the child while his parents were in school, allowing everyone involved in the baby's care a forum to discuss how responsibilities for care should be divided and to negotiate issues such as discipline.

Jamal graduated from high school during his probationary period and obtained work. He, Latifa, and their son moved into an apartment. The conflict between Jamal and Latifa increased with the stresses of independent living. Although there were no further incidents of violence, the child–parent psychotherapist reported to the team that they were arguing more and more, regardless of the obvious adverse impact of their discord on their baby. The court responded by providing six additional couples sessions and by encouraging Jamal and Latifa to take advantage of the child care that Latifa's mother offered so that they could have time for themselves when they were not working or in school. Jamal also attended the Kids' Turn class and said that it helped him understand his anger at his own father, who had been violent with his mother. He vowed to give his own partner and child a different life from the one he had grown up in.

By the end of 18 months, Jamal's probation was terminated. He had committed no further acts of violence, had finished high school, was working, and attending a class at the local community college. He and Latifa said that their relationship felt stable. They voluntarily continued with child–parent psychotherapy.

FAMILY-LAW-BASED COLLABORATIONS FOR YOUNG CHILDREN

Family law is different from delinquency and dependency law in one critical way. In family court parents have the right to make decisions for their children. In her position as supervising judge of the Unified Family Court, however, Hitchens has firsthand experience with parents who are too embroiled in conflict to place their children's interest first. Although the court cannot intervene in these families as directly as it can in families where the children are delinquent or dependent, it can collaborate with community agencies to make services readily available to these families and their children. The court can also make referrals designed to benefit young children, can assist families in contacting and connecting with service providers, and can schedule follow-up conferences to monitor whether the family is taking advantage of services and finding them helpful.

San Francisco's Safe Start Initiative[1] is the broadest collaborative project of the Unified Family Court. Supervising Judge Hitchens worked with city departments and agencies (San Francisco's Department of Children, Youth and Their Families, the San Francisco Unified School District, the San Francisco Police Department, the Department of Human Services, the Department on the Status of Women) and community-based child advocacy groups and domestic violence service providers to pull together a broad safety net for children under the age of 6 and their families affected by violence. A family services provider employed by the court and funded by Safe Start serves two functions. The first function is to help the court identify families with multiple legal needs—families who may be appearing in criminal court as well as in the departments of the Unified Family Court. The second function is to facilitate the referral of these families to Safe Start's network of advocates and mental health providers, located in neighborhood-based family resource centers and mental health clinics.

Case Example

Susan petitioned the Family Court for a domestic violence restraining order, alleging that her husband, Albert, had beaten her. She asked for custody of her year-old daughter, Anna, and asked the court to limit Albert's contact to supervised visitation. The Safe Start family services provider searched the court databases and discovered that several years earlier Albert's 5-year-old son from a prior relationship had been made a dependent of the court after Albert beat him. At the hearing on the request for the restraining order, the judge told both Albert and Susan that he had been advised of the dependency action. He granted the orders that Susan requested and told Albert that he would not consider permitting Albert to have unsupervised contact with Anna until he completed a 52-week batterers treatment program. The judge also recommended that Susan obtain an assessment of her baby's functioning. He asked the Safe Start family services provider to help Albert find and sign up for an appropriate program, to give Susan referrals for support groups, and to introduce Susan to the court-based assessor (see the following section). He also scheduled a chambers conference 2 months later to give Albert and Susan the opportunity to report back about the availability and quality of the services to which they had been referred.

COURT-BASED EVALUATIONS OF CHILDREN[2]

The court's newest collaboration for children has placed a clinician employed by the CTRP of the University of California, San Francisco, and supervised by Van Horn directly in the court. The clinician meets with children 5 years old and younger and their parents at the recommendation of either bench officers or mediators. She performs a developmental screening assessment, collects information from both parents regarding the kinds of difficult life experiences to which the child may have been exposed and the child's behavioral and emotional functioning. She also observes the child in interaction with each parent. After the assessment is complete, she gives confidential feedback to the parents and recommends services to them where appropriate. All of the meetings take place in the courthouse or in community sites that are convenient to the parents. Although the assessments are voluntary in almost all cases, if the judge or commissioner hearing the case is concerned that the parents are unable to focus on their children's needs, he or she may order them to attend the assessment. Even in cases where the assessment is ordered, only very limited information is given to the court after the assessment. The court is advised whether the parties took part in the assessment, what services were recommended for their child or children, and whether the assessor believes that the court should order participation in services.

Case Example

Levon was 12 months old when his parents came to the Unified Family Court to seek the dissolution of their marriage. There were no allegations of violence between them, but the mediator with whom they worked noted that there was a high level of conflict and hostility. They agreed on a shared parenting plan that gave both parents legal custody of Levon but made his mother the primary physical custodian. They agreed that Levon would spend three afternoons each week with his father, who worked nights. Because the mediator was concerned about the impact of their hostility and discord on Levon's development, he recommended that they seek a court-based assessment. Both parents were willing to take part in the assessment, and both came for their separate appointments with Levon. The assessor noted that although Levon was developing typically and that neither of his parents had concerns that reached a clinical level about his emotional and behavioral functioning, the father, who had been only minimally involved in Levon's care prior to separation, seemed at a loss about what to do during his times with Levon. He was too angry with his ex-wife to engage her in a conversation about Levon's likes and dislikes. The assessor was able to offer both parents reassurance about how well Levon was doing. She also gave the father the numbers of several single-father support groups so that he could meet with other dads and get support for his efforts to parent Levon. The assessor gave both parents referrals to the Kids' Turn "Early Years" program in the hope that the psychoeducational groups would help them understand Levon's needs and help them find ways to communicate with one another with less anger. On follow-up several weeks later, the assessor learned that both parents had enrolled in a Kids' Turn group and that they both felt they were benefiting from the experience.

Case Example

When Carlos was 3 years old and his little sister Juanita was 14 months old, his mother sought a restraining order against his father from the Unified Family Court, alleging domestic violence. At the hearing on the restraining order, the father was loud and threatening. Based on his demeanor, the judge ordered the parents to attend the court-based assessment and explained that it would give them information that they needed to know whether the conflict between them had influenced their children's development. The father declined the assessment and refused to see the children after the court ordered that all of his contact with them be supervised. The mother came to the assessment with both of her children. Both of them, by the mother's report, had been exposed to high levels of domestic violence and to some violence in their community. Both of them suffered from sleep and eating disturbances, and Carlos was aggressive with his mother and with his peers. The assessor observed that Carlos and Juanita could not calm themselves sufficiently to take part in even a simple developmental assessment. The mother was concerned about her children's functioning and eager for referrals. The assessor gave her referrals to agencies that served young children, and reported back to the court that she had made the referrals and that she believed that the mother would follow through with them without an order. On follow-up, she learned that the mother had taken both children for treatment

The advocacy and assessment services have raised complex issues because they are offered primarily to families appearing in the family law departments. Because of the breadth of the Safe Start collaboration, advocates and others had a forum at the Safe Start Advisory Council to express their concerns directly to the supervising judge, who is the chairman of the Advisory Council. Before the assessment services began, the present authors met with legal advocates to hear their concerns. The advocates' primary concern was that information from the assessment would not be kept confidential but would be communicated to the court outside the presence of counsel and used to make decisions regarding custody or visitation. The court was able to reassure legal advocates that this was not the intent: the court's purpose in offering the assessment service was to give families, particularly those embroiled in violence or high conflict, information that they needed to make the best decisions for their young children. To further ensure the confidentiality of assessment information, protocols were developed that required the assessments to be offered after custody and visitation decisions had already been made.

CONCLUSION

Involving courts in service collaborations is complex. The power of the court is such that often litigants hear even a suggestion from a judge as an order. Especially in family law matters, care must be taken to ensure that services intended to be voluntary truly are. Difficult issues are presented to bench officers as well. It is against judicial ethics for judges and commissioners to discuss or to hear communications outside the courtroom regarding cases that are pending before them. In meetings between a judge and potential collaborators, particularly community members, there is a risk that pending cases will be discussed to illustrate a point. If this happens, the judge who hears the communication will no longer be able to serve in that case.

If, however, care is taken to address these kinds of issues, involving a family court in a collaboration of community agencies can be a powerful tool to serve families most in need of assistance. Courts can help service providers reach families that might otherwise not come to their attention. Providers can make it possible for courts to offer more than orders and punishments to families. In San Francisco we have seen dozens of cases like those described in this chapter where the court, working with a cooperating agency, has intervened to protect our youngest children and to break the cycle of violence in families.

NOTES

1. The services described in this section are funded by the Office of Juvenile Justice and Delinquency Prevention of the U.S. Department of Justice.
2. The services described in this section are funded by the Substance Abuse and Mental Health Services Administration of the U.S. Department of Health and Human Services.

REFERENCES

Centers for Disease Control and Prevention [CDC]. (2001). *Web-based injury statistics query and reporting system (WISQARS)* [On-line]. Atlanta, GA: CDC, National Center for Injury Prevention and Control (producer). Available from URL:*www.cdc. gov/ncipc/wisqars*

Children's Defense Fund. (2002). *The state of children in America's union: A 2002 action guide to leave no child behind.* Washington, DC: Author.

Cichetti, D., & Cohen, D. J. (1995). *Manual of developmental psychopathology.* New York: Wiley.

De Bellis, M. D., Baum, A. S., Birmaher, B., Keshavan, M. S., Eccard, C. H., Boring, A. M., et al. (1999a). Developmental traumatology: Part I. Biological stress systems. *Biological Psychiatry, 45,* 1259–1270.

De Bellis, M. D., Baum, A. S., Birmaher, B., Keshavan, M. S., Eccard, C. H., Boring, A. M., et al. (1999b). Developmental traumatology: Part II. Brain development. *Biological Psychiatry, 45,* 1271–1284.

Groves, B. M., & Zuckerman, B. (1997). Interventions with parents and caregivers of children who are exposed to violence. In J. D. Osofsky (Ed.), *Children in a violent society* (pp. 183–201). New York: Guilford Press.

Marans, S., & Adelman, A. (1997). Experiencing violence in a developmental context. In J. D. Osofsky (Ed.), *Children in a violent society* (pp. 202–222). New York: Guilford Press.

Office of Juvenile Justice and Delinquency Prevention. (2000). Juvenile justice system structure and process. *Juvenile offenders and victims: 1999 national report* (Chapter 4). Washington, DC: U.S. Department of Justice.

Osofsky, J. D. (1997). Children and youth violence: An overview of the issue. In J. D. Osofsky (Ed.), *Children in a violent society* (pp. 3–8). New York: Guilford Press.

Osofsky, J. D., & Scheeringa, M. S. (1997). Community and domestic violence exposure: Effects of development and psychopathology. In D. Cichetti & S. Toth (Eds.), *Rochester Symposium on Developmental Psychopathology: Vol 8. Developmental perspectives on trauma* (pp. 155–180). Rochester, NY: University of Rochester Press.

Pynoos, R. S., Steinberg, A. M., & Piacentini, J. C. (1999). A developmental psychopathology model of childhood traumatic stress and intersection with anxiety disorders. *Biological Psychiatry, 46,* 1542–1554.

Thornton, T. N., Craft, C. A., Dahlberg, L. L., Lynch, B. S., & Baer, K. (2002). *Best practices of youth violence prevention: A sourcebook for community action.* Atlanta, GA: Centers for Disease Control and Prevention, National Center for Injury Prevention and Control.

U.S. Department of Health and Human Services. (2001). *Youth violence: A report of the Surgeon General.* Rockville, MD: Author.

Windom, C. S., & Maxfield, M. G. (1996). A prospective examination of risk for violence among abused and neglected children. *Annals of the New York Academy of Science, 794,* 224–237.

CHAPTER 11

WORKING WITH TRAUMATIZED INFANTS AND TODDLERS IN THE CHILD WELFARE SYSTEM

ANNA T. SMYKE
VALERIE WAJDA-JOHNSTON
CHARLES H. ZEANAH, JR.

Traumatized infants and toddlers in the child welfare system present with a multitude of issues different from those of older children in the child welfare system (Silver, Amster, & Haecker, 1999). While many of the basic needs of children in the system may be similar (e.g., stable placement, recovery from trauma), the unique developmental circumstances of infants and toddlers and the implications for the subsequent developmental trajectory must be understood (Clyman, Harden, & Little, 2002). This chapter consists of a brief review of types of trauma seen in infants and toddlers who have come into foster care, followed by a discussion of the important components of the child welfare system and the ways in which they impact the very young child. Specific types of treatment useful in the management of traumatized infants and toddlers will then be provided with case vignettes that will demonstrate the techniques in action and be thought provoking as well as helpful.

The organizing principle of our work is the best interest of the child; that is, the needs of these very young traumatized children are first and foremost. The adults in the young child's life, including the biological parents, foster parents, child protection case workers, judges, and child-care workers are asked to consider the emotional and physical needs of young children in every interaction that they have with the child and in every decision that they make regarding the child. We appreciate the realities and the different conceptual framework of the legal system, which does not always support the healthy development of very young children; however, we consistently focus our assessments and intervention on one primary goal: the infant's and toddler's recovery from significant abuse and neglect.

TRAUMA AND THE VERY YOUNG CHILD

Physical Abuse

The effects of physical abuse on infants and toddlers are particularly devastating. Children under 1 year of age, who comprise 44% of all child fatalities from abuse and neglect, represent the most at-risk segment of the population. Children under age 6 account for 85% of children killed by child abuse (National Clearinghouse on Child Abuse and Neglect Information, 2002). In addition, young children who have been abused are more likely to be placed in foster care than older children (U.S. Department of Health and Human Services, Administration on Children, Youth, and Families, 2001; Wulczyn, Hislop, & Harden, 2002).

Traumatic brain injury from shaking an infant or toddler can range from subclinical tears in the periphery of the retina, through retinal hemorrhages and subdural bleeding, to death (Palmer, 1998; Ricci, 2000). Shaken baby syndrome is particularly devastating for the very youngest infants (Showers, 1998). The shearing of blood vessels that takes place as the child is violently shaken causes differential damage to brain tissue based in large part on the "stiffness" of the involved brain areas and the velocity with which they are shaken. Injuries may cause visual deficits or blindness from retinal hemorrhages and motor deficits such as cerebral palsy (Palmer, 1998; Wharton, Rosenberg, Sheridan, & Ryan, 2000).

Small children also are at higher risk for bone fractures. A pattern of multiple fractures at various stages of healing is often indicative of abuse. Similarly, spiral fractures of long bones, particularly in young children who are not yet mobile, have been associated with nonaccidental trauma (Christian, 1999, 2003). Skull fractures that traverse the sutures of the skull rather than following suture lines are associated with nonaccidental injury and may result in a variety of sequelae depending on the location and severity of the fracture and the age at which the fracture is sustained. Long-term effects on cognitive development may require special educational services, while deficits in gross and fine motor skills must be addressed with ongoing physical and occupational therapy.

Parents often report that persistent crying is an important precipitating factor for abuse of infants and toddlers (Showers, 1998). There is some evidence that early, less vigorous shaking of infants, which does not result in extreme injury, may cause subclinical damage that is signaled by irritability and crying (Palmer, 1998; Showers, 1998).

Neglect

Chronic neglect refers to the failure of the primary caregiver to provide for the basic needs of the young child. Reports of neglect account for the majority of referrals to the child welfare system for very young children, and neglect is the single greatest reason that infants and toddlers are placed in foster care (National Clearinghouse on Child Abuse and Neglect Information, 2001). Neglect appears to have a particularly deleterious effect on the development of infants and toddlers (Hildyard & Wolfe, 2002), and its effects may be as marked as those of physical and sexual abuse.

Neglect may be present in a chaotic environment in which the child does not receive needed support or supervision. Usually, lack of emotional support or emotional abuse is not sufficient cause to bring a child into foster care, but it is often noted in the context of other neglecting circumstances. Some parents leave small children alone for extended periods of time or fail to monitor the child's whereabouts so that the child is found wandering the neighborhood. Others leave their infants or toddlers with a succession of neighbors or friends as they engage in substance abuse, making it difficult for the child to establish attachment relationships. Parents who fail to appropriately monitor their small children, either because of substance abuse or their own previous trauma, may fail to recognize individuals and situations which pose a risk to their child.

Sexual Abuse

Infants and toddlers account for approximately 10% of validated sexual abuse cases in the United States, while another 28% of victims are between 4 and 7 years of age (Putnam, 2003). Unlike older children, who may be capable of informing an adult of the trauma, very young children, who lack adequate language development, are unable to definitively inform their caregivers of the exact nature of their sexual abuse experiences (Kaufman & Henrich, 2000). Young children sometimes display sexualized behaviors that raise concern that sexual abuse has occurred. Without specific medical evidence, however, there is often uncertainty about the nature or extent of sexual abuse. Such behaviors are more likely to occur among younger children or children abused at younger ages (Putnam, 2003). Sexualized behavior is upsetting for caregivers who may require support to manage this behavior in young children and to manage their own feelings about the behavior. Foster parents may attribute intent or knowledge to the sexualized behaviors of young children. Young children who demonstrate sexualized behavior typically have no "adult" understanding of its meaning but quickly become aware that the adults around them are quite agitated when they see such behavior.

Exposure to Domestic Violence

The co-occurrence of child abuse and domestic violence has been well documented (National Clearinghouse on Child Abuse and Neglect Information, n.d.; Osofsky, 1998, 2003) and has significant implications for young children. Exposure to domestic violence takes many forms and results in confusing and chaotic feelings for young children. For example, the child who witnesses his or her mother being beaten has witnessed a significant threat to the person to whom they would turn for comfort and protection. The mother, however, is unable to protect herself and, by extrapolation, unable to protect her children. Women who are victims of domestic violence may in turn abuse their children, either from the stress and anger following their own beating or in an effort to force the children to "be quiet" and to comply so that they do not draw the ire of the batterer (National Clearinghouse on Child Abuse and Neglect Information, n.d.)

Regardless of whether children witness the abuse of their mother or whether they are actively abused by her (or the batterer), chaos and disorganization result. At the very least, the mother is not available to comfort and protect her child during this frightening time. In addition, she is at significant risk of severe injury or death. Domestic violence clearly violates the mother's essential role as protector of the child and may present a risk for serious relationship disturbance (see Lieberman & Van Horn, Chapter 4, this volume).

Many foster children have been exposed to domestic violence (see Lieberman & Van Horn, Chapter 4, this volume). Child protection personnel may not be aware of this exposure, as many victims are ashamed of their abuse and feel that they are responsible for it or have returned to the batterer because he has sworn that such abuse will never be repeated. The "honeymoon phase" following battering is a well-documented phase of the battering cycle and represents another confusing situation for the young child, who is compelled to put aside the hurt and confusion of the incident with little opportunity to understand or work through it.

It is not surprising, then, that the sequelae of exposure to domestic violence may be long lasting and may affect a number of developmental domains. Children exposed to violence in the home may display anxiety or aggression toward adults and peers (Margolin, 1998; Osofsky, 1998), be disorganized in their attachment to their parents (Zeanah et al., 1999), and display symptoms consistent with posttraumatic stress disorder (PTSD).

Attachment Disruption

One of the inevitable traumas of placement in foster care is attachment disruption (see Hinshaw-Fuselier, Heller, & Boris, Chapter 2, this volume, for a full discussion of this important issue). Infants are biologically predisposed to begin the task of developing a focused attachment to a caregiver at 6–9 months of age (Boris, Aoki, & Zeanah, 1999), even in the most extreme of circumstances (Smyke, Dumitrescu, & Zeanah, 2002). Although they may have begun the process of developing a preference earlier, the real task of developing a focused attachment begins in earnest once infants have developed object permanence and have formed the rudiments of a representational scheme (Boris et al., 1999). The exception to this scenario is the child who has had multiple, inconsistent, unpredictable caregivers. The child may have failed to develop a focused attachment with any of his or her caregivers and may approach strangers indiscriminately for interaction, comfort, and support (Hinshaw-Fuselier, Boris, & Zeanah, 1999).

For those children who have developed an attachment relationship, albeit insecure or disorganized (Barnett, Ganiban, & Cicchetti, 1999; Carlson, Cicchetti, Barnett, & Braunwald, 1989), their first steps into the child welfare system represent a disruption of attachment. This problem is compounded by moving children from foster home to foster home, often after they have managed to form an attachment with a subsequent caregiver (American Academy of Pediatrics, Committee on Early Childhood, Adoption, and Dependent Care, 2000). Specific intervention to foster a secure attachment relationship with the foster parent may be necessary (Dozier, Higley, Albus, & Nutter, 2002; Stovall & Dozier, 2000).

Until recently, foster parents were advised not to get "too close" to their foster children to protect themselves and the children from the pain of disruption. Although some foster parents manage to keep such infants and toddlers at arm's length, others recognize that they are "falling in love" with the child and risk disappointment and sadness if the child is removed from their home. The young foster child may appear indifferent to the attempts of the foster parent to establish a loving relationship with him or her, in part because of prior experience and repeated disruptions (Dozier et al., 2002).

COMPONENTS OF THE CHILD WELFARE SYSTEM

The young foster child is imbedded in a variety of contexts as he or she enters the child welfare system. We will discuss the ways in which the young child's development and well-being can be affected by each component of the system. Ideally, the child welfare system has all aspects of the child's well-being in mind: physical, mental, emotional, and educational. The following facets of the system are discussed in this section: the child's family of origin, Child Protective Services (CPS), foster care, mental health clinicians, the legal system, medical providers, and the educational system. Each of these entities has the potential to support or to negatively impact the abused and/or neglected child.

The Child's Family of Origin

The child's biological family may consist of the child's parents, siblings, grandparents, aunts, uncles, and cousins. Each family has its own history of interactions, values, norms, health, and—particularly important for the abused or neglected child—pathology. Regardless of the reasons for which a child and family have come into contact with the child welfare system, the parents of the child have demonstrated a clear inability to raise the child in a safe and effective manner. More specifically, a child who is removed from his or her parents and placed in foster care is taken from a situation in which the child was in imminent danger of harm.

To ensure a child's healthy development, parents should have as their priority the nurturance and protection of their children. In healthy families, this expectation has been met by parents through several generations, with each generation of parents teaching their offspring how to raise children, in part by modeling appropriate behaviors. Parents whose children are placed in foster care often come from families with few resources within the family to provide positive role models. Further, family members capable of supporting their choices to implement healthier, safer treatment of their children are rare.

Parents who are substance abusers may have diminished capacity to parent due to their substance abuse, placing their children at risk or actively maltreating them (Tomison, 1996). They may recognize the ways in which their substance abuse has affected their ability to parent prior to their involvement with the child welfare system but be unable to change. Such individuals may have family members who have successfully parented their own children and are willing to assist them in changing their parenting practices so that they can regain custody of their children. Others may have promised "to quit" or "get their lives together" and manipulated relatives so often that relatives are no longer willing to try to assist them.

Child Protective Services

The family's initial contact with the child welfare system is with an investigator who responds to a report that a child is not being cared for properly. When possible, the investigator interviews the parents, witnesses, and other family members, as well as the maltreated child or children. The investigator may also inspect the home of the child to ensure that the child has adequate food, clothing, and shelter. If the investigator decides that the claim of child abuse or neglect is valid, the investigator then must decide if the child can remain with one or both of the parents, often with additional services being put into place, if the child should be placed with a relative, or if the child should be taken into the state's custody. If the decision is made to remove the child from the parents, the investigator determines whether or not a family member is able, willing, and adequate to care for the child. Some parents whose children have come into foster care readily suggest alternative caregivers whereas others seem completely unwilling to do so. Placement in the "least-restrictive" environment, if possible with a relative, is one of the hallmark provisions of the Adoption and Safe Families Act (ASFA, 1997). In order to find the least-restrictive placement, it is not uncommon for child protection workers to do repeated searches for biological fathers or relatives. If a family member is not available, the child is placed in a foster home.

After a child is taken into custody and either placed with a family member or in a foster home, a caseworker from CPS is assigned to the child and his or her parents. The caseworker assists the family in completing a case plan that is designed to correct the problems that lead to the child being placed in foster care. Such a plan may include concrete objectives for the parent(s) such as obtaining job training or employment, obtaining stable housing, entering a drug treatment program, or attending counseling. The caseworker is also charged with monitoring the child's well-being while in the state's custody. This entails seeing the child on a regular basis and making sure that the child's physical and psychological needs are met by the foster parents. The caseworker should have an understanding of child development, especially for children under the age of 3 years. Infants and toddlers are unable to speak for themselves, making it essential for caseworkers, who make pivotal decisions regarding young children, to understand the impact that early relationships and maltreatment can have on children's development.

This is particularly important when decisions are made about moving a child, whether from foster home to foster home or from foster home back to the family. Recently, we have begun to pay special attention to the ways in which transitions occur for young children. If the biological parents have been able to learn to safely care for their young children and the decision is made to return the child to their home, we develop a systematic plan aimed at adding attachment figures for the child rather than disrupting the attachment relationship between the foster parent and the foster child. In some cases, foster parents have remained a resource to biological families for respite care, as the biological parents have come to appreciate the child's connection to the foster parent and realize that children are capable of developing attachments to several important caregivers. In turn, foster parents are relieved to know that children are returning to a safe home environment and that they may be able to remain in the child's life.

The Foster Family

Individuals who become foster parents agree to provide a home for children whose parents are unable to safely care for them. Children placed with foster parents vary in age, types of abuse or neglect that they have experienced, and sequelae associated with the abuse or neglect. Training and experience of foster parents may vary from state to state, and even within states from county to county (Zukoski, 1999). The foster parent often must manage a variety of behaviors from a child as the child attempts to adapt to new surroundings and new people. The challenges that foster parents face may be extensive and varied, and the foster parents may or may not feel supported by the child welfare system itself, by their own families, or by their communities (see Heller, Smyke, & Boris, 2002, for a review of the systems challenges and the personal challenges that foster parents face). The reasons that foster parents enter the field vary, as do the reasons that foster parents stop fostering children (Denby, Rindfleisch, & Bean, 1999). Foster families may be single- or two-parent families and may contain other children. The other children in the family may be the biological children of the foster parents, children adopted by the foster parents, or other foster children. As with any family, foster families are dynamic systems, with each member contributing to the experience of other members in the family. Foster siblings, who have experienced their own traumas, may be able to assist a newly placed foster child in adapting to the family and the foster care system. Conversely, those same siblings may have their own untreated behavioral and emotional problems, and therefore may be the cause of further trauma to the newly placed foster child (Johnson, 1997). In addition, biological children of the foster family may report significant concerns regarding the new, often transient members of the family and the time that their parents must spend on foster children (Poland & Groze, 1993).

It is the responsibility of foster parents to monitor the children in their home and to intervene as necessary. Foster parents often find themselves advocating for the appropriate treatment for children (Ross & Crawford, 1999) and carefully monitoring the interactions of the children in their home. Foster parents, additionally, are responsible for meeting the child's physical and psychological needs. This usually begins with taking the child for physical and dental examinations, and may continue with other appointments, such as speech and language assessments and therapy (Amster, 1999), as well as psychotherapy appointments (Ross & Crawford, 1999).

Foster parents also must be realistic in judging the number of children that they can manage. They may find that they must actively resist pressure from caseworkers to place more children in their homes. Knowing when they have reached their physical and emotional limits, while still appearing to be "good" foster parents, is a delicate balance.

Finally, the foster parents may be required to have contact with the biological parents, depending on the child's age and the requirements of the state in which they live. Even if there is no active contact with the biological parents, foster parents must manage the foster child's reactions to being separated from his or her biological parents as well as the child's reactions to seeing (or not seeing) the biological parents during visits. It can be devastating for children when visits are scheduled repeatedly and biological parents do not attend, attend only sporadically, or make unrealistic or false promises regarding reunification. Children may act out anger, frustration, and confusion about their situation in a variety of challenging ways, all of which the foster parent must address in a patient, safe, and effective manner.

Foster parents have an extremely challenging job. They are asked to make a commitment to a child who has been abused and/or neglected, which entails nurturing the child and helping the child heal, often when the child seems completely unwilling to do so. They also are asked to make a psychological commitment to the child. Not only are they responsible for the child's physical and psychological welfare, but they often make an emotional commitment to the child as well. Foster parents sometimes promise themselves not to "fall for" another child, but they find that they often grow to care deeply for the child and love the child almost in spite of themselves. It is not uncommon, after making these commitments and working and living with a child, that foster parents must watch as the child returns to parents who have been deemed adequate to parent the child. Foster parents may or may not agree with the state's decision, but either way the child and the foster parents must separate. Foster parents do all this, knowing that the child can be removed from their home at any time. The essential paradox of foster parenting is that children whose foster parents accept psychological ownership for them do best. Yet, foster parents who take psychological ownership of their foster children are at significant risk of having their hearts broken (Heller et al., 2002).

A full discussion of foster parents' issues of loss is outside the scope of this chapter, but it is an important variable in foster parents' ability to establish a nurturing relationship with the young foster child (Smyke, Foster, & Keyes, 2003). This is yet another area in which we ask the adults in the child's life to accept the risk of emotional discomfort and pain in order to provide for the best interest of the child.

For the young child, life with the foster family may be the first time that the child has experienced stability, predictability, and nurturing. Despite this stability, a child of any age may have difficulty adjusting to a new environment. The child does not know the rules of her new home and may act out while trying to adjust to her new surroundings. Children form attachments even to the cruelest of abusive parents, and they will maintain such attachments even when placed away from their parents. The child may also become attached to the foster parents. This may cause confusion or distress for the child, who may feel the need to choose one parent over another, or who may feel disloyal to one parent if there are positive feelings for another caretaker.

Conversely, the child and foster parent may have difficulty forming an attachment relationship. Even foster parents with secure attachment representations may eventually become less nurturing toward the foster child who acts as if she does not need them. Recent recognition of this dynamic has resulted in an attachment-based approach to remedying the situation (Dozier et al., 2002). In this approach, foster parents are trained to recognize their own response to the young foster child's behavior because their initial reactions may cause them to fail to recognize the child's needs and also may prevent foster parents from meeting those needs even when they are recognized. In turn, the child may seek contact or comfort from strangers rather than the foster parents.

All foster parents are not equal in their abilities, interests, or motivations. Incidents in which foster parents abuse or neglect their foster children have been well publicized, and the potential for abuse should not be ignored. Clearly, inadequate foster homes can cause further harm to the children in them. It is the responsibility of the state, and therefore that of the child welfare system, to monitor foster parents and foster homes closely and to protect the children placed with them.

Clinicians

Clinicians such as social workers, psychologists, and psychiatrists have multiple roles in the child welfare system. They may be called upon to assess areas of strength and areas of concern for parents and children in the child welfare system. They also may make recommendations about what parents must do in order to be able to parent in an adequately safe manner. Clinicians also are asked to treat parents and children, either separately or together. Types of treatment are discussed later in this chapter.

When clinicians work with families involved in the child welfare system, they must be clear about who their clients are. In most cases, the client is the child, as the clinician is usually involved with the family in order to ensure the best interest of the child. There are times, however, when clinicians may work with one or both parents independently on individual or relationship issues. On those occasions, clinicians must make careful assessments regarding parents' abilities. For example, parents may make progress in some areas but not necessarily in areas that increase the likelihood that they will safely and effectively raise their children. Recommendations should be made only after carefully and systematically assessing the relationship between each parent and the child (Zeanah, Larrieu, Heller, & Valliere, 2000).

The Legal System

When a family enters the child welfare system, they also enter the legal system. Infants and toddlers are currently entering this system in ever-increasing numbers, and addressing the special needs of these most vulnerable children is a challenge that the legal system is just beginning to address (Lederman, Osofsky, & Katz, 2001). The interaction between the child welfare system and the legal system varies from state to state. In some states, criminal charges are filed separately from juvenile court proceedings and the cases are heard in different courts. Therefore, a juvenile court, for example, may have jurisdiction over the custody of the child, but criminal charges may not be filed against the parent (see Van Horn & Hitchens, Chapter 10, this volume).

The state's custody of a child is a legal issue, and ultimately a judge must rule on whether or not parents can regain custody of their children. Usually all parties, including the parents, the child, and the state, are represented by an attorney. Parents have an attorney assigned to them by the courts if they cannot obtain legal counsel themselves. Children also are represented by court-appointed attorneys. The attorney for the child and the state's attorney must have the child's best interest in mind, while the parent's attorney represents the interests of the parent. The judge must determine what is in the best interest of the child based on the evidence provided by the attorneys and within legal constraints.

Recent initiatives, grounded in an infant mental health framework, have proven particularly helpful in providing judges and other personnel in the legal system with a systematic approach to understanding the impact of child abuse and neglect on the development and behavior of infants and toddlers (Lederman et al., 2001). An understanding of child development, informed by a careful assessment of the child and the child in relationship with important caregivers, is essential for professionals involved with young children in the legal system (Lederman et al., 2001). Without an adequate understanding of child development, judges and attorneys cannot fully understand the impact of their decisions; then a system that is founded on the best interest of the child might well become a system that is more attentive to the best interest of the parents. Attorneys and judges in the child welfare system should be able to utilize information provided by clinicians who work with the family to understand the parents' capabilities. Knowledge of the parents' strengths and weaknesses is an essential component in determining the best interest of the child.

Medical and Educational Providers

Medical providers and educators may be the first individuals to observe signs or symptoms of abuse, particularly for very young children (Christian, 2003). It is important that educators and physicians know their states' laws regarding reporting of suspected abuse and that professionals follow the law. It is just as important for educators and medical providers to be trained in ways to interact with children and their biological and foster families so that the child's needs are recognized and met.

Children who have experienced physical abuse may have injuries or resulting problems that require ongoing treatment. For example, an infant or toddler who has a head injury may require physical therapy to address gross motor delays or problems (Orlin, 1999). Children who have experienced severe neglect often demonstrate receptive and/or expressive language delays and require speech and language therapy (Amster, 1999). Therapists and doctors who treat abused and neglected children may have to address more challenging behaviors from these children than from their other patients. Children who have experienced trauma may demonstrate increased anxiety during medical procedures and become extremely upset, even combative. The skill of the medical staff in preparing both the child and the caretaker who accompanies the child for a given procedure may determine the child's ability to tolerate and benefit from the procedure. In contrast, lack of preparation of the child or the caretaker could sabotage the medical procedure.

Educators also may face special challenges from students who are the victims of abuse and neglect. As a consequence of trauma, preschoolers and kindergartners may exhibit short attention spans, difficulty regulating emotions, impulsivity, and difficulty separating from caretakers (Morrison, Frank, Holland, & Kates, 1999). Teachers and administrators who are sensitive to these issues can be instrumental in helping their young students to have successful school experiences. When such students are viewed as simply disruptive or problematic, inappropriate disciplinary techniques may be utilized in a way that starts the child on the road to school failure (Spiker & Silver, 1999; Vig & Kaminer, 1999).

Vignette 1: Multifaceted Intervention with a 12-Month-Old Girl

Twelve-month-old Gina came into foster care after receiving a spiral fracture of the femur, a hallmark of abuse. A bone scan revealed that the child had suffered several fractures over time, including rib fractures, consistent with a highly suspect pattern of injuries. Gina's parents reported that they had left the child with a baby-sitter while they sought employment and had no idea of how she had been injured. Witnesses reported that the child had been left with a neighbor who was often seen using drugs with the parents.

We assessed each parent's relationship with Gina, and it was clear that she did not look to either parent for comfort or reassurance. Both parents demonstrated limited parenting skills, poor understanding of their child's development, and developmental expectations that far exceeded their young child's capabilities. They also both admitted to substance abuse, including crack cocaine and various prescription medications. Additionally, the child's mother displayed significant signs of anxiety and depression, which intensified with her decrease in drug use. The child was placed with a maternal aunt and uncle who had cared for her when she was between 4 and 8 months of age. During the assessment, the girl was observed to approach her uncle and aunt frequently for comfort and to interact playfully with them.

Both parents were referred for substance abuse treatment. Additionally, the mother was seen for individual therapy. Gina's father refused to participate in individual therapy but agreed to attend dyadic sessions with his daughter. Her aunt and uncle asked for assistance in parenting Gina, who often threw temper tantrums and could not be distracted or soothed at these times. Additionally, it was observed that Gina was not making any utterances and often did not respond to people when they spoke to her. She was referred for speech and language evaluation and treatment as well as for hearing assessment.

Although both parents began substance abuse treatment, Gina's father did not comply with the outpatient program and often tested positive for cocaine. Although he had agreed to participate in dyadic therapy with Gina, he attended only the first session and did not return. Gina's mother made a commitment to her drug treatment and completed the initial outpatient program. She opted to remain in maintenance treatment while she was working to regain custody of her daughter. In individual therapy, Gina's mother reported that she did not want to remain in a relationship with Gina's father due to his continued drug use. Additionally, Gina's mother revealed that Gina's father had been physically abusive to her throughout their relationship, but she denied that either of them had ever hurt Gina. Gina's mother admitted that she and Gina's father often left their daughter with different people and that she could not account for Gina's injuries due to that. Gina's mother slowly came to realize that she had failed to protect her daughter and that she had placed her daughter in danger on numerous occasions. Over time, Gina's interactions with her mother improved due in part to dyadic therapy and in part to her mother's newfound sobriety.

Gina's aunt and uncle supported Gina's mother by providing encouragement and holding her to the rules of her case plan. They also assisted her in getting a job and an apartment. Eventually, Gina and her mother were reunified in a gradual, planned process. Gina and her mother continued to benefit from emotional and practical support from Gina's aunt and uncle.

TYPES OF INTERVENTIONS

Infants and toddlers in foster care pose special challenges for clinicians. Most maltreated children, even those who are less than 4 years old, are not removed from their parents. Those who are removed likely have experienced more serious maltreatment and possibly more substantial relationship disturbances prior to their removal. These difficulties may be compounded by placement in foster care because of the added burden of a caregiving disruption. Attempting to enhance the birth parent–child relationship at a time when they are not living together creates additional challenges. Infants and toddlers require frequent contact with parents in order to develop or sustain meaningful relationships with them (American Academy of Pediatrics, Committee on Early Childhood, Adoption, and Dependent Care, 2000). Because young children are living with one set of caregivers even as we attempt to reunite them with another, there is often a need for the child to be treated in multiple relationships simultaneously. Also, because of requirements of ASFA, the Adoption and Safe Families Act of 1997, treatment is necessarily time limited. This means that families with complex problems must make substantial progress in a relatively short time. Therapy for young children in the context of maltreatment requires a thorough understanding of the multiple contexts in which these children are embedded, as well as the systems that impact their functioning. Given the complexity of problems, it is imperative to apply multimodal interventions selected to address specific problems that have been identified (Larrieu & Zeanah, 2004).

Dyadic Therapies

By its very nature, maltreatment involves a serious parent–child relationship disturbance. Furthermore, caregiving relationships are the most powerful influence on infant develop. For these reasons, relationship-based treatments are the core approach with young maltreated children (Lieberman & Van Horn, Chapter 4, this volume; Zeanah et al., 2000).

Dyadic treatments allow the infant–parent relationship to be addressed directly. Goals of such treatment are for parents to be able to see the child as a unique individual rather than as a split off or a repudiated aspect of the self, or as a reenactment of relationships from the parents' past. Parents also must develop an empathic appreciation of the children's experiences, as well as make a commitment to place the children's needs ahead of their own (see Wiehe, 2003). They must accept responsibility for their child's maltreatment and entrance into foster care and be able to recognize their failure to protect the child. Parents must be willing to change their behavior as parents to ensure the safety and protection of the child. For parents who themselves have had chaotic lives and been the victims of maltreatment as children, just establishing sufficient trust to enable them to believe that help and change are possible is challenging.

One model of dyadic therapy that is useful in the context of maltreatment is *infant–parent psychotherapy* (Lieberman, Silverman, & Pawl, 2000). In this model, the parent and infant are seen together and the focus is on links between the parents' experiences of their infant and their other relationship experiences, current and past. Parents' subjective experiences of themselves as a parent and of themselves as a child are explored. Observed interactions with the infant in the sessions are used by the clinician to help understand the parent's affective responses. The therapist often acts as a decoder of the parent and child's behavior. For example, the therapist highlights the issues and emotions that underlie angry remarks, helps the parent to clarify motives, and supports the parent in expressing conflicted feelings verbally rather than behaviorally.

Infant–parent psychotherapy is useful when the parent has the capacity for insight, curiosity about the self, and/or a pressing internal conflict about the circumstances in which she finds herself. In our view, infant–parent psychotherapy is indicated when parents display intense interpersonal affect, usually toward the child, or when parents have ready access to memories for past (usually traumatic) events but no affect associated with the memories. Therapeutic explorations may lead to new discoveries about the self as a parent and as a responsible adult, as well as discoveries about the infant. Changes in these perceptions provide the basis for constructive adaptations leading to improved interactions between the parent and baby (Larrieu & Zeanah, 2004).

Another particularly useful model of treatment with caregivers who have specific challenges, including young parents, cognitively limited parents, or parents who are emotionally unavailable due to chronic trauma, is McDonough's (2000) *interaction guidance* (Larrieu & Zeanah, 2004). This is a strengths-based model specifically designed for families with multiple risk factors, including poverty, substance abuse, mental illness, lack of social support, and minimal education. The therapist supports the parent in understanding the child's development and behaviors through interaction. The clinician's role is to guide and support the parent as a competent caregiver by focusing on observed here-and-now interactions between parent and child.

In this approach, the clinician first videotapes about 5 minutes of parent–child interaction and then reviews and discusses it with the parent during the session. This allows for immediate feedback to the parent about her behaviors with the infant, as well as her affect during play with the baby. The clinician points out only positive behaviors or satisfying interactions and elicits comments from the parent regarding her own experience of the baby. In addition to videotape review, parents are encouraged to reflect upon anything that they feel is impeding their relationship with their infant, especially stressors in the here and now. These reflections are discussed in the context of providing relevant material for strengthening the relationship between the parent and infant.

An important and distinctive component of dyadic therapy is that interactions between the therapist and child are visible and meaningful to the parent. The young child's presence in the sessions confers advantages by focusing the treatment and by making parent–child interactions immediately accessible. In addition, young children's presence conveys hope for change through their ongoing development, a feature that Selma Fraiberg referred to as "a little like having God on your side" (Fraiberg, Shapiro, & Cherniss, 1980, p. 53).

Nevertheless, the young child's presence also poses special challenges. Deciding when to address or engage the child, how to respond to overtures from the child, when and if to pick up the child—all must be considered through the lens of the meaning of these interactions for the parent. A desire to model healthy interactions must be balanced against the possibility of shaming parents who already feel intimidated and ineffective. If the parent is angry with the child, the therapist's engaging positively with the child may be experienced by the parents as a repudiation. Not colluding with parent's negative perceptions of the child while maintaining an appreciation of the child's challenging behavior is crucial to dyadic therapy, regardless of the type employed.

Individual Psychotherapy with Parents

Often, it is useful to supplement dyadic child–parent therapy with individual therapy with parents. Most parents present with complex difficulties that impede their ability to parent their children safely and effectively. Individual therapy is designed to address interpersonal or other difficulties that appear to be related to their parenting problems, including psychiatric disorders, particularly affective disorder and PTSD, substance use and abuse, and conflicted relationship histories (Larrieu & Zeanah, 2004). Even though the therapy is focused on the individual adult, it is focused primarily on the adult as a parent. Pairing individual therapy with dyadic therapy generally helps maintain the focus on the adult as parent.

Often, even before beginning dyadic treatment of infants and parents, we begin with individual therapy in order to allow parents to demonstrate a commitment to treatment, as evidenced, for example, by attending individual sessions consistently. We assess whether they have an investment in making lasting changes in the circumstances in which they find themselves. Once we feel that we have established the beginnings of a collaborative therapeutic relationship and parents have demonstrated a reasonable commitment to individual treatment, we introduce dyadic treatment.

It is crucial for parents to develop trust in their clinicians despite often having a history of disappointment and conflict with authority figures. Many parents have few reasons to trust professional helpers, and they enter treatment under scrutiny from CPS and the court. Therefore, establishing trust with parents is both challenging and critical for effective treatment.

Building trust begins with being reliable and dependable, by meeting with parents regularly, for example. The therapist must convey interest in their stories and respond to them in a nonjudgmental way in order to convey to parents that they are worthy of help and capable of changing. Offering concrete assistance for specific problems that interfere with effective parenting is another component of building trust. Crises are not uncommon, and providing crisis intervention at these times to help parents face challenges is also important.

More than acceptance is required, however. Therapists must also help parents face up to painful aspects of themselves and their own experiences. Being accepted by the therapist in spite of their shortcomings provides a healthy model that parents can apply to themselves. They may be able to forgive those who violated their trust and/or maltreated them. This is an important step in forgiving themselves which then can lead to positive changes with their children.

To enhance behavior changes, we may use behavior management techniques, developmental guidance, or skills training in addition to infant–parent psychotherapy. In the majority of cases, infant–parent therapy with foster parents is in the form of interaction guidance or behavior modification (Heller et al., 2002).

Ancillary Treatments

Referrals for ancillary treatments are necessary at times to help to remove barriers to effective parenting. For example, substance abuse counseling, special education services, battered women's programs, and vocational counseling may be necessary for parents. In addition, developmental delays are common among young foster children (Leslie, Gordon, Ganger, & Gist, 2002). Most maltreated infants and toddlers have both receptive and expressive language delays, and we refer them for speech and language evaluation and therapy as needed. Other services for which we refer young children include genetic and neurological evaluations and occupational and physical therapies.

Vignette 2

Daniel was 6 months old when his mother, Joann, who was a markedly depressed alcoholic, asked a friend to keep her son for the afternoon and did not return for him. Two days later, the friend called CPS and stated that she could no longer care for the child, who had a bad diaper rash and had run out of diapers and formula. Joann could not be located, nor were any relatives available to take the child, so Daniel was placed in the home of the Woods family.

When the case was referred to our team, Daniel had been in foster care for approximately 2 months. Daniel's foster mother reported one significant concern: during the rare visits when Daniel visited his mother, he began to tremble and cry as soon as he saw her and remained distraught through the remainder of the visit. Joann and the child protection worker who supervised the visit, and, of course, Daniel, were all stressed and exhausted by the situation. Visits were moved to our offices in order to work out a solution for Daniel's distress during the visits.

When we evaluated Daniel with his foster mother, it became clear that Daniel was attached to his foster mother and that she could serve as a "secure base" for him during the visit. Initially, his mother did not understand what purpose it would serve to have Ms. Wood in the room. She slowly began to understand that the foster mother's presence allowed Daniel to feel safe and that when he felt safe his interactions with his mother were much more relaxed. In addition, Joann's therapist was in the room during the visit to support her, and another clinician was in the room to "speak for the baby." The clinician verbalized the possible thoughts and feelings of the baby in the first person (e.g., "I think I'll play with this toy, Mommy"; "It's kind of scary when I bounce around"). This powerful intervention technique (Carter, Osofsky, & Hann, 1991) has proven useful in helping parents to empathize with their babies' feelings.

Joann was thrilled to have the opportunity to interact with her son in such a calm, playful way. Over the course of her treatment, she grew to be able to recognize her son's wants and needs and he became comfortable spending time with his mother. Joann developed a positive relationship with Ms. Wood, who encouraged Joann's relationship with her son. Joann and her son were eventually reunified. Ms. Wood's role has been transformed from that of primary attachment figure to favorite "auntie," and she takes him on Saturdays several times per month. This has allowed Daniel to add an attachment figure, rather than disrupting his attachment relationship with Ms. Wood. Over the years, Joann also has contacted the team for support when important decisions arise, such as Daniel's placement in preschool or their move to another state.

Developmental Intervention

When maltreated infants and toddlers experience significant injuries as a result of abuse, treatment of the parent–child relationship must be augmented with efforts to help the parents to understand the long-term sequelae of the injuries and the effects of the injuries on the young child's development.

Vignette 3

Alisha was 6 weeks of age when she entered the child welfare system. She had sustained multiple fractures during a violent altercation between her parents. Alisha's injuries required surgical intervention, and after a hospitalization she was placed in the home of her foster parents, the Burtons, at 8 weeks of age. Alisha's parents rarely visited her, and they seemed unaware of the impact of her injuries on her development. They also failed to understand the impact of their inconsistent visitation efforts on their relationship with their daughter and on their long-term possibility for reunification. Shortly after our initial contact with the family, we learned that Alisha's father had been arrested for assault and for distribution of heroin. He was jailed and later convicted.

Our team carefully monitored Alisha's development because of her serious injuries (Jaudes & Shapiro, 1999). We pay special attention to motor and language development in our young foster children because these problems are so common among foster children (Amster, 1999; Orlin, 1999). When Alisha first came to her foster parents, they noticed that she smiled expressively and cooed as she interacted with her them. At 5 months of age, Alisha had little head control and, in view of the injuries that she had sustained, a referral was made to evaluate her motor development. Results suggested significant fine and gross motor problems, and thus a long journey began for Alisha through multiple developmental assessments. She was diagnosed with cerebral palsy by her developmental pediatrician and was referred for evaluation of hearing and vision problems, which can co-occur with cerebral palsy (Gersh, 1998).

In addition to her motor problems, Alisha was easily overwhelmed and susceptible to overstimulation, another common characteristic of brain-injured children (Gersh, 1998). The caseworker had convinced Alisha's mother that she needed to visit regularly to establish a relationship with her daughter. She agreed to begin visits, and her therapist worked with her to assist her in noting when her daughter was withdrawn or dysregulated because she was overwhelmed. We again used the "speaking for the baby" technique (Carter et al., 1991) to convey cues to Alisha's mother regarding Alisha's experience during the visit. In addition, one of Alisha's foster parents typically attended the supervised visit in order to provide a secure base in the stressful setting of the visit.

Alisha's mother made limited progress as she learned, step by step, to manage her daughter's emerging motor and regulatory problems, but she seemed unable to spontaneously empathize with her daughter's experience. When parents and caregivers can empathize with their child's experience, it is less necessary to teach individual skills for appropriate caregiving. However, when psychological issues prevent caregivers from being able to take their child's perspective, risk to the child's well-being remains (Wiehe, 2003).

Alisha made progress in physical and occupational therapy, but the effects of her motor problems remained. Alisha was also referred for speech and language evaluation because of oral motor difficulties and delays in language development. The team maintained contact with rehabilitative professionals who provided services to Alisha, in order to monitor her progress as well as her attendance at her various therapy sessions.

The ultimate goal of ongoing visitation with Alisha's mother was the establishment of an attachment relationship between mother and daughter. Alisha's mother remained uncertain of effective ways in which to comfort her daughter and occasionally became agitated when her daughter became upset, typically using noisy toys to attempt to distract her or moving the baby in an agitated manner when she cried. Alisha's mother made gradual improvement, but concerns remained.

The team also provided guidance for Alisha's foster parents, particularly as they responded to her multiple needs and the various professionals who provided for those needs. They contacted the team often to discuss progress that Alisha was making and to voice concerns about her development. Alisha was enrolled in an intensive daily program that addressed a variety of developmental concerns with physical, occupational, and speech and language therapy. Although Alisha made significant progress in this developmentally stimulating setting, her attendance was not always consistent, and her foster parents were supported in their efforts to meet her educational needs.

Individual therapy also was provided to Alisha's mother. Goals included assisting her in accepting responsibility for her child's injuries. Parents are not expected to provide a "confession," but rather to identify and confront their failure to protect their young child. Referrals were also made for substance abuse treatment. Parents who are high on drugs or intoxicated by alcohol are unable to make sufficient progress in therapy because of their continued focus on the substance rather than their child (Tomison, 1996).

Battered women's treatment also was recommended for Alisha's mother because of the circumstances in which Alisha was injured. Alisha's mother continued to deny the effects of violence in her life and in the life of her child. Her difficulty in assuming responsibility for her failure to protect Alisha increased the risk that Alisha would not be safe with her. In addition, her continued denial of Alisha's injuries suggested that she might be unable or unwilling to provide her daughter with the treatments that Alisha needed in order to ameliorate her condition.

When it became clear that Alisha's mother was unlikely to regain custody of her, Alisha's grandmother came forward and requested that Alisha be placed in her home. Alisha's grandmother resided out of state, and after a home study was conducted a transfer of custody took place. In the view of the team it was essential that Alisha establish a relationship with her grandmother prior to placement, but the court ordered that the child be moved immediately.

CONCLUSION

Child abuse and neglect represent a particular threat to the physical, emotional, and developmental well-being of infants and toddlers. Young children represent a significant portion of youngsters in the child welfare system and are at greatest risk from the effects of child abuse and neglect. They account for the greatest percentage of fatalities, but there are other implications as well. In part because of their inability to talk, flee, or defend themselves, they enter foster care at greater rates than other age groups. The effects of abuse on the rapid developmental growth that is a hallmark of this period can be profound. For example, young children in the foster care system often have marked speech and language delays as well as delays in motor and cognitive development.

Children of all ages react when placed in the stressful environment of abuse and neglect at the hands of their caregivers. It is important for those working with infants and toddlers to recognize the distinctive patterns of behavior that provide evidence that young children are distressed by their experience. After all, the devastating effects of child abuse and neglect are caused, in part, by the fact that the very individuals upon whom the young child must rely for safety, comfort, and survival often violate that trust by actively physically abusing the child, by neglecting the child's needs for sustenance and nurturance, or by permitting others to harm the child. Infants and toddlers, unable to put voice to their feelings, respond to the chaos and fear engendered by child abuse and neglect by acting out in the most basic spheres of development, such as emotional regulation, sleep, and toileting.

It is the job of all professionals involved with young children in the child welfare system, including the judge, the child protection worker, the foster parent, and the therapist, to ameliorate the effects of abuse and neglect by providing consistency, structure, love, and patience for their youngest clients. The guiding principle must always be the best interest of the child. This principle should be implemented for infants and toddlers, whenever possible, in small and large ways, from limiting their travel time to visits with parents to careful assessment of their safety and well-being when plans for reunification are underway. Professionals working with young children in the child welfare system who approach decisions about young children carefully, remaining mindful of the special risks posed to infants and toddlers when we fail to consider the best interest of the child, are in a position to affect the developmental trajectory not only of the young child but also of his or her family, community, and nation.

REFERENCES

Adoption and Safe Families Act [ASFA]. (1997). PL 105-89, 42 USC §§ 670 *et seq.*

American Academy of Pediatrics Committee on Early Childhood, Adoption, and Dependent Care. (2000). Developmental issues for young children in foster care. *Pediatrics, 106,* 1145–1150.

Amster, B. J. (1999). Speech and language development of young children in the child welfare system. In J. A. Silver, B. J. Amster, & T. Haecker (Eds.), *Young children and foster care: A guide for professionals* (pp. 117–138). Baltimore: Brookes.

Barnett, D., Ganiban, J., & Cicchetti, D. (1999). Maltreatment, negative expressivity, and the development of Type D attachments from 12 to 24 months of age. *Monographs of the Society for Research in Child Development, 64,* 97–118.

Boris, N. W., Aoki, Y., & Zeanah, C. H. (1999). The development of infant–parent attachment: Considerations for assessment. *Infants and Young Children, 11,* 1–10.

Carlson, V., Cicchetti, D., Barnett, D., & Braunwald, K. (1989). Disorganized/disoriented attachment relationships in maltreated infants. *Developmental Psychology, 25,* 525–531.

Carter, S. L., Osofsky, J. D., & Hann, D. M. (1991). Speaking for the baby: A therapeutic intervention with adolescent mothers and their infants. *Infant Mental Health Journal, 12,* 291–301.

Christian, C. W. (1999). Child abuse and neglect. In J. A. Silver, B. J. Amster, & T. Haecker (Eds.), *Young children and foster care: A guide for professionals* (pp. 195–212). Baltimore: Brookes.

Christian, C. W. (2003). Assessment and evaluation of the physically abused child [Electronic version]. *Clinics in Family Practice, 5,* 1–19.

Clyman, R. B., Harden, B. J., & Little, C. (2002). Assessment, intervention, and research with infants in out-of-home placement. *Infant Mental Health Journal, 23,* 435–453.

Denby, R., Rindfleisch, N., & Bean, G. (1999). Predictors of foster parents' satisfaction and intent to continue to foster. *Child Abuse and Neglect, 23,* 287–303.

Dozier, M., Higley, E., Albus, K. E., & Nutter, A. (2002). Intervening with foster infants' caregivers: Targeting three critical needs. *Infant Mental Health Journal, 23,* 541–554.

Fraiberg, S., Shapiro, V., & Cherniss, D. S. (1980). Treatment modalities. In S. Fraiberg (Ed.), *Clinical studies in infant mental health: The first year of life* (pp. 49–77). New York: Basic Books.

Gersh, E. (1998). What is cerebral palsy? In E. Geralis (Ed.), *Children with cerebral palsy: A parents' guide* (pp. 1–34). Bethesda, MD: Woodbine House.

Heller, S. S., Smyke, A. T., & Boris, N. W. (2002). Very young foster children and foster families: Clinical challenges and interventions. *Infant Mental Health Journal, 23,* 555–575.

Hildyard, K. L., & Wolfe, D. A. (2002). Child neglect: Developmental issues and outcomes. *Child Abuse and Neglect, 26,* 679–695.

Hinshaw-Fuselier, S., Boris, N. W., & Zeanah, C. H. (1999). Reactive attachment disorder in maltreated twins. *Infant Mental Health Journal, 20,* 42–59.

Jaudes, P. K., & Shapiro, L. D. (1999). Child abuse and developmental disabilities. In

J. A. Silver, B. J. Amster, & T. Haecker (Eds.), *Young children and foster care: A guide for professionals* (pp. 213–234). Baltimore: Brookes.

Johnson, T. C. (1997). *Sexual, physical, and emotional abuse in out-of-home care: Prevention skills for at-risk children.* Binghamton, NY: Haworth Press.

Kaufman, J., & Henrich, C. (2000). Exposure to violence and early childhood trauma. In C. H. Zeanah (Ed.), *Handbook of infant mental health* (2nd ed., pp. 195–207). New York: Guilford Press.

Larrieu, J. A., & Zeanah, C. H. (2004). Treating parent–infant relationships in the context of maltreatment: An integrated systems approach. In A. J. Sameroff, S. C. McDonough, & K. L. Rosenblum (Eds.), *Treating parent–infant relationship problems* (pp. 243–264). New York: Guilford Press.

Lederman, C. S., Osofsky, J. D., & Katz, L. (2001). When the bough breaks the cradle will fall: Promoting the health and well-being of infants and toddlers in juvenile court. *Juvenile and Family Court Journal, 52,* 33–38.

Leslie, L. K., Gordon, J. N., Ganger, W., & Gist, K. (2002). Developmental delays in young children in child welfare by initial placement type. *Infant Mental Health Journal, 23,* 496–516.

Lieberman, A. F., Silverman, R., & Pawl, J. H. (2000). Infant–parent psychotherapy: Core concepts and current approaches. In C. H. Zeanah (Ed.), *Handbook of infant mental health* (2nd ed., pp. 472–484). New York: Guilford Press.

Margolin, G. (1998). Effects of domestic violence on child development: A review of research. In P. K. Trickett & C. J. Schellenbach (Eds.), *Violence against children in the family and the community* (pp. 57–101). Washington, DC: American Psychological Association.

McDonough, S. C. (2000). Interaction guidance: An approach for difficult-to-engage families. In C. H. Zeanah (Ed.), *Handbook of infant mental health* (2nd ed., pp. 485–493). New York: Guilford Press.

Morrison, J. A., Frank, S. J., Holland, C. C., & Kates, W. R. (1999). Emotional development and disorders in young children in the child welfare system. In J. A. Silver, B. J. Amster, & T. Haecker (Eds.), *Young children and foster care: A guide for professionals* (pp. 33–64). Baltimore: Brookes.

National Clearinghouse on Child Abuse and Neglect Information. (2001). *In focus: Acts of omission—An overview of child neglect* [On-line]. Available from *http://www.calib.com/nccanch/pubs/focus/acts.cfm*

National Clearinghouse on Child Abuse and Neglect Information. (2002). *National Child Abuse and Neglect Data System (NCANDS): Summary of key findings from calendar year 2000* [On-line]. Available from *http://www.calib.com/nccanch/pubs/factsheets/canstats.cfm*

National Clearinghouse on Child Abuse and Neglect Information. (n.d.). *In harm's way: Domestic violence and child maltreatment* [On-line]. Available from *http://www.calib.com/nccanch/pubs/otherpubs/harmsway.cfm*

Orlin, M. N. (1999). Motor development and disorders in young children. In J. A. Silver, B. J. Amster, & T. Haecker (Eds.), *Young children and foster care: A guide for professionals* (pp. 93–115). Baltimore: Brookes.

Osofsky, J. D. (1998). Children as invisible victims of domestic and community violence. In G. W. Holden, R. Geffner, & E. N. Jouriles (Eds.), *Children exposed to marital violence: Theory, research, and applied issues.* (pp. 95–117). Washington, DC: American Psychological Association.

Osofsky, J. D. (2003). Prevalence of children's exposure to domestic violence and child maltreatment: Implications for prevention and intervention. *Clinical Child and Family Psychology Review, 6*(3), 161–170.

Palmer, S. (1998). *Shaken baby syndrome* [On-line]. Available from *http://www.thearc. org/faqs/shaken.html*.

Poland, D. C., & Groze, V. (1993). Effects of foster care placement on biological children in the home. *Child and Adolescent Social Work Journal, 10,* 153–163.

Putnam, F. W. (2003). Ten-year research update review: Child sexual abuse. *Journal of the American Academy of Child and Adolescent Psychiatry, 42,* 269–278.

Ricci, L. R. (2000). Initial medical treatment of the physically abused child. In R. M. Reece (Ed.), *Treatment of child abuse: Common ground for mental health, medical, and legal practitioners* (pp. 81–94). Baltimore: Johns Hopkins University Press.

Ross, P. E., & Crawford, J. (1999). On the front lines: Foster parents' experiences in coordinating services. In J. A. Silver, B. J. Amster, & T. Haecker (Eds.), *Young children and foster care: A guide for professionals* (pp. 279–291). Baltimore: Brookes.

Showers, J. (1998). *Never shake a baby: The challenges of shaken baby syndrome.* Alexandria, VA: National Association of Children's Hospitals and Related Institutions. Available from *http://www.childrenshospitals.net/nachri/news/pdfs/sbs.pdf*

Silver, J. A., Amster, B. J., & Haecker, T. (Eds.). (1999). *Young children and foster care: A guide for professionals.* Baltimore: Brookes.

Smyke, A. T., Dumitrescu, A., & Zeanah, C. H. (2002). Attachment disturbances in young children: I. The continuum of caretaking casualty. *Journal of the American Academy of Child and Adolescent Psychiatry, 41,* 972–982.

Smyke, A. T., Foster, R., & Keyes, A. W. (2003, February). *Fostering young children: Addressing issues of love and loss.* Paper presented at the annual meeting of Prevent Child Abuse Louisiana, Baton Rouge, LA.

Spiker, D., & Silver, J. A. (1999). Early intervention services for infants and preschoolers in foster care. In J. A. Silver, B. J. Amster, & T. Haecker (Eds.), *Young children and foster care: A guide for professionals* (pp. 347–371). Baltimore: Brookes.

Stovall, K. C., & Dozier, M. (2000). The development of attachment in new relationships: Single subject analyses for ten foster infants. *Development and Psychopathology, 12,* 133–156.

Tomison, A.M. (1996). *Child maltreatment and substance abuse* [On-line]. Melbourne: Australian Institute of Family Studies, National Child Protection Clearinghouse. Available from *http://www.aifs.org.au/nch/discussion2.html*

U.S. Department of Health and Human Services, Administration on Children, Youth and Families. (2003). *Child maltreatment 2001.* Washington, DC: U.S. Government Printing Office.

Vig, S., & Kaminer, R. (1999). Training professionals to work with young children with developmental disabilities. In J. A. Silver, B. J. Amster, & T. Haecker (Eds.), *Young children and foster care: A guide for professionals* (pp. 455–471). Baltimore: Brookes.

Wharton, R. H., Rosenberg, S., Sheridan, R. L., & Ryan, D. P. (2000). Long-term medical consequences of physical abuse. In R. M. Reece (Ed.), *Treatment of child abuse: Common ground for mental health, medical, and legal practitioners* (pp. 117–134). Baltimore: Johns Hopkins University Press.

Wiehe, V. R. (2003). Empathy and narcissism in a sample of child abuse perpetrators and a comparison sample of foster parents. *Child Abuse and Neglect, 27,* 541–555.

Wulczyn, F., Hislop, K. R., & Harden, B. J. (2002). The placement of infants in foster care. *Infant Mental Health Journal, 23,* 454–475.

Zeanah, C. H., Danis, B., Hirshberg, L., Benoit, D., Miller, D., & Heller, S. S. (1999). Disorganized attachment associated with partner violence: A research note. *Infant Mental Health Journal, 20,* 77–86.

Zeanah, C. H., Larrieu, J. A., Heller, S. S., & Valliere, J. (2000). Infant–parent relationship assessment. In C. H. Zeanah (Ed.), *Handbook of infant mental health* (2nd ed., pp. 222–235). New York: Guilford Press.

Zukoski, M. (1999). Foster parent training. In J.A. Silver, B. J. Amster, & T. Haecker (Eds.), *Young children and foster care: A guide for professionals* (pp. 473–490). Baltimore: Brookes.

CHAPTER 12

HOW LAW ENFORCEMENT AND MENTAL HEALTH PROFESSIONALS CAN PARTNER TO HELP TRAUMATIZED CHILDREN

Joy D. Osofsky
Jill Hayes Hammer
Nancy Freeman
J. Michael Rovaris

Police officers are "first responders" and are on the scene of violent events long before other people arrive to help. Children are often the "silent, invisible" victims who are exposed to violence but overlooked. Yet, in our 10 years of working with the New Orleans Police Department through the Violence Intervention Program, we have learned that police officers can become sensitive to the presence of children and helpful in making immediate appropriate interventions and referrals for consultation and services. This program is based on the premise that early actions taken by police officers may well be crucial in helping traumatized young children. Very often the referral time for a traumatized child receiving consultation and/or treatment can be weeks, months, or even years with their behaviors becoming increasingly disruptive, so that help at this particularly vulnerable time when the trauma occurs is critical.

The premise is that successful prevention and intervention efforts for children who witness violence require creative strategies and collaboration

285

in order to identify and reach the children soon after exposure to the trauma. It is much easier to intervene and make a difference in children's lives earlier for a number of different reasons. First, when intervention takes place earlier, children's symptoms are usually less severe and their behaviors may not yet be out of control or may often improve more quickly. In addition, there may still be supportive caretakers in their environment who are not yet overwhelmed by the child's reactions to the trauma and their own concurrent traumatization.

Research and clinical evidence indicates that exposure to violence contributes to negative outcomes for children, including posttraumatic stress symptoms, and is a significant risk factor for later violent behavior. Because of the prevalence of everyday violence in our society, children witness violence in their neighborhoods, at school, and at home to an extent that can interfere with their normal development. Unfortunately in the past few years in the United States there have been unusual traumatic events including terrorism and war that have contributed to traumatization and retraumatization. As has been emphasized by Judge William E. Gladstone, former administrative judge of the Miami/Dade Juvenile Court, "if we truly value our children and want to prevent the development of violent behaviors and consequent delinquency, it is vital that we put in place supports and prevention programs that address children's exposure to violence" (personal communication, July 16, 2001).

DEVELOPMENT OF THE VIOLENCE INTERVENTION PROGRAM FOR CHILDREN AND FAMILIES

In a response to the violence in New Orleans reflecting a national increase in youth violence in the early 1990s, the Violence Intervention Program (VIP) was initiated in 1992 (Osofsky, 1997). The Department of Psychiatry at Louisiana State University Health Sciences Center (LSUHSC) partnered with the New Orleans Police Department (NOPD) in an effort to prevent and reduce the negative effects of witnessing violence on children. The first step in this partnership was to identify the needs of the community and develop strategies to broaden and heighten the sensitivity of police officers' responses to children exposed to violence. Mental health professionals in the VIP program partnered with the NOPD to educate police officers about child development and traumatization and to learn from them about what can be done at the scene of a violent incident in order to reach traumatized children much earlier. As part of that process, NOPD officers learned more about the effects of violence on children and were provided information about available crisis intervention and other services to support their work when intervening with traumatized children and families.

The philosophy behind the VIP, based on both clinical evidence and a growing body of research, is that crisis intervention and follow-up psychological treatment, combined with family and community support, can decrease the severity of children's problems following traumatization. The program utilizes a systems approach to violence prevention working at a variety of levels involving raising awareness, education, training, referrals, and services to decrease children's exposure to violence and to help children and families who are exposed to violence.

The program has evolved and grown based on our conviction that early identification and intervention following violence exposure ultimately can be helpful in preventing future violence. While some research supports the idea that early exposure to trauma, including abuse and neglect, can lead to later serious problems (Widom, 1989, 1999), clinical experiences are also informative. During the 10 years of the VIP, we have learned a great deal about the impact of violence exposure on young children by following those who have been referred shortly after the traumatic event as compared with those referred after some delay, sometimes of several years. In a sample of approximately 100 seriously traumatized children referred to our program in the past 3 years, 30% were referred within the first 1½ years after the trauma and 70% were referred later. We are seeing interesting differences between these two groups of children, as well as some symptom patterns that tend to characterize children who are referred several years after an experience of violence. While many of the children live in chaotic environments, not all of our referrals lack family and community support. What is striking about these children is that many who are referred long after the trauma occurred are having significant problems despite their living with loving caregivers who also provide for their basic needs. Children who have been exposed to violence as infants, toddlers, and preschoolers but are referred to VIP 2 years or more after the incident tend to have significant learning problems. They are described as having trouble concentrating and paying attention in school. It is often reported that they are "not learning," sometimes act "spacey," and not infrequently have been retained. Behavior problems and acting out often accompany this picture. While many of these children evidence developmental delays, most have never received an evaluation and needed interventions. Some children referred later are intensely and unpredictably aggressive. They may attack siblings, peers, and even adults. Referral to VIP often comes when a child is asked to leave one or more day-care centers or after being expelled from school. Alternatively, some late-referred children tend to internalize acting withdrawn and depressed. They may be referred because they are doing poorly in school or because of adult concerns about their withdrawn behaviors. All of the children who have been referred to us have memories of the violence they witnessed or survived, even though the violence occurred some 4–5 years before when they were as young as 2 years of age. Even the youngest witnesses/survivors whom we have seen have memories of the events, though few ever shared their traumatic experiences previously (Gaensbauer, 2002).

HOW TO BUILD A PARTNERSHIP
WITH POLICE OFFICERS

Successful collaborations are effective because of the relationships that are built between individuals and the mutual trust that develops over time. A partnership between mental health professionals and police officers requires a twofold effort. First, mental health professionals need to learn to listen to police officers in order to ascertain their understanding of youth violence and their perspectives in approaching children exposed to violence. Second, police officers need to learn about what they can do beyond "policing" and how they can use available resources to support their work after intervening with children during violent incidents. Often police officers have commented to us that they feel better about doing their work when they know there are people and services available for the children. Previously, they would see children at a murder or other violent scene and believe that their job was to secure the scene and deal with the crime. Now they know that there is more support in the mental health and service communities for these families and that they can help them in other ways. An example of this expanded partnership is in the New Orleans Safe Start Program described below.

Evolution and Development of the Safe
Start Program

In 2000, we had the opportunity to expand the VIP to focus on younger children exposed to violence with a 2-year Safe Start service award from the Office of Juvenile Justice and Delinquency Prevention, U.S. Department of Justice. The Safe Start Initiative in New Orleans focused on young children's exposure to domestic violence and child abuse. Interventions included a crisis response team that provided 24-hour a day hotline, consultation, and service availability for children and families affected by domestic violence or child abuse.

Safe Start was designed as a collaborative endeavor that included several different groups including representatives from the NOPD, the New Orleans Police Foundation, the Juvenile Court, the Child Protection Agency, the Mayor's Office, and the Children's Collaborative, a local alliance of child service agencies. The group included a multidisciplinary staff of social work, psychology, and evaluation experts, as well as trainees.

The domestic violence component of the program focused on developing a partnership with an innovative police district, one of eight in New

Orleans. The captain of this district, Louis Dabdoub had previously taken the initiative to study the prevalence of domestic violence in New Orleans. From his study, he learned that 74% of those arrested in 2000 for domestic violence had prior violent crime arrests and convictions (Captain Louis Dabdoub, personal communication, March 31, 2003). He concluded that if perpetrators were willing to hurt the ones they "allegedly" loved, then they would not think twice about harming others. Captain Dabdoub and his colleagues also sampled a small number of domestic violence cases and found that 87% of domestic violence perpetrators had witnessed domestic violence as children. Using this information, he obtained funding to provide investigative staff devoted exclusively to the prosecution of domestic violence perpetrators and services for domestic violence victims. This new initiative for dealing with domestic violence cases by the police also included limiting dual arrests, training in determining who was the primary aggressor, and other victim-friendly approaches to the investigation of domestic violence cases.

One of the contributions of Safe Start was to help educate patrol officers as to the importance of recognizing the presence of children in domestic violence situations and, if possible, of providing a sensitive and appropriate intervention with the children on the scene. Included in the training materials was information about the effects of violence on children with a focus on domestic violence. Children who are exposed to domestic violence are more likely to be victims of physical abuse. Studies have indicated a co-occurrence rate ranging from 45 to 75% (Margolin, 1998). Some of the immediate steps that we suggested for officers with the children was providing them comfort during distress and accessing the Safe Start crisis response team described below.

The training offered at the New Orleans Police Academy and during roll call was supplemented by "ride-alongs" during which Safe Start staff joined police officers in their cars on patrol shifts. This activity served the dual function for the staff of sharing more of our knowledge while we learned from the officers. The staff learned about the range of activities and calls that police respond to, the complexity of the skill set required to function effectively as police officers, and the conflicting demands of their public safety responsibilities and their desire to respond in a human and caring way. One night while riding with an officer, a Safe Start staff member watched in amazement as the officer mediated a conflict between a middle-aged mother and her two adult daughters. The officer was able to get to the heart of the conflict amid shouts and name calling. In some ways, that officer showed outstanding sensitivity and clinical skills. Following the ride-alongs, the officers said that they were more aware of the previously "invisible" victims of violence and how often very young children were present when they responded to calls.

The second main component of the work of the Safe Start team with the NOPD focused on children's exposure to child abuse. For this work, the Safe Start team developed a relationship with the centralized child abuse unit serving the entire city of New Orleans. The initial intent was to provide training about working with child victims and witnesses after gaining information from focus groups about the division's needs. We found that officers felt they had adequate training in working with children; however, they requested assistance in managing the stress of their jobs. Therefore, we developed a series of training procedures, including experiential stress reduction sessions. This unexpected development emphasizes an important component of trauma work—that vicarious traumatization and burnout can occur in people who work in this area and that additional support for them may be very helpful.

For the child abuse unit, the Safe Start staff tried a different strategy to build a relationship and learn about what the unit's investigators and other officers do. In essence, Safe Start staff members "hung out" in the unit. If a call came in, at times the staff member would ride along with the officer, but not always. The goal of the time in the unit was to build trust and to increase the comfort level of the officers with the Safe Start staff members. One of the important components of this part of the program was that additional staff at LSUHSC would call the person at the child abuse unit periodically to check in and provide ongoing support and advise. The emotional availability of the staff and team support for crisis intervention work and traumatized children is crucial to the success of the work. At the request of the child abuse unit, we also provided training to child abuse detectives and patrol officers throughout the city on ways to respond to children during child abuse emergency calls.

The crisis response team, composed of social workers and psychologists, was available to both the selected district targeting domestic violence and the child abuse unit to provide on-site interventions. A portable response kit was developed to bring to the scene, containing referral information for the parents, booklets about the effects of violence on children, and play materials. Whenever possible, two staff members responded within 30 minutes so that one person could address the needs of the parents while the other person worked with the children.

Case Example of NOPD–Safe Start Collaboration

The following is an example of the use of the team by police officers. After taking three of her children to school, the mother of a 2-year-old and an 8-year-old left home to drive her partner to work. While she was gone, the house caught on fire. The police and fire officials responded to the scene and removed the two young children from the home. The 2-year-old was dead and the 8-year-old was dying. The identity of the family was learned from neighbors, and it was learned that older siblings were in school. At this point, police officers called the Safe Start hotline and a social worker responded to the call. While on her way to the school, the police located the mother and brought her to the school as well. The social worker met with the mother and notified her of the death of her youngest child and that her older child was in critical condition. She later assisted the mother in informing the younger children. The mother was taken to police headquarters, and the social worker rode with the three other siblings and a cousin in another patrol car. Upon arriving at the police station, the social worker provided therapeutic support for the children for 8 hours while the police continued the investigation. This support included feeding the children, playing with them, and engaging them in therapeutic activities. The police completed their investigation, and the local child protection agency found alternative housing for the children with family members. Ultimately, the parents were released from jail after being charged with criminal negligence. The social worker continued therapy, working with the family around issues of grief and loss.

While this intervention seems fairly simple (i.e., staying with the children and providing therapy), the social worker kept the situation from being unbearable for the family. She provided support for the mother in talking with the children about their sibling's death, support for the children in understanding what had happened both in terms of the loss of their siblings and the incarceration of their parents, and companionship and activities for the children in police headquarters until they could be placed with relatives. She also assisted the police in engaging the children so that the officers could complete their investigation of the incident. The social worker was a constant factor in the family's struggle, from the immediate crisis to the family's beginning readjustment after the tragedy.

New Orleans Safe Start Initiative

Another focus of the work of Safe Start with the NOPD was to provide better documentation of children's exposure to violence and to share this information with the larger community. At the beginning of the initiative, law enforcement procedure called for officers to note the presence of children in domestic violence situations but did not require specifics such as their number, ages, gender, and the nature of their involvement. The NOPD agreed to require this additional information. The police also agreed to compare domestic violence data with child abuse data in an effort to determine the co-occurrence of these two crimes locally. This work was not completed within the Safe Start timeline; however, both initiatives continued with additional funding obtained from a national foundation.

TRAINING AND EDUCATION ISSUES WITH POLICE

To come in as an "expert" without knowing the people to whom you want to introduce ideas is a mistake, particularly if you are coming from another discipline and institution. Infusing a system with new ideas has to be done carefully and sensitively. Educating police officers about the effects of violence on children requires flexibility, patience, and creativity. When police are investigating a homicide, a domestic dispute, or another violent incident, attention to what is happening to the children on the scene is unlikely to play a prominent role. The officers need to establish order, determine if an arrest is needed, follow protocols regarding attention to the crime scene, and take care of other activities that demand police attention. Through the joint efforts of the VIP and the NOPD, we have found that after educating officers about the effects of violence on children, including information about the difference even a few words or a comforting touch can mean to a traumatized child, many police officers see their role with children at a violent scene as one of extreme importance. Now they often feel much more support in their role, as they previously often worried about the children but had little information about how to help them.

Over the past 10 years, the VIP has provided education and training on the effects of violence on children at the New Orleans Police Academy, to new recruits, for in-service training, to Community-Oriented Police Services, and to school liaison officers during roll call. Of the training sessions offered, it became increasingly clear after we talked with police officers in the districts that a more "experience-near" approach might be more effective and make a difference in the minds of officers in a stressed police department in a large city, facing a high level of violence. We proceeded to provide between 15 and 20 minutes of education and discussion during the three roll call sessions held each day before the officers assumed their daily duties on the street. When officers in the eight police districts in New Orleans report for their watches, they join with the other patrol and ranking officers—for 20–30 minutes, depending on the day—to review the events of the day, the calls they need to address, violent incidents that need to be pursued, and any other news that might affect their activities for that day. After building relationships with the police, ranking officers provided us with some of that time depending on the other pressing business of the day to present information on the VIP, the effects of community and domestic violence on children, and available referral sources. At roll call, it became quickly apparent that some of the officers welcomed the opportunity to share their recent experiences with children at crime scenes. These contributions from the police were invaluable, as they made the material presented by the VIP staff much more salient for the other officers.

The premise behind our work with the police rests on recent data regarding police work. Despite the assumption that a majority of police agencies routinely report cases of child maltreatment to their local Child Protective Service (CPS) (Martin & Bersharov, 1991), data from the Third National Incidence Study of Child Abuse and Neglect (U.S. Department of Health and Human Services, 1996) indicate that almost three-quarters of the cases investigated by CPS were reported by noninvestigatory agencies (e.g., hospitals, schools, day-care centers, mental health agencies, and social services agencies). This information points to a potential problem with the recognition and reporting of potential child maltreatment cases by law enforcement personnel, indicating that more training is needed (Portwood, Grady, & Dutton, 2000). In addition, the surveys suggest that officers may emphasize the importance of the sexual nature of an act of child maltreatment more than other professional groups including mental health, legal, and medical professionals and elementary school teachers and administrators (Portwood, 1999). Thus, it is crucial that police officers, often the first responders to children who have witnessed violence, recognize the risks and consequences of victimization of children through witnessing the violence and other less direct exposure. The VIP roll call training protocol for the NOPD uses a traditional didactic approach that is offered within the military "chain of command" system within which most police agencies operate. Ranking officers at each district advise the appropriate watch/platoon commanders of the scheduled presentation during roll calls that occur four times a year in each district. The presentations, while repeatedly emphasizing certain points, are also designed to reflect some of the specific needs in that district. For example, the Eighth District of the New Orleans Police Department is located in the French Quarter, an area with many tourists in addition to residents and businesses. Officers assigned to this district are provided with information regarding child victimization and need for early intervention; however, these officers are also informed about social services for tourists in need. Roll call for officers assigned to the Second Police District, located in a more residential area of New Orleans with a mix of upper- and lower-income families and college students, includes additional information on abuse and domestic violence exposure.

The VIP information provided during roll call is integrated into the way the officers think about and do police work. When we first started education for police during roll call, we heard their concerns and soon learned that emphasizing what a difference just a word or concern from an officer could make for a traumatized child was key to gaining their trust and cooperation. We also learned that so many people come to talk to the officers about their programs that they tend to "tune out" when they come. We learned several years later that what made a difference for us and helped us gain their trust was that we kept coming back. We even returned when they didn't greet us that warmly. They said, "Since we really didn't treat you that well and you kept coming back, it made us think that you might be saying something important and we should pay attention."

During each roll call session, the following points were made:

I. *Contact Information and the Services Provided*
   A. The VIP has a 24-hour hotline for police and/or families to call for immediate consultation and referral for children and families who are traumatized. A mental health professional is always available on the line. The VIP distributes cards and pens to the officers with the contact information.
   B. A Community Resource List with referral information for different services has been developed with the collaboration of NOPD and is distributed to the officers.

II. *The Rationale for Early Identification and Intervention with Traumatized Children*
   A. The importance of prevention and turning intervention into prevention is discussed. Police are introduced to the data showing that children who are victimized by violence are at greater risk when they grow up to become either victims or perpetrators of violence.
   B. Discussion is included about the psychological and financial costs of prevention, intervention, and treatment as compared with the costs to the juvenile and criminal justice systems including incarceration.
   C. We emphasize that police officers are not "social workers"; however, we know that police are the first on the scene of violent incidents involving children with the goal of establishing and maintaining order. Therefore, while we recognize that police officers are indeed not social workers, we talk about the unique opportunity they have, after order is established, to approach the children, support them, or give them information. We stress that this is often a time when families may be looking for help.
   D. The information presented to the police is made more credible by describing data gathered by the VIP indicating that children, at least younger children age 8–12, are hopeful, trust the police, and are most likely to go to them if they are lost or need help.
   E. Information is reviewed on the effects of violence on children and posttraumatic stress behaviors. Posttraumatic stress disorder (PTSD), a common problem resulting from serious traumatization, is described. Ways to respond and treat children and families who have been traumatized are discussed.

III. *What You Can Do as a Police Officer*
   A. Give the VIP contact information cards to family members with instructions to call if they need help.
   B. If possible, make the call to the VIP hotline before leaving the family.

C. Be aware of how trauma impacts on children and can create barriers in communicating with them.

IV. *Trauma Education*

    A. A brief discussion is included about the effects of exposure to trauma and vicarious traumatization for professionals, including police offices, caregivers, teachers, parents, and therapists.

    B. A review of the importance of self-care for those who work with trauma is included.

    C. Information on services available to officers and their families is presented.

What We Do: A Second Case Example of VIP–NOPD Collaboration (Presented by J. Michael Rovaris)

A call was received by the VIP crisis response team from the police at 10:25 P.M. for assistance regarding three children, ages 7, 5, and 4, who had just witnessed their mother's shooting by her boyfriend. The man then turned the gun on himself, blowing off half of his head in front of the children as they held their dying mother. The officers stated they were transporting the children to the district station to get them away from the crime scene. However, the children's mother was taken to the local trauma center for emergency treatment. The staff at the emergency room told officers that the mother's wounds were likely to be fatal.

While driving to the scene, the social worker (J.M.R.) called another team member to meet him at the station. Teamwork and support for crisis intervention is a program policy for the VIP. In our experience with this work with traumatized children, we have learned that having more than one therapist present at crisis intervention scenes is critically important. When we work as a team, at no point are the children left alone while one of us is gathering information or attending to the needs of the adults. As a matter of course, the team member always has an "intervention kit" with him or her. The kit contains several blank sheets of paper, coloring pens, Play-Doh, card games, stickers, a small pack of cleansing tissues and wipes, and a small blanket and pillow. As some interventions require work around biohazards such as blood and body fluids, the team member usually carries a second kit containing rubber gloves, shoe covers, a surgical mask, and a paper gown for use in such situations.

When the social worker arrived at the police station, the officers quickly brought him to the children. Here is his report:

> "The three children were seated at a table in an interview room. They were dressed in their pajamas, all of which had stains of dried blood.

The officers immediately left the room. The children sat silently at first. Once the officers left the room and I greeted the children, the two younger ones started to talk about how their mother was shot by 'Red.' The children's speech patterns were rapid and disjointed. After about 30 seconds, the eldest child stood up and placed one hand on each of his sibling's mouths and told them they should not be talking to me because they did not know me and I did not have on a police uniform. At that point, I explained to these frightened children why I was there, telling them that our team works with children and that the police often call us when children need help who have seen bad things. Following this explanation, the eldest boy was satisfied and sat back in his chair. He then said that his name was Kevin but his family called him 'Slugger.' Slugger then introduced his brother, John, and his sister, Janet. Although he was small for his age, Slugger was in many ways overly mature for 7 years. John and Janet, having seen that their brother was now more at ease with me, continued to talk about what happened. Both John and Janet moved from their seats and stood so close to me that they were able to each sit on one of my legs. The children were able to draw a couple of pictures as they talked about what had happened. They both drew themes of a family that was centered around Mommy. When I told them that another social worker was on the way, they wanted to know if he was going to be nice. The second social worker arrived after 45 minutes, and the children wanted to play. Officers at the district were keeping up to date on the mother's medical status. All indications were that she was not going to survive. As it passed midnight, the children became sleepy but were unable to fall asleep. Officers who had talked to the children's maternal grandmother informed us that she would come to the station to pick them up once her daughter's condition had stabilized."

LESSONS LEARNED FROM THE VIOLENCE INTERVENTION AND SAFE START PROGRAMS

There is much that we have learned over the years from work with the VIP and the New Orleans Safe Start Program. We believe that these lessons learned may be helpful to others in building collaborative relationships with the police.

First, it is important to really be present and available to impact police officers' practice on a daily basis. While there are probably many ways to build a relationship with the police, we believe that developing a partnership involves mutual respect and attention to the expertise coming from each discipline. So, a major aspect of learning what police officers do and developing trust involves "hanging out" and spending time just being with them and being available to talk. Other ways to build a relationship while gaining valuable information is going on ride-alongs, providing education, and even offering skills for stress management that can be used to understand and cope with both the problems and the tensions that are ongoing elements of police work.

Second, it is crucial to secure involvement at all levels of the police department in order to build a partnership. Obviously, the chief of police needs to be informed about and supportive of such a program for it to work. However, it is equally important to gain the trust and support of the patrol officers who work day to day on the streets. They are the ones who meet the young children and come to learn what works and what doesn't in relation to them.

Third, we have found that success comes if we do not attempt to take on too big of a responsibility. It is important to do one or two things with the police consistently and well. For the duration of our program, we have been doing roll call training consistently with each district at least three times a years. We are also consistently available for crisis intervention when needed. Finally, when we are asked to assist the police with any activities or consultations, we are available to do so.

Other principles are important. It must be recognized that in order for a program to be accepted by the community and by law enforcement, it needs to be in effect for a number of years. The VIP has been ongoing for the past 10 years. Through that program, we have gained the trust of the police as it has become known and utilized often as a source of support and referral when police work interfaces with mental health. In contrast, for our Safe Start Program that was only funded for 2 years, it was more difficult to accomplish the objectives and become integrated into the domestic violence and child abuse programs. In fact, we are planning to develop a program with the police in these areas that is now structured differently, building on what we learned during the 2 years of that program. In any collaborative effort across disciplines, building relationships is an important part of the work—and relationship building leading to trust takes time. One of the things we learned through the Safe Start Program is to build flexibility into staff time so that is not too role defined. In order to do crisis intervention and to be available to police, it is difficult to have responsibilities for a job that requires regular hours and also be available for police emergency calls. Therefore, to meet these needs, it is important to be flexible as to job boundaries. Finally, we have learned that in order to do trauma work most effectively, it is important to have an integrated team that provides ongoing availability and support for everyone doing this difficult work.

CONCLUSION

In developing a program to work with law enforcement personnel to help young children exposed to violence, it is important first of all to develop a trusting relationship with police. These relationships and respect for the expertise of those coming from the other discipline are crucial in order to "infuse" a system with new ideas. Often, it may be helpful to identify someone who believes in the work and can become an "ambassador" for the program within the system. We have learned through our 10 years of working with the police that the programs are most successful if the focus is on a few things that are done consistently, sensitively, and thoroughly. Finally, it is important to be there for the long haul, which takes time and patience. It really is neither appropriate nor effective to expect to build a collaboration only for the tenure of a period of a grant. Rather, it behooves the mental health professional who is committed to developing collaborative programs to find a way to keep the program going once established, even if it is scaled down during leaner funding periods.

REFERENCES

Gaensbauer, T. J. (2002). Representations of trauma in infancy: Clinical and theoretical implications for the understanding of early memory. *Infant Mental Health Journal, 23*(3), 259–277.

Margolin, G. (1998). Effects of domestic violence on children. In P. K. Trickett & C. J. Shellenbach (Eds.), *Violence against children in the family and the community.* Washington, DC: American Psychological Association.

Martin, S. E., & Bersharov, D. J. (1991). *Police and child abuse: New policies for expanded responsibilities.* Washington, DC: U.S. Department of Justice, National Institute of Justice.

Osofsky, J. D. (1997). *Children in a violent society.* New York: Guilford Press.

Portwood, S. G. (1999). Coming to terms with a consensual definition of child maltreatment. *Child Maltreatment: Journal of the American Professional Society on the Abuse of Children, 4*(1), 56–68.

Portwood, S. G., Grady, M. T., & Dutton, S. E. (2000). Enhancing law enforcement identification and investigation of child maltreatment. *Child Abuse and Neglect, 24*(2), 195–207.

U.S. Department of Health and Human Services. (1996). *The third national incidence study of child abuse and neglect.* Washington, DC: U.S. Government Printing Office.

Widom, C. S. (1989). Does violence beget violence?: A critical examination of the literature. *Psychological Bulletin, 106*(1), 3–28.

Widom, C. S. (1999). Posttraumatic stress disorder in abused and neglected children grown up. *American Journal of Psychiatry, 156*(8), 1223–1229.

PART IV

DIRECTIONS FOR THE FUTURE

CHAPTER 13

HOW RESEARCH INFORMS CLINICAL WORK WITH TRAUMATIZED YOUNG CHILDREN

MICHELLE BOSQUET

In the history of psychology, there has often existed a chasm between the disciplines of research and clinical intervention. However, the relatively young field of infant mental health has intertwined the two disciplines since its earliest beginnings. The detailed observations of clinicians such as Selma Fraiberg, D. W. Winnicott, René Spitz, James Robertson, Erik Erikson, and John Bowlby, as well as the research findings of psychologists including Mary Ainsworth, Harry Harlow, and Sally Provence laid the groundwork for the emergence of a new area of psychology that recognized the specialized needs of children in the first 5 years of life. To this day, clinicians and researchers in infant mental health continue to inform each other's work and model the benefits of collaboration between the two disciplines for increasing our understanding of and improving our services for young children.

As noted in many of the chapters in this volume, research has begun to elucidate the issues facing traumatized children and their families. Studies have described the types of emotional and behavioral problems that are likely to emerge in young children who have experienced trauma and the ways in which trauma can interfere with normal development in early childhood. Research has also shown the critical role that caregivers play in fostering optimal development, especially in the first years of life, and their importance in promoting children's recovery from trauma.

The purpose of this chapter is twofold. The first is to highlight the ways in which research in developmental and clinical psychology, developmental psychopathology, and infant mental health can inform and improve clinical assessment and treatment with young traumatized children and their families. More specifically, guidelines are provided for conducting assessments and therapeutic interventions with traumatized children and their families that are informed by our current knowledge of normal child development, trauma, and developmental psychopathology. The second goal of this chapter is to consider issues regarding young children and trauma that the research literature has yet to address and to suggest objectives for future study.

ASSESSMENT

Research findings have demonstrated that children who have been traumatized may experience difficulties in multiple domains of development (see Part II of this volume, for a more complete review). Studies indicate that young traumatized children can experience serious emotional and behavioral symptoms, delays or regressions in the acquirement of developmental skills, and difficulties in cognitive and socioemotional functioning (Cicchetti & Lynch, 1995; Egeland & Sroufe, 1981; Farver, Natera, & Frosch, 1999; Huth-Bocks, Levendosky, & Semel, 2001; Main & George, 1985; Maughan & Cicchetti, 2002; Scheeringa, Zeanah, Drell, & Larrieu, 1995; Schneider-Rosen & Cicchetti, 1991). Data further show that numerous factors may moderate children's responses to and recovery from trauma (Kaufman & Henrich, 2000; Osofsky & Fenichel, 1994; Pynoos, Steinberg, & Wraith, 1995; Scheeringa & Gaensbauer, 2000; Scheeringa & Zeanah, 1995). These factors include (1) child-related variables, such as the child's age/developmental level, previous level of functioning, history of caregiving support, preexisting psychopathology, and past trauma history; (2) trauma-related variables, such as the type of trauma, level and duration of trauma exposure, exposure to traumatic reminders, and number and extent of secondary adversities and stressors; (3) caregiver-related variables, including caregivers' past and current psychopathology, trauma history, and representation of their own childhood; (4) caregiver–child relationship variables, including the quality of the dyadic relationship and the caregiver's representation of the child; and (5) contextual variables, such as the quality of the parents' marital relationship, the family's socioeconomic status (SES) and current life stress, and the level of support available within the family and to the family from the community.

These research findings point to the complexity involved in understanding a traumatized child's needs and the importance of a comprehensive assessment battery for evaluating the child's and family's functioning.

Below is a description of the important domains to assess and examples of measures that can be used to tap each of the domains described. This is not meant to be an exhaustive review of all the measures available in the relevant areas. Rather, the purpose of this section is to highlight the areas that research suggests clinicians should consider in their work with traumatized young children and to suggest possible measures that could be used in each of these areas. Many of these instruments were developed by researchers in developmental and clinical psychology and have a strong database supporting their reliability, validity, and clinical utility as well as a long history in the research literature.

Child Measures

A comprehensive psychological assessment of young children should include measures of their current developmental functioning, emotional and behavioral symptomatology, trauma history, and other relevant medical, social, and family history.

Current Developmental Functioning

Numerous measures are available to assess young children's developmental functioning. Developmental measures can generally be grouped into two categories, screeners and comprehensive assessments. Screeners require less time than comprehensive assessments to administer but offer less detailed information about the child's functioning.

The *Ages and Stages Questionnaires* (ASQ; Squires, Potter, & Bricker, 1999) is an example of a developmental screening system that can be used to identify children who may be developmentally delayed and in need of more in-depth assessment. The ASQ is composed of 19 questionnaires at multiple intervals from 4 to 60 months of age. The caregiver is asked to complete the questionnaire closest to the child's age. Each questionnaire contains 30 developmental items divided into five areas: communication, gross motor, fine motor, problem solving, and personal–social. Cutoff scores are used to determine if the child is at risk for delay and should receive further assessment. Research indicates that the questionnaires have high reliability and validity, distinguishing between children with and without developmental delays (Squires et al., 1999).

Several comprehensive assessment measures exist for testing young children. One of the most widely used measures of infant and toddler development in clinical and research settings is the *Bayley Scales of Infant Development–II* (BSID-II; Bayley, 1993). The BSID-II can be administered to children 1–42 months of age. The Mental Development Index reflects children's language and problem solving skills, and the Psychomotor Development Index indicates children's fine and gross motor skills. There is also an Infant Behavior Record that evaluators can use to rate children's attentional abilities, social engagement, affect regulation, and motor control during the test administration. The BSID-II has been heavily researched and widely validated (Gilliam & Mayes, 2000).

The *Wechsler Preschool and Primary Scale of Intelligence–R* (WPPSI-R; Wechsler, 1989) can be used for relatively older children (3 years, 0 months to 7 years, 3 months). The WPPSI-R assesses children's verbal and nonverbal cognitive skills and has shown excellent reliability and adequate validity (Sattler, 1992). An updated version, the WPPSI-III, recently became available, extending the age range down to 2 years, 6 months (Wechsler, 2002). The WPPSI-III has demonstrated initial validity and is continuing to undergo validity studies (Wechsler, 2002).

Symptomatology

Researchers and clinicians have recently begun to acknowledge that young children can experience significant psychiatric symptoms, though symptoms may be manifested differently among infants and toddlers than among older children and adults. In recognition of these differences in psychiatric symptomatology between younger and older children, Zero to Three's Task Force on Diagnostic Classification in Infancy developed the *Diagnostic Classification of Mental Health and Developmental Disorders of Infancy and Early Childhood* (DC: 0–3; Zero to Three/National Center for Clinical Infant Programs, 1994) to complement the fourth edition of the *Diagnostic and Statistical Manual of Mental Disorders* (DSM-IV; American Psychiatric Association, 1994) by extending downward to younger ages and focusing on problems not adequately addressed in DSM-IV. Of note is the addition of an axis for relationship disturbances in DC: 0–3 because the caregiver–child relationship plays such a critical role in young children's mental health. Clinicians working with young children should be familiar with DC: 0–3 as well as DSM-IV. Several measures are available that assess emotional and behavioral symptoms in young children that can assist clinicians in assessment and treatment planning.

The *Child Behavior Checklist for Ages 1½ to 5* (CBCL 1½ to 5; Achenbach & Rescorla, 2000) is a 100-item measure of young children's behavioral and emotional functioning completed by caregivers and others who see the child in a home setting. It provides standardized ratings and descriptive information of children's behavioral and emotional problems grouped into Internalizing and Externalizing scales. The Internalizing scales include Emotionally Reactive, Anxious/Depressed, Somatic Complaints, and Withdrawn scales. The Externalizing scales include Attention Problems and Aggressive Behavior. There is also a Sleep Problems scale. In addition, the CBCL 1½ to 5 includes five DSM-oriented scales that are linked to DSM-IV diagnoses: Affective Problems, Anxiety Problems, Pervasive Devel-

opmental Problems, Attention Deficit/Hyperactivity Problems, and Oppositional Defiant Problems. There is an optional two-page language development survey for 18- to 35-month-olds. Multiple studies have demonstrated
the reliability, validity, and clinical utility of the CBCL 1½ to 5 (Achenbach
& Rescorla, 2000). The language development survey has also demonstrated acceptable reliability and validity (Achenbach & Rescorla, 2000).

The *Infant–Toddler Social and Emotional Assessment* (ITSEA; Carter
& Briggs-Gowan, 2000) is a 166-item caregiver-report measure of socioemotional problems and competencies in infants and toddlers. It provides
standardized scores on several Externalizing scales, including Activity/
Impulsivity, Aggression/Defiance, and Peer Aggression; on several Internalizing scales, including Depression/Withdrawal, General Anxiety, Separation
Distress, and Inhibition to Novelty; and on Dysregulation, including Sleep,
Negative Emotionality, Eating, and Sensory Sensitivity. The ITSEA also in-
cludes several Competency scales, including Compliance, Attention, Imitation/
play, Mastery Motivation, Empathy, and Prosocial Peer Relations. In addi-
tion, the ITSEA provides scores on a number of indices, including a
Maladaptive index, Social Relatedness index, and Atypical Behavior index.
The authors have demonstrated acceptable reliability and validity for the
ITSEA (Briggs-Gowan & Carter, 1998; Carter, Little, Briggs-Gowan, &
Kogan, 1999).

The *Trauma Symptom Checklist for Young Children* (TSCYC; Briere
et al., 2001) is a 90-item caregiver-administered measure designed to assess
trauma-related behaviors, experiences, and feelings in children, ages 3–12
years. The TSCYC yields two validity scales, Response Level and Atypical
Response, and nine clinical scales, Posttraumatic Stress-Intrusion, Posttraumatic Stress-Avoidance, Posttraumatic Stress-Arousal, Posttraumatic Stress-
Total, Sexual Concerns, Anxiety, Depression, Dissociation, and Anger/
Aggression. The TSCYC has been shown to be reliable and valid and to be
associated with exposure to childhood sexual abuse, physical abuse, and
witnessing domestic violence (Briere et al., 2001).

Trauma History

Research has demonstrated that a child's response to trauma may be mod-
erated by trauma-related variables, including the type of trauma, the age at
which the child was exposed, the child's history of previous trauma exposure and loss, and exposure to traumatic reminders (Kaufman & Henrich,
2000; Osofsky, 1995, 1997; Pynoos et al., 1995; Scheeringa & Zeanah,
1995). Therefore, clinicians should gather detailed information about the
child's recent and past trauma exposure.

The *Traumatic Events Screening Instrument—Parent Report Form—
Revised* (TESI-PRF-R; Ghosh Ippen et al., 2002) is 24-item measure designed to screen for trauma history and the presence of traumatic responses

in young children. The TESI-PRF-R assesses a wide range of potentially traumatic events, including accidents, abuse, witnessing community/domestic violence, natural disasters, and traumatic loss. The parent report form asks the caregiver whether or not the child has experienced specific traumatic events and, if so, when the child experienced the event(s) and if the child was negatively impacted by the experience(s). The TESI-PRF-R is a revised form of the Traumatic Events Screening Instrument (TESI), a reliable and valid measure designed to assess trauma history in older children (Carlson, 1997; Ribbe, 1996). The TESI-PRF-R was revised to be developmentally sensitive to the types of trauma that young children may experience. After administering the TESI-PRF-R, clinicians should interview the caregiver for more detailed information about the traumatic events that the child experienced (e.g., specific circumstances surrounding the event, exposure to traumatic reminders since the event).

Other Relevant History and Demographic Information

As part of a comprehensive assessment, clinicians should gather information on the child's developmental, medical, social, and family history, as these factors may impact the child's current functioning and determine appropriate treatment interventions. Important areas to explore are the following:

- Child's prenatal and delivery history
- Developmental history, including achievement of developmental milestones
- Developmental disabilities
- Past and current interventions (e.g., occupational therapy, special education, early intervention, Head Start)
- Medical history, including any serious past and current illnesses, past and current medications, and history of head injury
- Psychiatric history, including previous assessments and psychotherapeutic and pharmacological interventions that were or were not successful
- Child-care and school history
- Past and current living arrangements, including moves
- Safety of the home, including exposure to domestic and/or community violence
- Exposure to traumatic reminders, including contact with the perpetrator in cases in which there was a perpetrator
- Past and current involvement with child protection agencies
- Strengths, including individual strengths (e.g., intelligence, social skills, strong peer relationships), familial strengths (e.g., family support, consistent and sensitive caregivers), and community strengths (e.g., good school, caring teachers/child-care providers, safe neighborhood, involvement in religious/spiritual community).

Caregiver Measures

There is very strong evidence in the research literature that caregiver history and functioning significantly impacts young children's mental health (Appleyard & Osofsky, 2003; Osofsky & Fenichel, 1994, 2000). Therefore, it is imperative that clinicians working with young children obtain a thorough assessment of caregivers' history and past and present functioning. More specifically, clinicians should assess caregiver psychopathology/ symptomatology, trauma history, life stressors, and other relevant history. Clinicians should offer to include all of the child's relevant caregivers in the assessment and treatment process unless contraindicated by therapeutic concerns (e.g., a perpetrator who continues to represent a threat).

Psychopathology/Symptomatology

When a child presents for treatment due to trauma exposure, the clinician should consider assessing the caregiver(s) for past and present psychopathology. First, the caregiver may be suffering symptoms from exposure to the same trauma that has affected the child. Second, the caregiver may be experiencing psychiatric symptoms that are unrelated to the trauma but that impact the caregiver's parenting abilities and the caregiver–child relationship.

Clinicians interested in detailed past and present diagnostic information may consider administering a structured interview, such as the *Structured Clinical Interview for DSM-IV* (SCID; First, Spitzer, Gibbon, & Williams, 1996, 1997). The advantage of interviews like the SCID is that they provide very detailed information about past and present Axis I and Axis II diagnoses. However, these instruments are very time consuming to administer and usually require trained interviewers.

An alternative to conducting a lengthy structured interview is to administer paper-and-pencil self-report measures that assess symptoms likely to be prevalent in a trauma population and to impact the child negatively. Research has shown that maternal depression, anxiety, dissociative symptoms, and posttraumatic symptoms are associated with negative parenting behaviors and poor outcome among young children (Goodman & Gotlib, 1999; Lyons-Ruth & Block, 1996; Manassis, Bradley, Goldberg, Hood, & Swinson, 1995; Scheeringa & Gaensbauer, 2000).

The *Beck Depression Inventory–II* (BDI-II; Beck, 1987) is a 21-item self-report instrument measuring the presence and severity of DSM-IV depressive symptoms in individuals aged 13 years and older. Research has shown the BDI-II to be a reliable measure with high internal consistency and convergent and criterion validity and has demonstrated that it discriminates between depressed and nondepressed individuals (Beck, 1987; Beck, Steer, & Garbin, 1988).

The *Beck Anxiety Inventory* (BAI; Beck, 1990) is a 21-item self-report instrument measuring the presence and severity of anxious symptoms in adults and adolescents aged 17 years and older. Research has shown the BAI to be reliable and to have high convergent and discriminant validity, discriminating between anxious and nonanxious diagnostic groups (Beck, 1990; Osman, Kopper, Barrios, Osman, & Wade, 1997; Steer, Ranieri, Beck, & Clark, 1993).

The *Davidson Trauma Scale* (DTS; Davidson, 1996) is a self-report measure designed to assess posttraumatic stress disorder (PTSD) and aid in the treatment of adults. The scale consists of 17 symptoms, answered on two 5-point scales (frequency and severity). The items closely mirror the diagnostic criteria of PTSD contained in DSM-IV. The respondent is asked to identify the trauma that is most disturbing to him or her and then indicate how often and how severely he or she has experienced each of the 17 symptoms during the past week. One summary score (sum of the frequency and severity ratings) and three cluster scores are derived: intrusion, avoidance/ numbing, and hyperarousal. Research indicates that the measure is internally consistent, reliable, and valid and that it distinguishes between groups with and without PTSD diagnoses (Davidson, 1996; Davidson et al., 1997; Davidson, Tharwani, & Connor, 2002).

Stress and Trauma History

The Life Stressor Checklist—Revised (LSC-R; Wolfe & Levin, 1991) is a 31-item self-report measure for adults that assesses lifetime exposure to trauma and the incidence and impact of stressful life events on current functioning. The respondent is asked to indicate whether he or she has experienced the described stressful life events and to indicate the impact that the event has had on him or her, both at the time of the event and in the past year. The LSC-R includes a number of items that are particularly relevant to traumatized populations and that do not appear on other popular stressor measures (e.g., "Have you every been emotionally abused or neglected?"; "When you were young did you ever see violence between family members?"; "Were you ever put in foster care or put up for adoption?"). Initial data support the validity of the LSC-R (Kimerling et al., 1999; Wolfe & Kimerling, 1997).

State of Mind with Regard to Attachment

An adult's state of mind with regard to attachment—that is, the subjective meaning the individual makes about his or her childhood experiences and the relationship with his or her parents—has been found to have a significant influence on parenting behavior and child outcome (Crowell & Feldman, 1988; Eiden, Teti, & Corns, 1995). The *Adult Attachment Interview* (AAI; George, Kaplan, & Main, 1984; Main & Goldwyn, 1984) is a semistructured interview designed to assess adult states of mind expressed in individuals' discussions about their childhood attachment experiences and reflections on how these experiences influence their personality and parenting. Questions were designed to elicit general descriptions of subjects' attachment relationships, specific memories to support their descriptions, and descriptions of upsetting or traumatic experiences, and to assess subjects' understanding of how their early experiences affect their current personality and parenting. The scoring system assesses the subjects' coherency in discussing their attachment experiences and assigns a measure of their current state of mind with respect to attachment issues. Though the AAI was developed as a research instrument, the interview can be used to obtain valuable information about the caregiver's current state of mind regarding his or her own childhood and trauma and loss history. Research indicates that caregivers' AAI categorizations are associated with their parenting behaviors, their children's attachment status, and their children's behavior. Compared to adults who are classified as autonomous/secure, adults who are classified as insecure on the AAI are more likely to be negative and insensitive with their children and to have children who demonstrate more emotional and behavioral difficulties and who are categorized as insecure in the Strange Situation (Cohn, Cowan, Cowan, & Pearson, 1992; Crowell & Feldman, 1988; Crowell, O'Connor, Wollmers, Sprafkin, & Rao, 1991; Eiden et al., 1995; Pearson, Cohn, Cowan, & Cowan, 1994; van IJzendoorn, 1992, 1995; Ward & Carlson, 1995).

Other Relevant History and Demographic Information

Clinicians should gather information on caregiver's history that may be relevant to the caregiver–child relationship and the caregiver's ability to parent the child sensitively. Relevant information includes the caregiver's medical history, including any serious past and current illnesses, and past and current medications; psychiatric history, including past and current diagnoses, and past and current psychotherapeutic and pharmacological treatment; past and current substance use; and relationship history, including involvement in domestic violence, separations and divorces, and current romantic relationship status/marital quality. Clinicians should also inquire about the caregiver's other children (e.g., psychiatric history), the family's past and present involvement with child protection agencies, and familial history of psychiatric illness. Clinicians should ascertain the family's current level of social support and access to community resources.

Child–Caregiver Relationship Measures

Given the significance of the caregiver–child relationship to the young child's functioning, a proper psychological assessment of a young child must include an examination of the quality of that dyadic relationship. Researchers have developed several measures to examine the quality of the relationship from several perspectives. Many of these measures can be adapted for clinical purposes. Crowell and Fleischmann (1993) noted that, though there are no structured observational assessments used to diagnose young children, semistructured assessment procedures of young children and their caregivers may be useful in characterizing patterns of behaviors and planning appropriate interventions.

The *Clinical problem-solving procedure/Crowell procedure* (Crowell & Feldman, 1988) is an adaptation of a research procedure developed by Matas, Arend, and Sroufe (1978). The Crowell procedure was originally created for children 24–54 months of age. Zeanah and colleagues (1997) made minor modifications to the procedure to extend it down to children 12 months of age. The 45-minute procedure consists of nine episodes designed to elicit various caregiver and child behaviors. More specifically, the procedure includes a 10-minute free-play session, a cleanup session, a session when the caregiver and child blow bubbles, a series of four teaching tasks of increasing difficulty, and a brief separation and reunion. Numerous caregiver and child behaviors can be assessed from the procedure. For example, Zeanah and colleagues (Zeanah et al., 1997; Zeanah, Larrieu, Heller, & Valliere, 2000) observed that the Crowell procedure taps the caregiver domains of emotional availability, nurturance/valuing/empathic responsiveness, comforting/response to distress, teaching, play, and discipline/limit setting, and the child domains of emotion regulation, security/trust/self-esteem, comfort seeking, learning/curiosity/mastery, play/imagination, and self-control/cooperation. Zeanah et al. (2000) noted that, though the formal Crowell procedure was not designed to be administered to children younger than 12 months of age, components of the procedure may be relevant. For example, the free-play and appropriate teaching tasks may be observed. Though there is a scoring system for the procedure that requires training, the procedure was designed to be useful in clinical settings (Crowell & Fleischmann, 1993). Clinicians knowledgeable about young children can make direct observations of the dyadic interactions and of caregiver and child behaviors that they find clinically useful (Crowell & Fleischmann, 1993). Also clinicians may develop their own scales that assess behaviors of interest to track changes over the course of therapy. For example, Osofsky, Bosquet, Kronenberg, and Costa (2003) recently modified scales developed by Heller et al. (1998) to evaluate the effects of a relationship-based intervention on parent and child behaviors.

A procedure that can be administered to infants younger than 9 months of age is the *"still-face"* (or *"face-to-face"*) *procedure* (Tronick, Als, Adamson, Wise, & Brazelton, 1978; Tronick, Cohn, & Shea, 1985). For the still-face procedure, the infant is seated in an infant seat across from his or her caregiver. The procedure consists of three segments: free play at the beginning and end of the session, and the still-face segment in the middle, during which the caregiver is instructed to maintain a neutral face and not to talk to or react to the infant. Microcoding techniques have been used to code the still-face procedure in research settings (Crowell & Fleischmann, 1993). However, the clinician can observe the interactions for relevant caregiver and child behaviors, including turn-taking behavior, eye contact versus gaze avoidance, caregiver responsiveness, and the dyad's ability to return to mutually enjoyable interactions after the still-face disruption (Crowell & Fleischmann, 1993).

Though assessing the quality of the attachment relationship would be of obvious importance, the standard attachment measures are not specific or sensitive enough to be used in clinical settings (Zeanah & Boris, 2000). The original attachment procedure, the Strange Situation (Ainsworth, Blehar, Waters, & Wall, 1978), was designed for research purposes to identify correlates of different attachment patterns. The Strange Situation should not be used as a clinical procedure to identify specific children's attachment patterns. Also, coding the Strange Situation requires considerable time and training that makes it impractical as a clinical tool. The Attachment Q-sort (Waters & Deane, 1985) is a procedure for assessing attachment behaviors in infants, toddlers, and preschoolers. The Attachment Q-sort can be administered by the caregiver or a trained observer. However, it is a time-intensive procedure and has not been well validated in clinical populations (Zeanah & Boris, 2000).

The *MacArthur Story Stem Battery* (Bretherton, Ridgeway, & Cassidy, 1990) has been used to assess preschoolers' internal representations of attachment. The task involves the examiner narrating and acting out the beginning of six stories, then the child is asked to show how the story ends. The story stems include themes relevant for preschoolers that are meant to elicit attachment representations (e.g., separation from and reunion with caregiver, fear, hurt). Research has shown that children's responses to the story stem task relate to other measures of attachment security (Bretherton et al., 1990). Unlike the Strange Situation, the story stem task can be used in clinical settings (Lieberman, Van Horn, Grandison, & Pekarsky, 1997).

Recognizing the lack of applicability of the standard attachment research procedures to the clinical setting, Zeanah and colleagues developed a caregiver attachment interview that could be used in both research and clinical work (Zeanah & Benoit, 1995; Zeanah, Benoit, Hirshberg, Barton, & Regan, 1994). Zeanah et al. (1994) created the Working Model of the Child Interview (WMCI) to elicit caregivers' internal representations of their young children. The WMCI asks caregivers questions about their past and current impressions of their child's personality and behaviors, and their anticipations about their child's future development (Zeanah et al., 1994). Numerous aspects of the caregiver's response can be coded including (1) narrative features such as richness of perceptions, openness to change, coherence, intensity of involvement, acceptance of the child, caregiving sensitivity, infant's degree of difficulty, and fear of loss; (2) affective tones; and (3) narrative organization or classification (balanced, disengaged, or distorted). Research has shown that ratings on the WMCI are associated with infant attachment classification and clinic status (Benoit, Zeanah, Parker, Nicholson, & Coolbear, 1997; Zeanah et al., 1994). Crowell and Fleischmann (1993) noted that the WMCI "clinically . . . provides a fascinating look into how a parent thinks about his or her child and the relationship with the child; it has the potential to provide an excellent foundation for intensive therapy with the parent and infant" (p. 218). Zeanah and Benoit (1995) cautioned that the WMCI should only be considered one component of an assessment and should be administered in conjunction with behavioral observations (e.g., the Crowell procedure).

Summary

Research has demonstrated that young children can experience numerous difficulties following a traumatic event and that several factors influence children's reaction to and recovery from trauma. Clinical assessment procedures should be guided by our current research knowledge. More specifically, study findings suggest that a comprehensive assessment of a young traumatized child should include measures of the following: the child's current developmental functioning, child symptomatology, child trauma history, caregiver symptomatology, caregiver trauma history, caregiver life stress, and quality of the child–caregiver relationship. Researchers have developed various reliable and valid measures that can be used in clinical settings to assess these domains.

TREATMENT INTERVENTIONS

Though there are numerous published case descriptions of successful therapeutic interventions with traumatized infants and toddlers (e.g., Drell, Gaensbauer, Siegel, & Sugar, 1995; Gaensbauer & Siegel, 1995; Osofsky, Cohen, & Drell, 1995; Osofsky & Fenichel, 1996), there is little systematic research examining the effectiveness of clinical interventions with young traumatized children. However, clinicians and researchers in the field, based on our current knowledge of infant mental health and trauma in early childhood, have suggested a number of treatment principles that should be considered when treatment interventions are designed for families affected by trauma.

Based on their examination of published clinical reports of treatment of PTSD in infants and toddlers, Scheeringa and Gaensbauer (2000) identified six essential goals for therapeutic work with traumatized children: (1) establish a sense of safety, both within the child's life and within the therapeutic setting; (2) reduce the intensity of the overwhelming affect associated with the traumatic experience; (3) help the child to develop a coherent narrative about the traumatic event from the memories, which are often fragmented; (4) help the child to integrate the traumatic events psychologically and to gain a sense of mastery over them; (5) address the numerous "ripple" effects from the traumatic experience (e.g., behavioral problems, developmental disturbances); and (6) provide support and guidance to the child's family so that they can help the child and cope with their own reactions to the trauma.

Kaufman and Henrich (2000) recommended targets for intervention with traumatized children that were based on their review of the literature on the effects of trauma exposure and mediating factors impacting children's outcomes. Recommended targets included (1) clinical symptomatology; (2) developmental deficits; (3) caregiver problems, including partner violence, substance abuse, and psychiatric disturbances; (4) social factors, including provision of concrete resources; and (5) trauma-specific interventions. They noted that trauma-specific interventions may include restructuring of cognitive appraisal of the trauma, survey and restriction of exposure to trauma-related triggers, interventions for secondary adversities, support through court proceedings, grief work for losses associated with the trauma, and facilitation of permanency planning efforts (Kaufman & Henrich, 2000). The authors also pointed out that, because there is significant variation in the clinical, developmental, family, and social characteristics of trauma victims, it is unlikely that one treatment approach will be effective with all clients.

Recognizing the importance of the caregiver on young children's functioning, many clinicians and researchers have examined the effectiveness of dyadic/relationship-based interventions with infants, toddlers, and preschoolers. For example, numerous programs have had some success in producing positive outcomes among young children and mothers by promoting the development of secure attachment relationships (for a review, see Egeland, Weinfield, Bosquet, & Cheng, 2000). The interaction guidance treatment approach has also demonstrated some success (McDonough, 2000). However, these interventions have generally not been conducted with traumatized populations.

Lieberman and colleagues (1997) have applied the infant–parent psychotherapy model to the treatment of preschoolers (36–75 months) who have witnessed domestic violence and their mothers. The theoretical basis for this child–parent psychotherapy is an integration of psychoanalytic/ attachment theory and social-learning paradigms, particularly those involving social coercion (Lieberman & Van Horn, 2003; Zuckerman & Lieberman, 2002). The treatment is an adaptation of the classic infant–parent psychotherapy model, driven by the child's play (Lieberman et al., 1997; Lieberman & Van Horn, 2003). The goals of the therapy are (1) to enable the mother to appreciate and enter the child's inner world; (2) to help the mother and child jointly construct a narrative of their experiences; and (3) to give the mother and child a safe space in which to reenact their conflicts and to resolve them in more adaptive ways. Target areas for change include punitive parenting practices and unmodulated and dysregulated caregiver and child behaviors, including externalizing and internalizing problems (Zuckerman & Lieberman, 2002). The intervention supports and reinforces caregiver and child perceptions, attitudes, and behaviors that indicate positive affect, age-appropriate assertion or discipline, reciprocal play, joint exploration of the world, and constructive conflict resolution. Child–parent psychotherapy uses six intervention modalities: (1) use of play, physical contact, and language to promote healthy exploration, contain overwhelming affect, clarify feelings, and correct misperceptions; (2) unstructured developmental guidance; (3) modeling of appropriate protective behaviors; (4) interpretation, particularly to link the caregiver's affective responses with current parenting practices; (5) emotional support and empathic communication; and (6) concrete assistance with problems of living (Lieberman & Van Horn, 2003; Zuckerman & Lieberman, 2002). Preliminary analyses suggest that child–parent psychotherapy may be an effective method for treating traumatized children. In Lieberman and colleagues' sample, they found improvement in the quality of child–mother interactions and in child cognitive performance and decreases in child internalizing, externalizing, and total behavior problems and maternal PTSD symptoms (Lieberman, Silverman, & Pawl, 2000; Zuckerman & Lieberman, 2002).

IMMEDIATE VERSUS DELAYED RESPONSE TO YOUNG CHILDREN WHO HAVE BEEN TRAUMATIZED: WHY EARLY INTERVENTION IS CRITICAL

Research findings from several areas of psychology suggest the importance of devising effective early intervention techniques for children who have been traumatized. Developmental psychopathology research suggests that individuals must negotiate stage-salient tasks to achieve developmental competence (Cicchetti & Cohen, 1995; Masten & Braswell, 1991; Waters & Sroufe, 1983). Researchers further posit that earlier developmental structures are incorporated into later developmental structures, so that early competence tends to foster later competence, and early incompetence tends to promote later incompetence (Cicchetti & Cohen, 1995; Waters & Sroufe, 1983). Though change in functioning is possible at each transitional point in development, the longer an individual is on a maladaptive pathway, the more difficult it will be to move onto a normal developmental pathway (Cicchetti & Cohen, 1995; Sroufe, 1990; Sroufe, Egeland, & Kreutzer, 1990). Therefore, traumatized children who do not receive early intervention will be at risk for greater and greater difficulties throughout childhood and adolescence, and these difficulties will become increasingly difficult to treat successfully as maladaptive behaviors and coping responses become more and more entrenched.

Evidence from the neurobiology literature indicates that trauma produces psychobiological changes that can negatively impact the development of the brain and biological stress regulatory systems (DeBellis et al., 1999; Kaufman & Henrich, 2000). Very young children may be particularly vulnerable to the toxic psychobiological effects of trauma, perhaps because of the rapid rate of neurological development and experience-related changes in neural circuitry that occur in the first 3 years of life (DeBellis et al., 1999; Galvin, Stilwell, Shekhar, Kopta, & Goldfarb, 1997; Gunnar, 1998; Kaufman & Henrich, 2000; Nelson & Bosquet, 2000). Furthermore, these changes may become more severe the longer the child experiences chronic stress and adversity and the longer the trauma symptoms persist without treatment (DeBellis et al., 1999; Kaufman, 1991; Kaufman et al., 1997; Osofsky & Dickson, 2000; Perry, Pollard, Blakley, Baker, & Vigilante, 1995).

In summary, research indicates that young children who experience trauma should receive immediate intervention; delays in treatment may result in more severe biological and psychological changes that are resistant to later intervention.

FUTURE RESEARCH DIRECTIONS: WHAT DO WE STILL NEED TO KNOW? WHERE SHOULD WE GO FROM HERE?

Though there is increasing recognition of the specialized needs of young children who have experienced trauma, much more research is needed. Studies have only begun to elucidate the types of difficulties facing young traumatized children and their families and the ways in which clinicians can be most effective in working with them. Numerous issues and questions remain.

The introduction of the *Diagnostic Classification of Mental Health and Developmental Disorders of Infancy and Early Childhood* (DC: 0–3; Zero to Three/National Center for Clinical Infant Programs, 1994) marked significant progress in infant mental health, as researchers and clinicians recognized the specialized psychological characteristics of very young children. However, many of the diagnoses in DC: 0–3 have yet to be validated. Research should examine the validity of the DC: 0–3 diagnoses. Validating the traumatic stress disorder diagnosis has particular significance for clinical work with young traumatized children.

More research needs to be conducted on the specific symptoms and diagnoses that occur among traumatized young children. Much of our current knowledge about young traumatized children's symptom pictures comes from clinical reports. Systematic research is needed to determine the types of difficulties that traumatized children most commonly experience and the ways in which the symptom picture may change over the course of development. This knowledge may better equip clinicians to recognize signs of trauma in young children and to design appropriate treatment interventions.

Understanding the factors moderating children's response to trauma is also critical for designing effective assessment batteries and treatment interventions. Studies should attempt to answer the following questions: Which characteristics (of the child, of the trauma, of the family, of the environment, etc.) place children at risk for developing severe and/or long-term difficulties? Are there child characteristics and/or environmental factors that protect children from developing significant symptoms following a traumatic event? Are there child, family, or other environmental factors that help a traumatized child to recover more quickly and completely? More fully understanding the moderating effects of individual and environmental factors on children's responses to trauma can inform clinical work in multiple ways. It can help clinicians to determine the most important variables to measure when conducting assessments and to design more effective treatment interventions. Clinicians may choose to target their outreach to populations that research indicates are most at risk for poor outcomes. Also, knowledge of risk and protective factors can be used to design preventive interventions, particularly in high-risk communities/groups.

Research may also play a critical role in demonstrating the need for early intervention for young traumatized children to prevent long-term difficulties that impact not only the child but also his or her family, community, and the larger society. There has been growing recognition of the importance of the first 3 years of life for long-term development, supported by research findings that early experiences and the quality of the early environment have a significant impact on brain development and functioning. Such research findings have led to an increased recognition of the value of early prevention and intervention. However, there still exists in our society a reluctance to recognize that infants, toddlers, and preschoolers can be seriously affected by exposure to violence and other forms of trauma. For many people, accepting that our youngest, most vulnerable children can experience such anguish is too painful to conceive. Many believe that infants and toddlers are too young to remember traumatic experiences and they will "get over it" or "grow out of it" with time. Research can play a critical role in demonstrating the short- and long-term effects of trauma on children's biological, cognitive, and socioemotional functioning and in showing the effectiveness of early intervention services in preventing later problems. Research may demonstrate that early intervention is not only more effective therapeutically than later intervention but also more cost effective, not to mention more humane. Consequently, more mental health dollars may be channeled toward clinical services for young children. This may include more resources for direct clinical services as well as for training programs to educate more professionals in the specialized field of infant mental health.

Though there is recognition of the need for immediate intervention, very limited research is currently available on effective treatment interventions with young traumatized children. Studies are beginning to emerge on the efficacy of different interventions with older children and adolescents who have experienced trauma. However, many of the treatments have used cognitive-behavioral techniques (Cohen, 1998), which are often inappropriate for very young children due to their limited cognitive abilities. Also, though pharmacological interventions may be successful in treating traumatized adults, adolescents, and older children, infant mental health experts are often reluctant to prescribe drugs to very young children because of the unknown effects of the drugs on the rapidly developing brain.

New treatment designs should be guided by principles learned from developmental psychology, developmental psychopathology, and effective infant mental health interventions in nontrauma populations (e.g., attachment-based interventions, infant–parent psychotherapy, interaction guidance) as well as by knowledge about the impact of trauma on child development and the child–caregiver relationship. Researchers could compare different treatment approaches/modalities to see which work best. Important questions to consider are the following: What are the necessary components of an effective treatment approach with young traumatized children? Which issues/factors must be addressed for a positive treatment outcome? Do children/families with different characteristics respond differently to different types of interventions? Which interventions work best with which children/families? What effect does including caregivers in the treatment have on the child's mental health and on the caregivers' mental health? Can children with various levels of trauma exposure and different levels of symptom severity all return to a level of "normal" functioning? Which baseline measures show change over time, and which changes are associated with improvement in the child's and the caregiver's symptoms and functioning? This information might be used to guide subsequent interventions. For example, if a reduction in caregiver psychiatric symptoms is strongly related to child recovery, then future treatments should include as a treatment goal reducing caregiver symptoms.

Finally research may reveal the obstacles that prevent traumatized children from receiving the services they need. Clinicians should then attempt to eliminate these barriers to make services more accessible to and effective with families. Removing treatment barriers may be particularly important for families with multiple stressors and risk factors, who may be in the most need of treatment and the least able to access it.

Awareness of the need for improved clinical services for traumatized children has been growing. Recently, the Substance Abuse and Mental Health Services Administration (SAMHSA) of the U.S. Department of Health and Human Services funded the National Child Trauma Stress Initiative (NCTSI) to improve treatment and services for all children and adolescents in the United States who have experienced traumatic events. Through this initiative, the National Child Traumatic Stress Network (NCTSN) was established. The NCTSN is a nationwide collaborative network of organizations involved in the evaluation, treatment, and support of children and their families impacted by traumatic stress. The NCTSN's mission is to develop and implement the first national initiative to improve access to services and raise the standard of care for traumatized children, adolescents, and their families.

In recognition of the importance of early intervention and the need for more research on clinical assessment and treatment for very young traumatized children, the Early Trauma Treatment Network (ETTN) was established within NCTSN. The ETTN is a four-site clinical research collaborative that includes the University of California at San Francisco Child Trauma Research Project, the Child Witness to Violence Project at Boston Medical Center, the Early Trauma Treatment Program at Louisiana State University Health Sciences Center in New Orleans, and the Infant Team at Tulane University Medical Center in New Orleans. The ETTN is working to contribute to the expansion and systematization of the treatment of trauma in children from birth to age 6, to add to the basis of scientific knowledge on assessment and treatment, and to disseminate knowledge about trauma and young children to others across the country. In order to accomplish these goals, the ETTN sites are providing child–parent psychotherapy to an ethnically and culturally diverse group of children, ages birth to 6 years, who have been traumatized by interpersonal violence and/or loss. The ETTN sites have developed an assessment battery to administer to young traumatized children and their caregivers to inform clinicians and researchers about the characteristics and needs of such children, to monitor the effectiveness of the intervention, and to determine the characteristics that influence the effectiveness of the intervention so that improved services can be developed. The assessment battery described in this chapter emerged out of the work of the ETTN. By participating in this collaboration, the ETTN members endeavor to add to our knowledge about trauma and young children and expand and improve the services available to traumatized children in their communities and across the United States.

In conclusion, research has provided important directions for clinicians working with young traumatized children and their families. More specifically, study findings point to relevant domains for assessment and suggest treatment goals and modalities for intervention. However, much more research is needed to improve clinical services available to traumatized infants, toddlers, preschoolers, and their families. Fortunately, there is a growing recognition of the need for improved services for traumatized children. We hope this recognition will continue to increase and research efforts will continue to be funded so that clinicians will have the most effective tools possible to serve their clients.

REFERENCES

Achenbach, T. M., & Rescorla, L. A. (2000). *Manual for the ASEBA Preschool Forms and Profiles*. Burlington: University of Vermont, Department of Psychiatry.

Ainsworth, M. D. S., Blehar, M., Waters, E., & Wall, S. (1978). *Patterns of attachment*, Hillsdale, NJ: Erlbaum.

American Psychiatric Association. (1994). *Diagnostic and statistical manual of mental disorders* (4th ed.). Washington, DC: Author.

Appleyard, K., & Osofsky, J. D. (2003). Parenting after trauma: Supporting parents and caregivers in the treatment of children impacted by violence. *Infant Mental Health Journal, 24,* 111–125.

Bayley, N. (1993). *Bayley Scales of Infant Development* (2nd ed.). San Antonio, TX: Psychological Corporation.

Beck, A. T. (1987). *Beck Depression Inventory* (2nd ed.). San Antonio, TX: Psychological Corporation.

Beck, A. T. (1990). *Beck Anxiety Inventory* (2nd ed.). San Antonio, TX: Psychological Corporation.

Beck, A. T., Steer, R. A., & Garbin, M. G. (1988). Psychometric properties of the Beck Depression Inventory: Twenty-five years of evaluation. *Clinical Psychology Review, 8,* 77–100.

Benoit, D., Zeanah, C. H., Parker, K C. H., Nicholson, E., & Coolbear, J. (1997). Working Model of the Child Interview: Infant clinical status related to maternal perceptions. *Infant Mental Health Journal, 18,* 107–121.

Bretherton, I., Ridgeway, D., & Cassidy, J. (1990). Assessing internal working models of the attachment relationship: An attachment story completion task for 3–year-olds. In M. T. Greenberg, D. Cicchetti, & E. M. Cummings (Eds.), *Attachment in the preschool years: Theory, research, and intervention* (pp. 273–308). Chicago: University of Chicago Press.

Briere, J., Johnson, K., Bissada, A., Damon, L., Crouch, J., Gil, E., Hanson, R., & Ernst, V. (2001). *Child Abuse and Neglect, 25,* 1001–1014.

Briggs-Gowan, M. J., & Carter, A. S. (1998). Preliminary acceptability and psychometrics of the Infant–Toddler Social and Emotional Assessment (ITSEA): A new adult-report questionnaire. *Infant Mental Health Journal, 19,* 422–445.

Carlson, E. B. (1997). *Trauma assessments: A clinician's guide*. New York: Guilford Press.

Carter, A. S., & Briggs-Gowan, M. J. (2000). *The Infant–Toddler Social and Emotional Assessment (ITSEA)*. New Haven, CT: Yale University, Department of Psychology.

Carter, A. S., Little, C., Briggs-Gowan, M. J., & Kogan, N. (1999). The Infant–Toddler Social and Emotional Assessment (ITSEA): Comparing parent ratings to laboratory observations of task mastery, emotion regulation, coping behaviors, and attachment status. *Infant Mental Health Journal, 20,* 375–392.

Cicchetti, D., & Cohen, D. J. (1995). Perspectives on developmental psychopathology. In D. Cicchetti & D. J. Cohen (Eds.), *Developmental psychopathology: Vol. 1. Theory and methods* (pp. 3–20). New York: Wiley.

Cicchetti, D., & Lynch, M. (1995). Failures in the expectable environment and their impact on individual development: The case of child maltreatment. In D. Cicchetti & D. J. Cohen (Eds.), *Developmental psychopathology: Vol. 2. Risk, disorder, and adaptation* (pp. 32–71). New York: Wiley.

Cohen, J. A. (1998). Practice parameters for the assessment and treatment of children and adolescents with posttraumatic stress disorder. *Journal of the American Academy of Child and Adolescent Psychiatry, 37*(Suppl. 10), 4–26.

Cohn, D. A., Cowan, P. A., Cowan, C. P., & Pearson, J. (1992). Mothers' and fathers' working models of childhood attachment relationships, parenting styles, and child behavior. *Development and Psychopathology, 4,* 417–431.

Crowell, J. A., & Feldman, S. S. (1988). Mothers' internal models of relationships and children's behavioral and developmental status: A study of mother–child interaction. *Child Development, 59,* 1273–1285.

Crowell, J. A., & Fleischmann, M. A. (1993). Use of structured research procedures in clinical assessments of infants. In C. H. Zeanah (Ed.), *Handbook of infant mental health* (pp. 210–221). New York: Guilford Press.

Crowell, J. A., O'Connor, E., Wollmers, G., Sprafkin, J., & Rao, U. (1991). Mothers' conceptualizations of parent–child relationships: Relation to mother–child interaction and child behavior problems. *Development and Psychopathology, 3,* 431–444.

Davidson, J. R. T. (1996). *Davidson Trauma Scale*. Toronto, Ontario, Canada: Mental Health Systems.

Davidson, J. R. T., Book, S. W., Colket, J. T., Tupler, L. A., Roth, S., David, D., Hertzberg, M., Mellman, T., Beckham, J. C., Smith, R. D., Davison, R. M., Katz, R., & Feldman, M. E. (1997). Assessment of a new self-rating scale for posttraumatic stress disorder. *Psychological Medicine, 27,* 153–160.

Davidson, J. R. T., Tharwani, H. M., & Connor, K. M. (2002). Davidson Trauma Scale (DTS): Normative scores in the general population and effect sizes in placebo-controlled SSRI trials. *Depression and Anxiety, 15,* 75–78.

DeBellis, M. D., Keshavan, M., Clark, D., Casey, B. J., Giedd, J., Boring, A., Frustaci, K., & Ryan, N. (1999). Developmental traumatology: Part II. Brain development. *Biological Psychiatry, 45,* 1271–1284.

Drell, M. J., Gaensbauer, T. J., Siegel, C. H., & Sugar, M. (1995). Clinical round table: A case of trauma to a 21–month-old girl. *Infant Mental Health Journal, 16,* 318–333.

Egeland, B., & Sroufe, L. A. (1981). Developmental sequelae of maltreatment in infancy. *New Directions for Child Development, 11,* 77–92.

Egeland, B., Weinfield, N. S., Bosquet, M., & Cheng, V. K. (2000). Remembering, repeating, and working through: Lessons from attachment-based interventions. In

J. D. Osofsky & H. E. Fitzgerald (Eds.), *WAIMH Handbook of infant mental health: Vol. 4. Infant mental health in groups at high risk* (pp. 35–89). New York: Wiley.

Eiden, R. D., Teti, D. M., & Corns, K. M. (1995). Maternal working models of attachment, marital adjustment, and the parent–child relationship. *Child Development, 66,* 1504–1518.

Farver, J. M., Natera, L. X., & Frosch, D. L. (1999). Effects of community violence on inner-city preschoolers and their families. *Journal of Applied Developmental Psychology, 20,* 143–158.

First, M. B., Spitzer, R. L., Gibbon, M., & Williams, J. B.W. (1996). *Structured Clinical Interview for DSM-IV Axis I Disorders, Clinician Version (SCID–CV).* Washington, DC: American Psychiatric Press.

First, M. B., Spitzer, R. L., Gibbon, M., & Williams, J. B. W. (1997). *Structured Clinical Interview for DSM-IV Personality Disorders (SCID-II).* Washington, DC: American Psychiatric Press.

Gaensbauer, T. J., & Siegel, C. H. (1995).Therapeutic approaches to posttraumatic stress disorder in infant and toddlers. *Infant Mental Health Journal, 16,* 292–305.

Galvin, M. R., Stilwell, B. M., Shekhar, A., Kopta, S. M., & Goldfarb, S. M. (1997). Maltreatment, conscience functioning and dopamine beta hydroxylase in emotionally disturbed boys. *Child Abuse and Neglect, 21,* 83–92.

George, C., Kaplan, N., & Main, M. (1984). *Attachment interview for adults.* Unpublished manuscript, University of California, Berkeley.

Ghosh Ippen, C., Ford, J., Racusin, R., Acker, M., Bosquet, M., Rogers, K., Ellis, C., Schiffman, J., Ribbe, D., Cone, P., Lukovitz, M., Edwards, J., the Child Trauma Research Project of the Early Trauma Treatment Network, & the National Center for PTSD Dartmouth Child Trauma Research Group. (2002). *Traumatic Events Screening Inventory—Parent Report Revised.* San Francisco: University of California, San Francisco Early Trauma Treatment Network.

Gilliam, W. S., & Mayes, L. C. (2000). Developmental assessment of infants and toddlers. In C. H. Zeanah (Ed.), *Handbook of infant mental health* (2nd ed., pp. 236–248). New York: Guilford Press.

Goodman, S. H., & Gotlib, I. H. (1999). Risk for psychopathology in the children of depressed mothers: A developmental model for understanding mechanisms of transmission. *Psychological Review, 106,* 458–490.

Gunnar, M. R. (1998, March). *Bioprocesses in human development.* Paper presented at the Canadian Institute for Advanced Research, Vancouver, British Columbia.

Heller, S., Aoki, Y., Crowell, J., Chase-Landsdale, L., Brooks-Gunn, J., Schoffner, K., & Zamsky, E. (1998). *Parent–child interaction procedure: Coding manual.* Unpublished manuscript, Department of Psychiatry, Tulane University Health Sciences Center.

Huth-Bocks, A. C., Levendosky, A. A., & Semel, M. A. (2001). The direct and indirect effects of domestic violence on young children's intellectual functioning. *Journal of Family Violence, 16,* 269–290.

Kaufman, J. (1991). Depressive disorders in maltreated children. *Journal of the American Academy of Child and Adolescent Psychiatry, 30,* 257–265.

Kaufman, J., Birmaher, B., Perel, J., Dahl, R., Moreci, P., Nelson, B., Wells, W., &

Ryan, N. (1997). The corticotropin releasing hormone challenge in depressed abused, depressed nonabused and normal control children. *Biological Psychiatry, 44,* 973–981.

Kaufman, J., & Henrich, C. (2000). Exposure to violence and early childhood trauma. In C. H. Zeanah (Ed.), *Handbook of infant mental health* (2nd ed., pp. 195–207). New York: Guilford Press.

Kimerling, R., Calhoun, K. S., Forehand, R., Armistead, L., Morse, E., Morse, P., Clark, R., & Clark, L. (1999). Traumatic stress in HIV-infected women. *AIDS Education and Prevention,* 11, 321–330.

Lieberman, A. F., Silverman, R., & Pawl, J. H. (2000). Infant–parent psychotherapy: Core concepts and current approaches. In C. H. Zeanah (Ed.), *Handbook of infant mental health* (2nd ed., pp. 472–484). New York: Guilford Press.

Lieberman, A. F., & Van Horn, P. (2003, August). *Guide for child–parent psychotherapy for infant, toddler, and preschooler witnesses of domestic violence.* Unpublished manuscript, Child Trauma Research Project, University of California, San Francisco.

Lieberman, A. F., Van Horn, P., Grandison, C. M., & Pekarsky, J. H. (1997). Mental health assessment of infants, toddlers, and preschoolers in a service program and a treatment outcome research program. *Infant Mental Health Journal, 18,* 158–170.

Lyons-Ruth, K., & Block, D. (1996). The disturbed caregiving system: Relation among childhood trauma, maternal caregiving, and infant affect and attachment. *Infant Mental Health Journal, 17,* 257–275.

Main, M., & George, C. (1985). Responses of abused and disadvantaged toddlers to distress in agemates: A study in the day care setting. *Developmental Psychology, 21,* 407–412.

Main, M., & Goldwyn, R. (1984). *Adult Attachment Classification System.* Unpublished manual, University of California, Berkeley.

Manassis, K., Bradley, S., Goldberg, S., Hood, J., & Swinson, R. P. (1995). Behavioral inhibition, attachment, and anxiety in children of mothers with anxiety disorders. *Canadian Journal of Psychiatry, 40,* 87–92.

Masten, A. S., & Braswell, L. (1991). Developmental psychopathology: An integrative framework. In P. R. Martin (Ed.), *Handbook of behavior therapy and psychological science: An integrative approach* (pp. 35–56). New York: Pergamon Press.

Matas, L., Arend, R. A., & Sroufe, L. A. (1978). Continuity of adaptation in the second year: The relationship between quality of attachment and later competence. *Child Development, 49,* 547–556.

Maughan, A., & Cicchetti, D. (2002). Impact of child maltreatment and interadult violence on children's emotion regulation abilities and socioemotional adjustment. *Child Development, 73,* 1525–1542.

McDonough, S. C. (2000). Interaction guidance: An approach for difficult-to-engage families. In C. H. Zeanah (Ed.), *Handbook of infant mental health* (2nd ed., pp. 485–493). New York: Guilford Press.

Nelson, C. A., & Bosquet, M. (2000). Neurobiology of fetal and infant development: Implications for infant mental health. In C. H. Zeanah, (Ed.), *Handbook of infant mental health* (2nd ed., pp. 37–59). New York: Guilford Press.

Osman, A., Kopper, B. A., Barrios, F. X., Osman, J. R., & Wade, T. (1997). The Beck

Anxiety Inventory: Reexamination of factor structure and psychometric properties. *Journal of Clinical Psychology, 53,* 7–14.

Osofsky, J. D. (1995). The effects of exposure to violence on young children. *American Psychologist, 50*(9), 782–788.

Osofsky, J. D. (Ed.). (1997). *Children in a violent society.* New York: Guilford Press.

Osofsky, J.D., Bosquet, M., Kronenberg, M., & Costa, R. (2003). *Parent–Child Relationship Scale manual* (rev ed.). New Orleans: Louisiana State University Health Sciences Center.

Osofsky, J. D., Cohen, G., & Drell, M. (1995). The effects of trauma on young children: A case of two-year-old twins. *International Journal of Psychoanalysis, 76,* 595–607.

Osofsky, J. D., & Dickson, A. (2000). Treating traumatized children: The costs of delay. In J. D. Osofsky & E. Fenichel (Eds.), *Protecting young children in violent environments.* Washington, DC: Zero to Three/National Center for Infants, Toddlers, & Families.

Osofsky, J. D., & Fenichel, E. (Eds.). (1994). *Caring for infants and toddlers in violent environments: Hurt, healing, and hope.* Arlington, VA: Zero to Three/National Center for Clinical Infant Programs.

Osofsky, J. D., & Fenichel, E. (Eds). (1996). *Islands of safety: Assessing and treating young victims of violence.* Washington, DC: Zero to Three/National Center for Infants, Toddlers, and Families.

Osofsky, J. D., & Fenichel, E. (Eds.). (2000). *Protecting young children in violent environments.* Washington, DC: Zero to Three/National Center for Infants, Toddlers, & Families.

Pearson, J. L., Cohn, D. A., Cowan, P. A., & Cowan, C. P. (1994). Earned- and continuous-security in adult attachment: Relation to depressive symptomatology and parenting style. *Development and Psychopathology, 6,* 359–373.

Perry, B. D., Pollard, R. A., Blakley, T. L., Baker, W. L., & Vigilante, D. (1995). Childhood trauma, the neurobiology of adaptation, and "use-dependent" development of the brain: How "states" become "traits." *Infant Mental Health Journal, 16,* 271–291.

Pynoos, R. S., Steinberg, A. M., & Wraith, R. (1995). A developmental model of childhood traumatic stress. In D. Cicchetti & D. J. Cohen (Eds.), *Developmental psychopathology: Vol. 2. Risk, disorder, and adaptation* (pp. 72–95). New York: Wiley.

Ribbe, D. (1996). Psychometric review of the Traumatic Events Screening Instrument for Parents (TESI-P). In B. H. Stamm (Ed.), *Measurement of stress, trauma, and adaptation* (pp. 386–387). Lutherville, MD: Sidran Press.

Sattler, J. M. (1992). *Assessment of children* (3rd ed.). San Diego, CA: Author.

Scheeringa, M. S., & Gaensbauer, T. J. (2000). Posttraumatic stress disorder. In C. H. Zeanah (Ed.), *Handbook of infant mental health* (2nd ed., pp. 369–381). New York: Guilford Press.

Scheeringa, M. S., & Zeanah. C. H. (1995). Symptom expression and trauma variables in children under 48 months of age. *Infant Mental Health Journal, 16,* 259–270.

Scheeringa, M. S., Zeanah, C. H., Drell, M. J., & Larrieu, J. (1995). Two approaches to the diagnosis of posttraumatic stress disorder in infancy and early childhood. *Journal of the American Academy of Child and Adolescent Psychiatry, 34,* 191–200.

Schneider-Rosen, K., & Cicchetti, D. (1991). Early self-knowledge and emotional development: Visual self-recognition and affective reactions to mirror self-image in maltreated and non-maltreated toddlers. *Developmental Psychology, 27*, 471–478.

Squires, J., Potter, L., & Bricker, D. (1999). *The ASQ User's Guide* (2nd ed.). Baltimore: Brookes.

Sroufe, L. A. (1990). Considering normal and abnormal together: The essence of developmental psychopathology. *Development and Psychopathology, 2*, 335–347.

Sroufe, L. A., Egeland, B., & Kreutzer, T. (1990). The fate of early experience following developmental change: Longitudinal approaches to individual adaptation in childhood. *Child Development, 61*, 1363–1373.

Steer, R. A., Ranieri, W. F., Beck, A. T., & Clark, D. A. (1993). Further evidence for the validity of the Beck Anxiety Inventory with psychiatric outpatients. *Journal of Anxiety Disorders, 7*, 195–205.

Tronick, E. Z., Als, H., Adamson, L., Wise, S., & Brazelton, T. B. (1978). The infant's response to entrapment between contradictory messages in face-to-face interaction. *Journal of the American Academy of Child Psychiatry, 17*, 1–13.

Tronick, E. Z., Cohn, J., & Shea, E. (1985). The transfer of affect between mothers and infants. In T. B. Brazelton & M. Yogman (Eds.), *Affective development in infancy* (pp. 11–25). Norwood, NJ: Ablex.

van IJzendoorn, M. H. (1992). Intergenerational transmission of parenting: A review of studies in nonclinical populations. *Developmental Review, 12*, 76–99.

van IJzendoorn, M. H. (1995). Adult attachment representations, parental responsiveness, and infant attachment: A meta-analysis on the predictive validity of the Adult Attachment Interview. *Psychological Bulletin, 117*, 387–403.

Ward, M. J., & Carlson, E. A. (1995). Associations among adult attachment representations, maternal sensitivity, and infant–mother attachment in a sample of adolescent mothers. *Child Development, 66*, 69–79.

Waters, E., & Deane, K. (1985). Defining and assessing individual differences in attachment relationships: Q-methodology and the organization of behavior in infancy and early childhood. In I. Bretherton & E. Waters (Eds.), Growing points of attachment theory and research. *Monographs of the Society for Research in Child Development, 50*(1–2, Serial No. 209), 41–65.

Waters, E., & Sroufe, L. A. (1983). Social competence as a developmental construct. *Developmental Review, 3*, 79–97.

Wechsler, D. (1989). *Wechsler Preschool and Primary Scale of Intelligence—Revised.* San Antonio, TX: Psychological Corporation.

Wechsler, D. (2002). *Wechsler Preschool and Primary Scale of Intelligence—3rd edition.* San Antonio, TX: Psychological Corporation.

Wolfe, J., & Kimerling, R. (1997). Gender issues in the assessment of posttraumatic stress disorder. In J. Wilson & T. M. Keane (Eds.), *Assessing psychological trauma and PTSD* (pp. 192–238). New York: Guilford Press.

Wolfe, J., & Levin, K. (1991). *Life Stressor Checklist.* Unpublished instrument, National Center for PTSD, Boston.

Zeanah, C. H., & Benoit, D. (1995). Clinical applications of a parent perception interview in infant mental health. *Child and Adolescent Psychiatric Clinics of North America, 4*, 539–554.

Zeanah, C. H., Benoit, D., Hirshberg, L., Barton, M. L., & Regan, C. (1994). Mothers' representations of their infants are concordant with infant attachment classifications. *Developmental Issues in Psychiatry and Psychology, 1,* 9–18.

Zeanah, C. H., & Boris, N. W. (2000). Disturbances and disorders of attachment in early childhood. In C. H. Zeanah (Ed.), *Handbook of infant mental health* (2nd ed., pp. 353–368). New York: Guilford Press.

Zeanah, C. H., Boris, N. W., Heller, S. S., Hinshaw-Fuselier, S., Larrieu, J., Lewis, M., Palomino, R., Rovaris, M., & Valliere, J. (1997). Relationship assessment in infant mental health. *Infant Mental Health Journal, 18,* 182–197.

Zeanah, C. H., Larrieu, J. A., Heller, S. S., & Valliere, J. (2000). Infant–parent relationship assessment. In C. H. Zeanah (Ed.), *Handbook of infant mental health* (2nd ed., pp. 222–235). New York: Guilford Press.

Zero to Three/National Center for Clinical Infant Programs, National Center for Clinical Infant Programs. (1994). *Diagnostic classification of mental health and developmental disorders of infancy and early childhood.* Arlington, VA: Author.

Zuckerman, B. S., & Lieberman, A. F. (2002). In B. S. Zuckerman, A.F. Lieberman, & N. A. Fox (Eds.), *Emotional regulation and developmental health: Infancy and early childhood* (pp. 339–361). Skillman, NJ: Johnson & Johnson Pediatric Institute.

CHAPTER 14

PERSPECTIVES ON WORK WITH TRAUMATIZED YOUNG CHILDREN

How to Deal with the Feelings Emerging from Trauma Work

JOY D. OSOFSKY

> Sometimes the Judge should stop changing us from house to house. They should listen to what kids have to say in their heart.
> —STATEMENT BY 12-YEAR-OLD LAZARO, who then drew a picture of a "heart with ears" for Judge Cindy Lederman of the 11th Circuit Juvenile Court, Miami

Traumatized children "pull" many different reactions and responses from therapists, first responders, and nontraditional first responders. In this volume, many different clinical approaches to work with traumatized children have been described. The goal has been to include "state-of-the-art" strategies for evaluation and treatment for very young traumatized children so that practitioners, first responders, and others interested in learning more about children exposed to trauma and helping them will find useful information in this book. While different evaluation and treatment strategies have been presented, one area that has not yet been covered relates to the intense feelings that can emerge for therapists or other intervenors when working with traumatized children and families. Recently, a talented mental health professional who works in a supervisory capacity for a community mental health agency commented about how difficult it is to maintain consistency of staff when working in settings serving traumatized children, especially those under supervision of child protective service agencies and those in foster care. In response to her concerns, we spent some time discussing both the lack of preparation for therapists related to the difficulties of working with this high-risk often traumatized population as well as the often limited support available to those who work in this field. As is well illustrated in the diverse chapters in this book, it is not only therapists who may be traumatized by working with young children who are suffering, but also traditional "first responders" such as police officers, firefighters, emergency medical technicians, and nontraditional first responders such as teachers, judges, and even members of the media. As a part of their everyday jobs, all of these individuals may continually be exposed to trauma for which they rarely received support, help, or even someone to talk to about the intense feelings that often accompany trauma exposure. Juvenile court judges, particularly those who must decide the fate of very young abused and neglected children in dependency court, with caseloads that are frequently as large as 150 children each week, have shared how difficult it is to see and hear horrific stories every day about parents or caregivers who are supposed to protect and nurture their children. Police officers also must respond to domestic violence calls and deal with the needs of the victims and the aggression of the perpetrators; most often they do not have the time, knowledge, or resources to attend to the needs of the children who witness or are victimized by the violent incidents. Rarely are any of these professionals provided time to talk about how this work makes them feel; there is barely enough time to meet with these high-risk families and attend to their immediate needs.

In this chapter, I focus on the areas that are often not discussed concerning those who work with traumatized children and are particularly important when intervening or treating very young children who may pull even more from therapists and first responders due to their vulnerability and helplessness. The areas include vicarious traumatization, burnout, compassion fatigue, and countertransference, all of which impact by bringing up very strong feelings and emotions in the therapist or intervenor that are frequently an integral part of the work. When not addressed, however, such reactions can interfere with and even sidetrack the therapeutic progress.

VICARIOUS TRAUMATIZATION, BURNOUT, AND COMPASSION FATIGUE

Vicarious traumatization, the experiencing of posttraumatic symptoms similar to those experienced by victimized patients, can occur in therapists (Neumann & Gamble, 1995). They may experience somatic symptoms such as nausea, headaches, intrusive thoughts, difficulty with sleep, emotional numbing, feelings of personal vulnerability similar to those of their patients, the victims of trauma. It is important to recognize, especially for therapists who have had less experience working with traumatized patients, that these signs and symptoms, though disturbing, may actually be expectable reactions to trauma work. McCann and Pearlman (1990) have defined vicarious traumatization as negative transformation in the therapist's internal experience that can result from exposure to the traumatic experiences shared by patients. When therapists suffer from vicarious traumatization, they may experience intrusive imagery that can be highly distressing and interfere with their ability to function in their work. Burnout, which is endemic to working with trauma victims, refers to the reduced effectiveness that is often accompanied by feelings of helplessness, hopelessness, frustration, anger, or cynicism. Burnout most commonly results from repeated exposure to traumatic situations with the accompanying human suffering and injuries. Treaters do not want to turn down calls, and yet over time they may become aware that they are functioning less well, both in their work and in their personal lives. With chronic exposure to trauma, especially when young children are involved, treaters may eventually find it difficult to continue with the work as they begin to feel helpless and hopeless themselves. These feelings may be exacerbated for therapists who themselves are parents of young children. It is recognized that burnout is more likely when the therapist is isolated, overwhelmed with work, has little supervision and/ or consultation, and experiences little progress or success with the work. All of these reactions are prevalent in work with trauma victims as well as in the aftermath of a large-scale disaster or terrorist attack. Individuals need time off, the ability to talk about their experiences, support from peers and colleagues, supervision related to difficult and painful encounters, and recognition of the quality of their work.

Compassion fatigue, another component of vicarious traumatization and burnout, is defined as a form of caregiver burnout among psychotherapists related to caring, empathy, and emotional investment in helping those who suffer (Figley, 2002; McBride, 2003). To avoid compassion fatigue, self-care is necessary that includes more effectively managing caseloads, limiting compassion stress, and dealing with traumatic memories. Wilson and Lindy (1994) thoughtfully described the empathic strains—including tendencies for overidentification and avoidance—for therapists working with torture victims and other patients with severe posttraumatic stress disorder (PTSD; see also Nader, Dudley, & Kriegler, 1994). Some of their findings are directly relevant to work with children and families exposed to community and domestic violence. At times, the stories told by the children and families are so painful that therapists may wish to prematurely solve problems and bring closure to the work, which can result in limited success, failure, or early termination of the therapeutic work. The desire to "rescue" the family, while unrealistic, often interferes with the effectiveness of the therapeutic interventions. In contrast, the therapist may feel so overwhelmed and helpless that he or she withdraws emotionally from the patient, again leading to limited treatment success, treatment failure, or premature termination.

COUNTERTRANSFERENCE

Countertransference is defined as the therapist's emotional reaction to the patient based on his or her unconscious needs and conflicts as distinguished from conscious response to the patient's behavior. Countertransference may interfere with the therapist's ability to understand the patient and may adversely affect the therapeutic technique (American Psychiatric Association, 1994, p. 32). When first beginning work with traumatized young children, most intervenors and therapists are altruistically motivated by wishes to be of help. In the case of young children, therapists work with the children to help them process the trauma and support their normal development so that they are able to cope with and, as they grow older, understand events to which they should not have been exposed. At the same time, while doing this therapeutic work, many therapists experience their own strong feelings about the children's traumatization that may include fear, anger, sadness, confusion and even, as mentioned above, a sense of helplessness and hopelessness similar to that experienced by the children. For children exposed to community and family violence, intervenors or therapists must be able to be available and listen, as it is difficult to predict what will be shared. It is crucial to keep an open perspective in order to gain an understanding of the causes of the violence, what can be accomplished, and how much the children's futures have already been compromised. There may be complex feelings of vulnerability that alternative with those of optimism and pessimism. Frequently, there may be uncertainty about the child's future, especially if the family is violent and chaotic. Thus for the therapist, mixed with the wish to help can be feelings of fear, danger, and (at times) helplessness.

Many people do not want to think about countertransference issues with traumatized children. One of the main reasons is that they may be painful to consider and difficult to discuss. Almost 10 years ago, shortly after we began the Violence Intervention Program for Children and Families (VIP) and had started our work with the New Orleans Police Department (see Osofsky et al., Chapter 12, this volume), twin boys, almost 3 years old, were referred to our child clinic at Louisiana State University Health Sciences Center and brought in by their maternal grandparents, who had been given custody of the children by Child Protective Services (CPS) after their father shot and killed their mother. These little boys had witnessed their mother's murder by their father and, as a result, showed disorganized, aggressive, "out-of-control" behaviors. They showed little ability to control their behaviors, and even in the playroom they were "all over the place." Typically, we observe children in the playroom and videotape their play with permission for purposes of supervision and to review the progress of the case. As I observed the little boys and reviewed the videotape, I found myself becoming more and more angry and realized that it was because I was distressed that these little children had to go through something as horrible as witnessing their mother being shot by their father. I also realized immediately, however, that such feelings would not be very helpful for either the treatment or the supervisory process. I wondered further if the therapist might also be experiencing a similar range of emotions as she provided treatment for the little boys and helped to support the grandparents who had lost their daughter. Being aware of the feelings engendered in me as well as the helplessness and hopelessness that sometimes accompanies work with traumatized young children, I was able to use my feelings to help understand the current inner confusion and distress of the boys and provide more effective supervision and guidance to the therapist.

Countertransference can work in different—sometimes unexpected—ways to influence responses. A number of years ago, the VIP team was working with a group of mothers, all of whom had sons who had been murdered. We were helping them start a group called "Moms Against Violence" with the goal of outreach into the community to help other mothers who had lost children to violence. We started by meeting as a group during which each person shared her own experiences of previous losses in her life. I realized as the discussion went on that some of the stories were difficult to hear and I recognized that, for me, losing a child was one of the worst things I could imagine. And so I listened to the stories, supported people as they shared their stories of loss and their grief, and at the end of the day went home and said to my family, "I'm going to bed." I had young children myself and recognized (in a way that ultimately proved useful to them) that, at that time in my life, it was difficult to hold and process the grief of so many mothers. Interestingly, a few years later, one of my colleagues responded to a call from a school where a 6-year-old child had been killed by an automobile that raced right through the school zone. This social worker often responded to crises in the school. However, he came to me later in the day and said that he felt shaky and thought someone else should follow up on this situation. As we discussed it further, we both realized that one of his three children was 6 years old and that the tragedy hit "too close to home" for him to be able to hold and process the loss and grief in that school. These two personal examples illustrate how powerful our own countertransference reactions may be with trauma survivors and how important it is to be sensitive to these reactions.

Other countertransference issues are important and unsettling at times to the therapist. For example, when therapists feel helpless, they may be reflecting their patient's sense of being helpless and pessimistic about the future. Winnicott (1964/1987), in describing objective and subjective forms of interaction, emphasized hate in the countertransference and the importance of recognizing such hate if one is to do effective work. Especially when children's behaviors are disruptive and aberrant, when parents are unappreciative and insensitive to their children's needs, and when individual reactions of grief remain refractory to the therapist's interventions and dismissive of the therapist, he or she may experience anger even though reluctant to acknowledge it. Poggi and Ganzarain (1983) have described how the recognition and use of countertransference hate can be helpful in the treatment of difficult patients. Recognition of such reactions and their antecedents can similarly be useful in working with victims of violence and other traumatic experiences.

TERMINATION ISSUES FOR CHILDREN EXPERIENCING PREVIOUS LOSSES AND TRAUMATIZATION[1]

It is important to understand the "meaning" of termination for children experiencing previous losses and trauma. Termination is planned for children at a time that seems appropriate related to the symptoms, conflicts, and concerns of the child and—for the young child—of the parents or caregivers. However, there is usually an understanding that treatment may be resumed at a later stage in development if these issues or new ones should arise. Because development may be fluid, patterns of growth or "derailment" may occur again and may need to be addressed when the child is older. Termination may occur quickly or slowly depending on the needs of the child, or at times, because the child or therapist may be leaving. In our training program, often therapists are in training for 1 year and must terminate their patients by necessity. While we are mindful of this timing in assigning cases, disruptions occur every year. From the outset of treatment it is crucial to sustain the parent or caregiver and the child in their relationship, and this goal may become even more important with termination.

In child therapy, the therapist works in tandem with other significant caregivers to achieve positive outcomes. The child's relationship with the therapist replicates (and often repairs) aspects of other relationships. The therapist must also take into account other influences on the child, including school, child-care settings, extended family members, etc. Ultimately, the parent or caregiver is the most significant ongoing relationship for the child and will provide guidance and direction. Often individual therapy and parental guidance may be needed to strengthen that relationship and help support it in the course of the termination process.

It is very important to recognize and support the developmental needs of young children in the course of termination. Many children, especially at times of stress, are extremely vulnerable to changes in routine. They also are highly sensitive to changes in their primary caregiver and the other significant relationships in their lives. Multiply stressors may have a cumulative effect on children with the number of risk factors and stressor decreasing children's competence and ability to cope.

For high-risk children who have experienced previous losses and/or trauma, termination may re-create feelings that have emerged with earlier loss of relationships, loss of safety, and loss and stability and reliability. Losing a significant relationship early in life can impact profoundly on a child, especially if such a loss results in continuing instability. Children may experience loss of relationships through death of a parent or primary caregiver, or through parental abandonment, divorce, separation, long-term illness, incarceration, or other disruptions due to substance abuse or mental illness. Children may experience a loss of safety if they are exposed to community and/or domestic violence at a young age. Children may also be traumatized if they have serious illness including hospitalization with painful procedures themselves, experience or witness abuse or are involved in an automobile accident. Loss of stability or reliability can result from experiences of loss, especially if they result in disruption in routines or in their environment. Their routines and environment can be disrupted with changes in residence, changes in day-care staff or location, as well as neglectful caregiving without established routines. With loss of stability, children's sense of security is threatened and they may feel an overwhelming sense of helplessness.

Therapeutic work and termination with foster children and others with significant loss experiences involves helping them work through conflicts about earlier relationships, helping them deal with the trauma that accompanies loss, mourning the loss of the biological parent (even if this parent was not a great parent), and recognizing and re-creating early life experiences in the therapeutic relationship. Within a developmental perspective, the therapist can help the child work through conflicts and feelings, help to develop a sense of trust and stability, deal with the feelings of emptiness, despair, anxiety, and grief that emerge in many cases, and help the child understand these or cope with them at the time of termination. It is important at the time of termination to support the child's ego functions to deal with the loss by helping the child mourn the loss of previous caregivers, work on restoring developmental integrity, help her work through her trauma, including reexperiencing the trauma, and work on developing trust in new relationships. The goals are to help her develop enough inner stability to cope adequately with future loss and stress, recognize, depending on her age, that she may not have completely mourned the loss of her biological parents and may not be able to complete that process until she is older. For the young child and for child–parent psychotherapy, during termination the therapist may acquire the role of surrogate attachment figure providing both a haven of safety and being a transference object (Lieberman & Van Horn, 2003).

The end of treatment and also the end of sessions represent a valuable opportunity for providing the child with corrective emotional experiences of separation and loss. Through the therapist's responses, the child learns that the image of the loved person can be kept when that person is no longer present. The image and associated memories can be brought back to mind at times of emotional need and used for comfort and support. At the end of treatment, it is often useful to go through a brief review of how things were at the beginning of treatment and how they are now. Preschoolers often need concrete reminders of how much time is left before the final session. Finally, it is crucial to use parental support to help the preverbal and young child with the sadness of good-byes.

Termination is a crucial time for children who have experienced multiple losses. First, it may provide both the child and parent with their first experience of nontraumatic loss. Further, a good and supportive termination process can provide the child with a new "script" and a way to face and navigate the losses he or she will inevitably face in the future.

THE NEED FOR REFLECTIVE SUPERVISION

An important way to provide support and guidance for therapists and intervenors working with traumatized children and families is through reflective supervision (Shahmoon-Shanok, Gilkerson, Eggbeer, & Fenichel, 1995). Reflective supervision, a process requiring reflection, collaboration, and regularity, provides an opportunity for therapists or intervenors to deepen and broaden knowledge, discuss reactions to experiences, discuss individual goals and progress, and develop and refine their individual style through self-understanding. Reflective supervision is carried out regularly in a safe and trusting environment. Through this type of supervision, the therapist learns how to understand and provide relationship-based treatment for infants and toddlers in the context of their families, as well as different ways to build on the capacities, resilience, and resourcefulness of children and families. In reflective supervision, the supervisor introduces and reinforces the idea that emotions and feelings are crucial to understand work with infants and families. Further, by recognizing our own emotional responses, it is possible to recognize, understand, and respect the emotional responses of infants, toddlers, and their families. The trusting environment allows the supervisee to feel free to express anxieties, concerns, and feelings that may arise in the course of the work, which with traumatized children and families may be very intense. By sharing and discussing the feelings in a safe environment, the therapist will then be in a better position to understand and to "hold," if needed, the intense feelings that arise in the course of treatment of the young children and family.

Dealing with countertransference issues is an integral part of reflective supervision. Often working with traumatized children and families brings up for the supervisee strong feelings toward the young traumatized child and, even more often, the parent. Reflective supervision allows the therapist to express and better understand these feelings so that they will not interfere with the development of a working alliance and impede the progress of the treatment. Issues of vicarious traumatization, burnout, and compassion fatigue will also come up in the course of this type of supervision, especially if the supervisor is attuned to these issues. Examples of such problems were illustrated earlier in this chapter. With this type of supervision, the supervisor and supervisee can step back from the immediate intense experience of the work in order to better conceptualize what is being observed and what may be happening. The supervisor also encourages the supervisee to talk about what he or she "thought" and "felt" when a particular event occurred. This type of supervision takes into account ambiguity that may come up in the course of the work as well as areas of confusion for both the supervisee and the supervisor. An important part of the work with young traumatized children and families is to just "be there," and this type of supervision helps support the therapist in this role. The open communication that occurs in supervision can be a model for communication between professionals and parents, as well as parents and children.

CONCLUSION

Work with traumatized young children and families pulls a great deal from the therapist as well as others in the child's environment. Therapists who work with children and families exposed to community and family violence, and those who have suffered at a young age from many disruptions and losses, may repeatedly suffer from vicarious traumatization, burnout, compassion fatigue, and strong and confusing countertransference. Powerful feelings may be evoked in therapists working with trauma victims, and in some situations the therapist may also be traumatized. They may also find themselves feeling very sorry for the children—wanting to rescue them—and, at the same time, angry with the abusive, neglectful, or just unfeeling parents. Supervisors of new trainees seeing traumatized young children become familiar quickly with the feelings that emerge in these therapists, who want to protect and care for them, thinking that these children would be better off it they could take them home with them. They may feel frustrated as they work with the caregivers to help them become more sensitive and responsive parents. Some trainees may feel that if they could just get the child out of the situation, everything would be much better. Countertransference responses can inform and enrich treatment, and unacknowledged or unexamined responses can damage both the client and the therapist.

It is important to recognize that many survivors of traumatic exposure do well. Their involvement with the trauma may be minimal and their symptoms, if any, may be relatively short lived. Others may be severely traumatized, having witnessed horrendous scenes and having lost loved ones. Therapists must be prepared to listen, to absorb the traumatized children's concerns, to "hold" them, and to help them emotionally to "get back on track" and to return to their normal developmental functions. Ann Masten (personal communication, May 2003) discussed resilience as the ability of the child, often with intervention, to return to a normal developmental trajectory after having experienced trauma. In an earlier publication, I have discussed violence exposure for children as derailing their normal developmental trajectory and the therapeutic work being helpful to them to be able to get back on track (Osofsky, 1995). They cannot right the wrongs, nor can they erase the scars; however, they can be helped and supported in their development. As Selma Fraiberg (1987) so sensitively stated, working with children is a little like having God on your side. For clinicians who continually consult, treat, and supervise others who work with traumatized young children, dealing with issues of countertransference, burnout, and compassion fatigue is an integral part of the work. Each therapist must find his or her own way to deal with the overwhelming affects that are often aroused. Whether it takes working with a supportive team, self-care, or some other method, there must always be some type of support to be able to effectively do the work.

Nader (1994) provided important guidelines to help therapists with the strong feelings that can emerge and countertransference reactions when working with traumatized children. First, the therapist needs to develop a willingness to hear anything and to be able to "hold" the information and feelings to help the child. Second, it is crucial that the therapist recognize the phasic nature of trauma recovery. The healing will come over time, and there may be a need for occasional "time-outs" from direct focus on the trauma. Third, as has been emphasized in this chapter, it is crucial as part of the work that issues of burnout and countertransference be an integral part of training and supervision.

For clinical work with traumatized children other guidelines are also important:

- Don't be afraid to talk about the traumatic event.
- Provide consistency and predictability.
- Be nurturing and affectionate in appropriate ways and contexts.
- Discuss your expectations for behavior with the child.
- Talk with the child and explain things to him or her.

- Watch for signs of reenactment, avoidance and reactivity.
- Protect the child from traumatization if possible.
- Give the child choices and a sense of control.
- If you have questions, ask for help.
- Get supervision and consultation; do not work with trauma cases in isolation.

Mental health professionals and others who work with traumatized young children invariably have their own stories about a case or circumstance that was particularly difficult for them to deal with and that has "haunted" them over the years. Due to the nature of the work and often the personalities of the treaters, self-care is often something that people do not do for themselves. Although the United States continues to be a violent society where children are exposed to violence, many people continue to deny that even very young children are exposed and traumatized. Recently, I was talking with a little boy whose parents had just been divorced and who fought a great deal before they separated. I asked him what he did and how he felt when they fought. He said he tried to stop them. Then he said thoughtfully, "I used to be much braver then." He was 4 years old when they separated. Although many would prefer to deny it, even very young children are traumatized by violence exposure. The behavioral reactions, symptom picture, intensity, and severity vary depending on developmental and situational factors, including the age of the child, proximity to the event, familiarity with the victim or perpetrator, and—perhaps most important—the presence of an emotionally available parent or caregiver. Thus, caring for the caregivers when trauma occurs is an important and crucial component to help support the child. For very young children, traumatization of caregivers means that is may be more difficult for them to listen to their child, hear their story, and provide support. Further, parents may have less patience when they too are traumatized and may become more easily irritated as well as less resourceful in handling their children's stress. Treatment approaches that are effective in helping traumatized young children and families are varied. They may include working individually with the parents or caregivers to support them and help them deal with and process their trauma and, at the same time, working individually with the young child most often through play. However, treatment will also need to be relationship based, recognizing that issues and conflicts emerging between the parent/caregiver and the child may be crucial for healing to occur. Finally, less frequently addressed problems are those of countertransference, burnout, and vicarious traumatization, all of which occur when working with victims of trauma. These issues have been overwhelmingly evident in recent years in our work with first responders, police, firefighters, and EMS (Emergency Medical Service) workers, as well as therapists—all trying to help the many traumatized children and families when they themselves have been traumatized by the horrific events that have occurred. Perhaps here the dicta "Heal Thyself" and "Do No Harm" are important for mental health professionals and others working with trauma victims.

NOTE

1. The ideas on termination in this section have been influenced by an unpublished paper by Michele Many, LCSW, Department of Psychiatry, Louisiana State University Health Sciences Center, New Orleans.

REFERENCES

American Psychiatric Association. (1994). *American Psychiatric Association glossary* (p. 32). Washington, DC: Author.

Figley, C. (2002). Compassion fatigue: Psychotherapists' chronic lack of self care. *JCLP/In Session: Psychotherapy in Practice, 58,* 1433–1441.

Fraiberg, L. (Ed.). (1987). *Selected writings of Selma Fraiberg.* Columbus: Ohio State University Press.

Fraiberg, S., Adelson, E., & Shapiro, V. (1975). Ghosts in the nursery: A psychoanalytic approach to the problems of impaired mother-infant relationships. *Journal of the American Academy of Child Psychiatry, 14,* 378–421.

Lieberman, A. F., & Van Horn, P. (2003, August). *Guide for child–parent psychotherapy for infant, toddler, and preschooler witnesses of domestic violence.* Unpublished manuscript, Child Trauma Research Project, University of California, San Francisco.

McBride, S. A. (2003, July). *Secondary traumatic stress.* Paper presented to the Infant Mental Health Training Program, West Palm Beach, FL.

McCann, I. L., & Pearlman, L. A. (1990). Vicarious traumatization: A framework for understanding the psychological effects of working with victims. *Journal of Traumatic Stress, 3,* 131–149.

Nader, K. O. (1994). Countertransference in the treatment of acutely traumatized children. In J. P. Wilson & J. D. Lindy (Eds.), *Countertransference in the treatment of PTSD* (pp. 179–205). New York: Guilford Press.

Nader, K. O., Dudley, D. B., & Kriegler, J. (1994). *Clinician-Administered PTSD Scale, Child and Adolescent Version (CAPS-C).* Boston: National Center for PTSD.

Neumann, D. A., & Gamble, S. J. (1995). Issues in the professional development of psychotherapists: Countertransference and vicarious traumatization in the new trauma therapist. *Psychotherapy, 32,* 341–347.

Osofsky, J. D. (1995). The effects of exposure to violence on young children. *American Psychologist, 50*(9), 782–788.

Poggi, R. G., & Ganzarain, R. (1983). Countertransference hate. *Bulletin of the Menninger Clinic, 47*(1), 15–35.

Shahmoon-Shanok, R., Gilkerson, L., Eggbeer, L., & Fenichel, E. (1995). *Reflective supervision: A relationship for learning*. Washington, DC: Zero to Three/National Center for Infants, Toddlers, and Families.

Wilson, J. P., & Lindy, J. D. (Eds.). (1994). *Countertransference in the treatment of PTSD*. New York: Guilford Press.

Winnicott, D. W. (1987). *The child, the family, and the outside world* (2nd ed.). Reading, MA: Addison-Wesley. (Original work published 1964)

INDEX